VETERINARY IMMUNOLOGY

VETERINARY IMMUNOLOGY
AN INTRODUCTION

Oliver Gagnon
Connor Murphy

Kruger Brentt
Publishers

2023

Kruger Brentt Publishers UK. LTD.
Company Number 9728962

Regd. Office: 68 St Margarets Road, Edgware, Middlesex HA8 9UU

ISBN: 978-1-78715-109-3

For information on all our publications visit our website at http://krugerbrentt.com/

PREFACE

The immune system represents a nodal point in the balance between animal health and disease. Functional parameters of immunity are central in the fight against infectious diseases. Unfortunately, deregulation of the complex regulatory networks that compose the immune system can also have dire consequences for the animal host such as those involved in allergic reactions, autoimmunity, and cancer. Despite the progress made in recent decades understanding the pathological basis of animal disease, comparatively little progress has been made to our understanding of the immune parameters associated with these ailments. The one clear exception is the mouse, for which significant resources have been spent to develop state of the art technologies and cutting-edge approaches that help us understand the fundamentals of its immune system, the intricacies of host-pathogen interactions, and the contributions of these to host defense mechanisms and disease. Ironically, a quick screen of the available literature on this species quickly yields highly effective approaches to defend against the most challenging of pathogens, unique methodologies to dissect the complex regulatory mechanisms behind effective immune responses, and even elegant procedures to regain immune competence when genetics or environmental factors compromise host immunity. Achieving equivalent levels of knowledge for all other animals in the short-term would be highly unrealistic. Yet, we continue to become increasingly aware of the dangers associated with underestimating the impact of veterinary issues on animal and human populations alike. New and re-emerging infectious diseases continue to appear, driven by socio-economic, environmental and ecological factors. Their impact continues to be felt globally, and among others, emphasizes the pressing need to critically evaluate the links between wild animal populations, domestic animals, and humans.

The present book contains 13 chapters covering all related disciplines. These chapters include An overview of the immune system: innate and adaptive immunity and the inflammatory response, diseases of immunity, antigens and antibodies, the complement system, serological testing , cells and tissues of the immune system, the major histocompatibility complex, antigen presentation and cytokine, red cell antigens and antibody-mediated hypersensitivity, regulation of adaptive immunity, allergy, immunodeficiency, cancer and vaccines immunotherapy treatment. Related terminology is given at the end for ready reference. This book provides a very helpful way of understanding the diagnostic tests, animal immunization and immune-mediated diseases. The book provides an excellent insight into the complexity of diseases caused by or prevented via innate and/or adaptive immunity. The book is also supported with a comprehensive glossary and index in the end. Veterinary Immunology will provide students with a good working knowledge of veterinary immunology that will serve them both in the completion of their curricula and in professional practice.

We are grateful to all those persons as well as various books, manuals, periodicals, magazines, journals etc. that helped in the preparation of this book. In spite of the best efforts, it is possible that some errors may have occurred into the compilation and editing of the book. Further queries, constructive suggestions and criticisms for the improvement of the book are always welcome and shall be thankfully acknowledged..

Oliver Gagnon

Connor Murphy

CONTENTS

CHAPTER

1

AN OVERVIEW OF THE IMMUNE SYSTEM: INNATE AND ADAPTIVE IMMUNITY AND THE INFLAMMATORY RESPONSE

INTRODUCTION

Immunology deals with physiological functioning of the immune system in states of both health and disease as well as malfunctions of the immune system in immunological disorders like allergies, hypersensitivities, immune deficiency, transplant rejection and autoimmune disorders.

Immunology deals with physical, chemical and physiological characteristics of the components of the immune system in vitro, in situ, and in vivo. Immunology has a vast array of uses in several disciplines of science and medical science.

The immune system protects us from infection through various lines of defence. If the immune system is not functioning as it should, it can result in disease, such as autoimmunity, allergy and cancer. It is also now becoming clear that immune responses contribute to the development of many common disorders not traditionally viewed as immunologic, including metabolic, cardiovascular, and neurodegenerative conditions such as Alzheimer's.

Over the past decade, there have been numerous advances in our current understanding of the immune system and how it functions to protect the body from infection. Given the complex nature of this subject, it is beyond the scope of this article to provide an in-depth review of all aspects of immunology.

Rather, the purpose of this article is to provide medical students, medical residents, primary-care practitioners and other healthcare professionals with a basic introduction to the main components and function of the immune system and its role in both health and disease. This article will also serve as a backgrounder to the immunopathological disorders discussed in the remainder of this supplement. The topics covered in this introductory article include: innate and acquired immunity, passive and active immunization and immunopathologies, such as hypersensitivity reactions, autoimmunity and immunodeficiency.

THE IMMUNE SYSTEM: INNATE AND ADAPTIVE IMMUNITY

The immune system refers to a collection of cells and proteins that function to protect the skin, respiratory passages, intestinal tract and other areas from foreign antigens, such as microbes (organisms such as bacteria, fungi, and parasites), viruses, cancer cells, and toxins. The immune system can be simplistically viewed as having two "lines of defense": innate immunity and adaptive immunity. Innate immunity represents the first line of defense to an intruding pathogen. It is an antigen-independent (non-specific) defense mechanism that is used by the host immediately or within hours of encountering an antigen. The innate immune response has no immunologic memory and, therefore, it is unable to recognize or "memorize" the same pathogen should the body be exposed to it in the future. Adaptive immunity, on the other hand, is antigen-dependent and antigen-specific and, therefore, involves a lag time between exposure to the antigen and maximal response. The hallmark of adaptive immunity is the capacity for memory which enables the host to mount a more rapid and efficient immune response upon subsequent exposure to the antigen. Innate and adaptive immunity are not mutually exclusive mechanisms of host defense, but rather are complementary, with defects in either system resulting in host vulnerability.

INNATE IMMUNITY

The primary function of innate immunity is the recruitment of immune cells to sites of infection and inflammation through the production of cytokines (small proteins involved in cell-cell communication). Cytokine production leads to the release of antibodies and other proteins and glycoproteins which activate the complement system, a biochemical cascade that functions to identify and opsonize (coat) foreign antigens, rendering them susceptible to phagocytosis (process by which cells engulf microbes and remove cell debris). The innate immune response also promotes clearance of dead cells or antibody complexes and removes foreign substances present in organs, tissues, blood and lymph.

Numerous cells are involved in the innate immune response such as phagocytes (macrophages and neutrophils), dendritic cells, mast cells, basophils, eosinophils, natural killer (NK) cells and lymphocytes (T cells). Phagocytes are sub-divided into two main cell types: neutrophils and macrophages. Both of these cells share a similar function: to engulf (phagocytose) microbes. In addition to their phagocytic properties, neutrophils contain granules that, when released, assist in the elimination of pathogenic microbes. Unlike neutrophils (which are short-lived cells), macrophages are long-lived cells that not only play a role in phagocytosis, but are also involved in antigen presentation to T cells. Macrophages are named according to the tissue in which they reside. For example, macrophages present in the liver are called Kupffer cells while those present in the connective tissue are termed histiocytes

Dendritic cells also phagocytose and function as antigen-presenting cells (APCs) and act as important messengers between innate and adaptive immunity. Mast cells and basophils share many salient features with each other and both are instrumental in the initiation of acute inflammatory responses, such as those seen in allergy and asthma. Unlike mast cells, which generally reside in the connective tissue surrounding blood vessels, basophils reside in the circulation. Eosinophils are granulocytes that possess phagocytic properties and play an important role in the destruction of parasites that are too large to be phagocytosed. Along with mast cells and basophils, they also control mechanisms associated with allergy and asthma. NK cells (also known as large granular lymphocytes [LGLs]) play a major role in the rejection of tumours and the destruction of cells infected by viruses. Destruction of infected cells is achieved through the release of perforins and granzymes from NK-cell granules which induce apoptosis (programmed cell death).

Innate immunity can be viewed as comprising four types of defensive barriers: anatomic (skin and mucous membrane), physiologic (temperature, low pH and chemical mediators), endocytic and phagocytic, and inflammatory.

Cytokine Release Affect

The binding of PRRs with PAMPs triggers the release of cytokines, which signal that a pathogen is present and needs to be destroyed along with any infected cells. A cytokine is a chemical messenger that regulates cell differentiation (form and function), proliferation (production), and gene expression to affect immune responses. At least 40 types of cytokines exist in humans that differ in terms of the cell type that produces them, the cell type that responds to them, and the changes they produce. One type cytokine, interferon, is illustrated in Fig. 1.

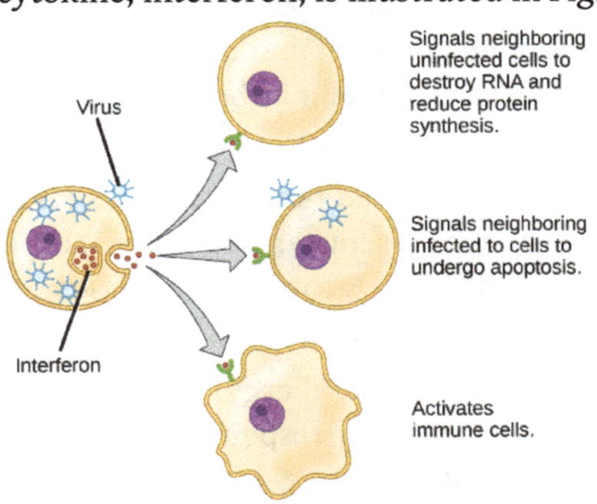

Fig. 1. Interferons are cytokines that are released by a cell infected with a virus.

One subclass of cytokines is the interleukin (IL), so named because they mediate interactions between leukocytes (white blood cells). Interleukins are involved in bridging the innate and adaptive immune responses. In addition to being released from cells after PAMP recognition, cytokines are released by the infected cells which bind to nearby uninfected cells and induce those cells to release cytokines, which results in a cytokine burst.

A second class of early-acting cytokines is interferons, which are released by infected cells as a warning to nearby uninfected cells. One of the functions of an interferon is to inhibit viral replication. They also have other important functions, such as tumor surveillance. Interferons work by signaling neighboring uninfected cells to destroy RNA and reduce protein synthesis, signaling neighboring infected cells to undergo apoptosis (programmed cell death), and activating immune cells.

In response to interferons, uninfected cells alter their gene expression, which increases the cells' resistance to infection. One effect of interferon-induced gene expression is a sharply reduced cellular protein synthesis. Virally infected cells produce more viruses by synthesizing large quantities of viral proteins. Thus, by reducing protein synthesis, a cell becomes resistant to viral infection.

Phagocytosis and Inflammation

The first cytokines to be produced are pro-inflammatory; that is, they encourage inflammation, the localized redness, swelling, heat, and pain that result from the movement of leukocytes and fluid through increasingly permeable capillaries to a site of infection. The population of leukocytes that arrives at an infection site depends on the nature of the infecting pathogen. Both macrophages and dendritic cells engulf pathogens and cellular debris through phagocytosis. A neutrophil is also a phagocytic leukocyte that engulfs and digests pathogens.

Neutrophils have a nucleus with two to five lobes, and they contain organelles, called lysosomes, that digest engulfed pathogens. An eosinophil is a leukocyte that works with other eosinophils to surround a parasite; it is involved in the allergic response and in protection against helminthes (parasitic worms).

Neutrophils and eosinophils are particularly important leukocytes that engulf large pathogens, such as bacteria and fungi. A mast cell is a leukocyte that produces inflammatory molecules, such as histamine, in response to large pathogens. A basophil is a leukocyte that, like a neutrophil, releases chemicals to stimulate the inflammatory response as illustrated in Fig. 2.

Basophils are also involved in allergy and hypersensitivity responses and induce specific types of inflammatory responses. Eosinophils and basophils produce additional inflammatory mediators to recruit more leukocytes. A hypersensitive immune response to harmless antigens, such as in pollen, often involves the release of histamine by basophils and mast cells.

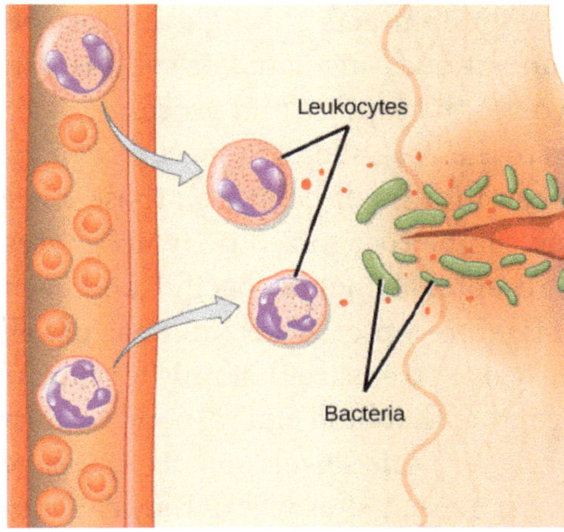

Fig. 2. In response to a cut, mast cells secrete histamines that cause nearby capillaries to dilate. Neutrophils and monocytes leave the capillaries. Monocytes mature into macrophages. Neutrophils, dendritic cells and macrophages release chemicals to stimulate the inflammatory response. Neutrophils and macrophages also consume invading bacteria by phagocytosis.

Cytokines also send feedback to cells of the nervous system to bring about the overall symptoms of feeling sick, which include lethargy, muscle pain, and nausea. These effects may have evolved because the symptoms encourage the individual to rest and prevent them from spreading the infection to others. Cytokines also increase the core body temperature, causing a fever, which causes the liver to withhold iron from the blood. Without iron, certain pathogens, such as some bacteria, are unable to replicate; this is called nutritional immunity.

ADAPTIVE IMMUNITY IN ANIMALS

Innate immune responses, although critical to the defense of the body, cannot guarantee protection. They lack the flexibility to respond optimally to a diverse set of microorganisms and they may cause significant tissue damage. A third layer of defense is required that can act automatically in response to microbial invasion, generate resistance proportional to the threat, and improve with experience. These are the key features of the adaptive immune system. Adaptive immune responses are of two major types, antibody (humoral) immunity directed against extracellular invaders and cell-mediated immunity directed against intracellular invaders.

Adaptive immune responses must be very carefully regulated. The immune defenses of the body constitute a potent weapon system whose use must be controlled to minimize collateral damage. As a result, much of the immune system is devoted to the production of regulatory cells and cytokines whose function is to ensure that immune responses only occur under appropriate circumstances. If these regulatory pathways fail, disease or death may result.

The adaptive immune system acts through a series of steps that must occur sequentially for either an antibody-mediated or cell-mediated immune response to occur. The first step involves the capture and processing of antigens (an antigen is a substance that is foreign to the host, such as a piece of a bacterium or a viral protein). Once processed (ie, broken into small peptides), these antigens are transported to cell surfaces, where they can be recognized by lymphocytes carrying receptors for antigens. Each antigen receptor is highly specific, and each lymphocyte expresses only a single form of antigen receptor. Thus, millions of cells have the potential to recognize millions of antigens. To ensure that only foreign antigens trigger adaptive immunity, cells with receptors that bind and respond to normal body "self" antigens are selectively killed early in their development. The surviving lymphocytes are situated within lymphoid organs at sites where they can most effectively encounter antigens on microbial invaders, triggering them to respond by mounting immune responses.

There are two major populations of lymphocytes:

- B cells - responsible for antibody responses, effector (or cytotoxic)
- T cells - responsible for cell-mediated immune responses

Within the population of T lymphocytes there are subpopulations: helper T cells, whose job it is to provide assistance to B cells for antibody production (these are T helper type 2 cells) and T helper cells that provide help to other T cells and macrophages by secreting certain cytokines (these are T helper type 1 cells); and T regulatory cells, whose job it is to regulate the immune response.

Antibody Responses

Antibodies are B cell antigen receptors that are synthesized in large quantities and secreted into the bloodstream where they circulate. Antibodies are produced by B cells and plasma cells. Antibodies bind to foreign molecules and mark them for destruction by phagocytic cells or complement-mediated lysis. Plasma cells are differentiated B cells optimized to synthesize and secrete enormous quantities of antibodies. Antibodies are critical to host defense against extracellular invaders such as most bacteria, some blood parasites, and viruses traveling between cells.

B cells originate in the bone marrow and reside in lymphoid tissues such as lymph nodes, bone marrow, Peyer's patches, and the spleen. Each B cell is covered by several thousand identical antigen receptors and can bind and respond to only a single antigen. When a microbe enters the body, it will inevitably encounter B cells that can bind to some of its surface antigens. As a result of this antigen binding, and with appropriate additional stimulation, these B cells will divide repeatedly and differentiate into two descendant populations.

One population, antibody-producing plasma cells, are the major sources of antibodies. The other B cell population becomes memory B cells that can persist within an animal for months or years. When an animal encounters an antigen for a second time, these memory B cells respond rapidly, producing large numbers of plasma cells (and yet more memory cells). As a result, the animal mounts a vastly improved antibody response, and the invader is rapidly eliminated. Subsequent exposure to a microbe leads in turn to the accumulation of more memory cells, resulting in better protection, virtually guaranteeing that the organism will never again be able to cause disease in that individual. This response is the basis of all vaccination programs. Although simple in concept, B cell responses and antibody production must be carefully regulated. Thus, a B cell is not usually able to respond to a bound foreign antigen unless it also receives "co-stimulation" in the form of a signal from helper T cells. These helper T cells in turn can only be activated if they, too, are presented with antigen under carefully controlled circumstances.

An antigen is a foreign or "non-self" macromolecule that reacts with cells of the immune system. Not all antigens will provoke a response. For instance, individuals produce innumerable "self" antigens and are constantly exposed to harmless foreign antigens, such as food proteins, pollen, or dust components. The suppression of immune responses to harmless macromolecules is highly regulated and typically prevents processes that could be damaging to the host, known as tolerance.

The innate immune system contains cells that detect potentially harmful antigens, and then inform the adaptive immune response about the presence of these antigens. An antigen-presenting cell (APC) is an immune cell that detects, engulfs, and informs the adaptive immune response about an infection. When a pathogen is detected, these APCs will phagocytose the pathogen and digest it to form many different fragments of the antigen. Antigen fragments will then be transported to the surface of the APC, where they will serve as an indicator to other immune cells.

Dendritic cells are immune cells that process antigen material; they are present in the skin (Langerhans cells) and the lining of the nose, lungs, stomach, and intestines. Sometimes a dendritic cell presents on the surface of other cells to induce an immune response, thus functioning as an antigen-presenting cell. Macrophages also function as APCs. Before activation and differentiation, B cells can also function as APCs.

After phagocytosis by APCs, the phagocytic vesicle fuses with an intracellular lysosome forming phagolysosome. Within the phagolysosome, the components are broken down into fragments; the fragments are then loaded onto MHC class I or MHC class II molecules and are transported to the cell surface for antigen presentation, as illustrated in Fig. 3. Note that T lymphocytes cannot properly respond to the antigen unless it is processed and embedded in an MHC II molecule. APCs express MHC on their surfaces, and when combined with a foreign antigen, these complexes signal a "non-self" invader. Once the fragment of antigen is embedded in the MHC II molecule, the immune cell can respond. Helper T- cells are one of the main lymphocytes that respond to antigen-presenting cells. Recall that all other nucleated cells of the body expressed MHC I molecules, which signal "healthy" or "normal."

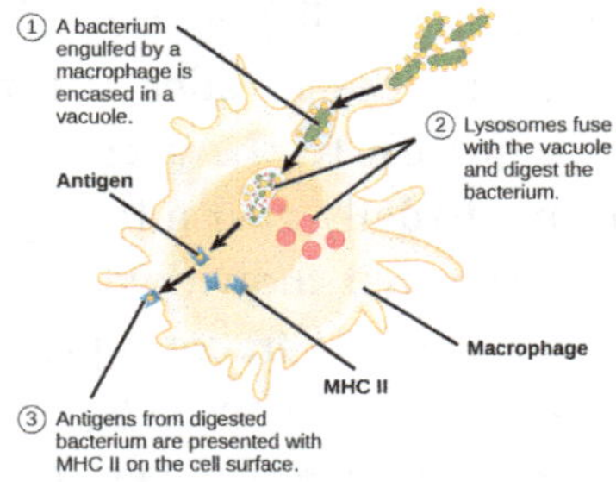

Fig. 3. An APC, such as a macrophage, engulfs and digests a foreign bacterium. An antigen from the bacterium is presented on the cell surface in conjunction with an MHC II molecule Lymphocytes of the adaptive immune response interact with antigen-embedded MHC II molecules to mature into functional immune cells.

T and B Lymphocytes

Lymphocytes in human circulating blood are approximately 80 to 90 percent T cells, shown in Fig. 4, and 10 to 20 percent B cells. Recall that the T cells are involved in the cell-mediated immune response, whereas B cells are part of the humoral immune response.

T cells encompass a heterogeneous population of cells with extremely diverse functions. Some T cells respond to APCs of the innate immune system, and indirectly induce immune responses by releasing cytokines. Other T cells stimulate B cells to prepare their own response. Another population of T cells detects APC signals and directly kills the infected cells. Other T cells are involved in suppressing inappropriate immune reactions to harmless or "self" antigens.

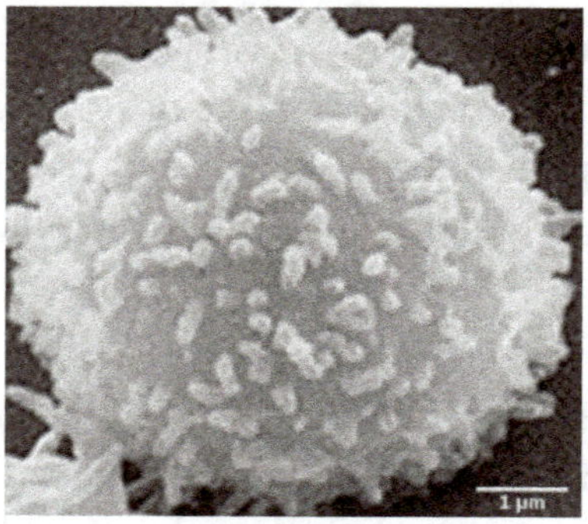

Fig. 4. This scanning electron micrograph shows a T lymphocyte, which is responsible for the cell-mediated immune response. T cells are able to recognize antigens. (credit: modification of work by NCI; scale-bar data from Matt Russell)

T and B cells exhibit a common theme of recognition/binding of specific antigens via a complementary receptor, followed by activation and self-amplification/ maturation to specifically bind to the particular antigen of the infecting pathogen. T and B lymphocytes are also similar in that each cell only expresses one type of antigen receptor. Any individual may possess a population of T and B cells that together express a near limitless variety of antigen receptors that are capable of recognizing virtually any infecting pathogen. T and B cells are activated when they recognize small components of antigens, called epitopes, presented by APCs, illustrated in Fig. 5.

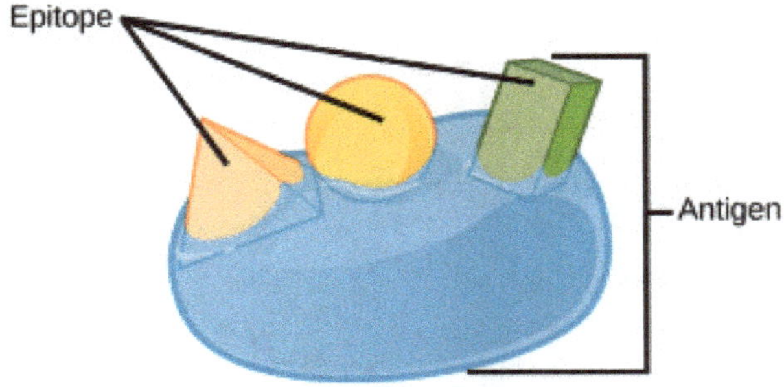

Fig. 5. An antigen is a macromolecule that reacts with components of the immune system. A given antigen may contain several motifs that are recognized by immune cells. Each motif is an epitope. In this figure, the entire structure is an antigen, and the orange, salmon and green components projecting from it represent potential epitopes

Note that recognition occurs at a specific epitope rather than on the entire antigen; for this reason, epitopes are known as "antigenic determinants." In the absence of information from APCs, T and B cells remain inactive, or naïve, and are unable to prepare an immune response. The requirement for information from the APCs of innate immunity to trigger B cell or T cell activation illustrates the essential nature of the innate immune response to the functioning of the entire immune system.

These molecules are important because they regulate how a T cell will interact with and respond to an APC. Naïve $CD4^+$ cells bind APCs via their antigen-embedded MHC II molecules and are stimulated to become helper T (T_H) lymphocytes, cells that go on to stimulate B cells (or cytotoxic T cells) directly or secrete cytokines to inform more and various target cells about the pathogenic threat. In contrast, $CD8^+$ cells engage antigen-embedded MHC I molecules on APCs and are stimulated to become cytotoxic T lymphocytes (CTLs), which directly kill infected cells by apoptosis and emit cytokines to amplify the immune response. The two populations of T cells have different mechanisms of immune protection, but both bind MHC molecules via their antigen receptors called T cell receptors (TCRs). The CD4 or CD8 surface molecules differentiate whether the TCR will engage an MHC II or an MHC I molecule. Because they assist in binding specificity, the CD4 and CD8 molecules are described as coreceptors.

Consider the innumerable possible antigens that an individual will be exposed to during a lifetime. The mammalian adaptive immune system is adept in responding appropriately to each antigen. Mammals have an enormous diversity of T cell populations, resulting from the diversity of TCRs. Each TCR consists of two polypeptide chains that span the T cell membrane, as illustrated in Fig. 6; the chains are linked by a disulfide bridge.

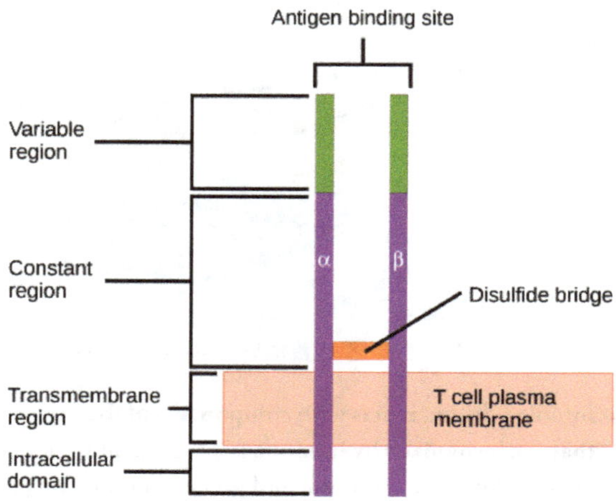

Fig. 6. A T cell receptor spans the membrane and projects variable binding regions into the extracellular space to bind processed antigens via MHC molecules on APCs.

Each polypeptide chain is comprised of a constant domain and a variable domain: a domain, in this sense, is a specific region of a protein that may be regulatory or structural. The intracellular domain is involved in intracellular signaling. A single T cell will express thousands of identical copies of one specific TCR variant on its cell surface. The specificity of the adaptive immune system occurs because it synthesizes millions of different T cell populations, each expressing a TCR that differs in its variable domain. This TCR diversity is achieved by the mutation and recombination of genes that encode these receptors in stem cell precursors of T cells.

The binding between an antigen-displaying MHC molecule and a complementary TCR "match" indicates that the adaptive immune system needs to activate and produce that specific T cell because its structure is appropriate to recognize and destroy the invading pathogen.

Helper T Lymphocytes

The T_H lymphocytes function indirectly to identify potential pathogens for other cells of the immune system. These cells are important for extracellular infections, such as those caused by certain bacteria, helminths, and protozoa. T_H lymphocytes recognize specific antigens displayed in the MHC II complexes of APCs. There are two major populations of T_H cells: T_H1 and T_H2. T_H1 cells secrete cytokines to enhance the activities of macrophages and other T cells. T_H1 cells activate the action of cyotoxic T cells, as well as macrophages. T_H2 cells stimulate naïve B cells to destroy foreign invaders via antibody secretion. Whether a T_H1 or a T_H2 immune response develops depends on the specific types of cytokines secreted by cells of the innate immune system, which in turn depends on the nature of the invading pathogen.

The T_H1-mediated response involves macrophages and is associated with inflammation. Recall the frontline defenses of macrophages involved in the innate immune response. Some intracellular bacteria, such as *Mycobacterium tuberculosis*, have evolved to multiply in macrophages after they have been engulfed. These pathogens evade attempts by macrophages to destroy and digest the pathogen. When *M. tuberculosis* infection occurs, macrophages can stimulate naïve T cells to become T_H1 cells. These stimulated T cells secrete specific cytokines that send feedback to the macrophage to stimulate its digestive capabilities and allow it to destroy the colonizing *M. tuberculosis*. In the same manner, T_H1-activated macrophages also become better suited to ingest and kill tumor cells. In summary; T_H1 responses are directed toward intracellular invaders while T_H2 responses are aimed at those that are extracellular.

B Lymphocytes

When stimulated by the T_H2 pathway, naïve B cells differentiate into antibody-secreting plasma cells. A plasma cell is an immune cell that secrets antibodies; these cells arise from B cells that were stimulated by antigens. Similar to T cells, naïve B cells initially are coated in thousands of B cell receptors (BCRs), which are membrane-bound forms of Ig (immunoglobulin, or an antibody). The B cell receptor has two heavy chains and two light chains connected by disulfide linkages. Each chain has a constant and a variable region; the latter is involved in antigen binding. Two other membrane proteins, Ig alpha and Ig beta, are involved in signaling.

The receptors of any particular B cell, as shown in Fig. 7 are all the same, but the hundreds of millions of different B cells in an individual have distinct recognition domains that contribute to extensive diversity in the types of molecular structures to which they can bind. In this state, B cells function as APCs. They bind and engulf foreign antigens via their BCRs and then display processed antigens in the context of MHC II molecules to T_H2 cells. When a T_H2 cell detects that a B cell is bound to a relevant antigen, it secretes specific cytokines that induce the B cell to proliferate rapidly, which makes thousands of identical (clonal) copies of it, and then it synthesizes and secretes antibodies with the same antigen recognition pattern as the BCRs. The activation of B cells corresponding to one specific BCR variant and the dramatic proliferation of that variant is known as clonal selection. This phenomenon drastically, but briefly, changes the proportions of BCR variants expressed by the immune system, and shifts the balance toward BCRs specific to the infecting pathogen.

T and B cells differ in one fundamental way: whereas T cells bind antigens that have been digested and embedded in MHC molecules by APCs, B cells function as APCs that bind intact antigens that have not been processed. Although T and B cells both react with molecules that are termed "antigens," these lymphocytes actually respond to very different types of molecules. B cells must be able to bind intact antigens because they secrete antibodies that must recognize the pathogen directly, rather than digested remnants of the pathogen. Bacterial carbohydrate and lipid molecules can activate B cells independently from the T cells.

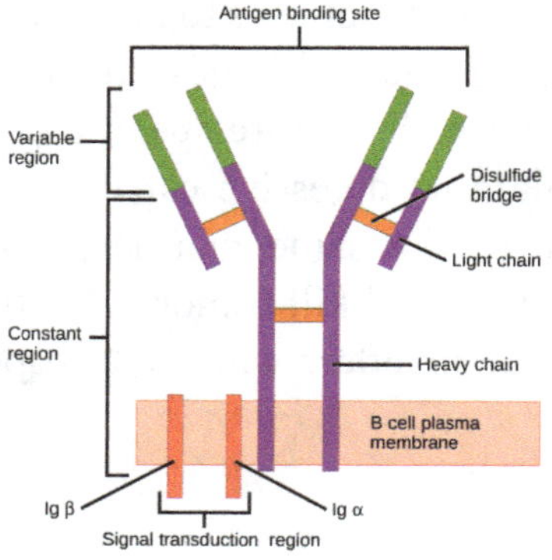

Fig. 7. B cell receptors are embedded in the membranes of B cells and bind a variety of antigens through their variable regions. The signal transduction region transfers the signal into the cell.

Cytotoxic T Lymphocytes

CTLs, a subclass of T cells, function to clear infections directly. The cell-mediated part of the adaptive immune system consists of CTLs that attack and destroy infected cells. CTLs are particularly important in protecting against viral infections; this is because viruses replicate within cells where they are shielded from extracellular contact with circulating antibodies. When APCs phagocytize pathogens and present MHC I-embedded antigens to naïve CD8$^+$ T cells that express complementary TCRs, the CD$^+$8 T cells become activated to proliferate according to clonal selection. These resulting CTLs then identify non-APCs displaying the same MHC I-embedded antigens (for example, viral proteins)—for example, the CTLs identify infected host cells.

Intracellularly, infected cells typically die after the infecting pathogen replicates to a sufficient concentration and lyses the cell, as many viruses do. CTLs attempt to identify and destroy infected cells before the pathogen can replicate and escape, thereby halting the progression of intracellular infections. CTLs also support NK lymphocytes to destroy early cancers. Cytokines secreted by the T_H1 response that stimulates macrophages also stimulate CTLs and enhance their ability to identify and destroy infected cells and tumors.

CTLs sense MHC I-embedded antigens by directly interacting with infected cells via their TCRs. Binding of TCRs with antigens activates CTLs to release perforin and granzyme, degradative enzymes that will induce apoptosis of the infected cell. Recall that this is a similar destruction mechanism to that used by NK cells. In this process, the CTL does not become infected and is not harmed by the secretion of perforin and granzymes. In fact, the functions of NK cells and CTLs are complementary and maximize the removal of infected cells.

If the NK cell cannot identify the "missing self" pattern of down-regulated MHC I molecules, then the CTL can identify it by the complex of MHC I with foreign antigens, which signals "altered self." Similarly, if the CTL cannot detect antigen-embedded MHC I because the receptors are depleted from the cell surface, NK cells will destroy the cell instead.

CTLs also emit cytokines, such as interferons, that alter surface protein expression in other infected cells, such that the infected cells can be easily identified and destroyed. Moreover, these interferons can also prevent virally infected cells from releasing virus particles.

Based on what you know about MHC receptors, why do you think an organ transplanted from an incompatible donor to a recipient will be rejected?

Plasma cells and CTLs are collectively called effector cells: they represent differentiated versions of their naïve counterparts, and they are involved in bringing about the immune defense of killing pathogens and infected host cells.

ANTIBODIES IN ANIMALS

Antibodies are proteins called immunoglobulins. Mammals use five different classes of antibodies: immunoglobulin G (IgG), IgM, IgA, IgE, and IgD. The class of immunoglobulin secreted by B cells and plasma cells depends on their location. Cells located in lymphoid organs within the body secrete IgM and IgG, whereas cells located on mucosal surfaces mainly secrete IgA and/or IgE.

IgG is the most abundant immunoglobulin found in the bloodstream and plays the major role in eliminating organisms that succeed in penetrating deep into the body. IgM is usually confined to the bloodstream because it is a very large molecule with much more antigen binding capacity compared with the smaller IgG, which can easily go into interstitial spaces. IgM is produced early in the antibody response, when its high effectiveness compensates for its low quantity.

IgA is produced by B cells and plasma cells located on mucosal surfaces. As a result, IgA is produced and secreted in large amounts into the upper respiratory tract, the GI tract, tears, sweat, etc. On those surfaces, it complements the physical barriers of the body and prevents microbial invasion. IgE is produced locally by plasma cells and then binds with a very high affinity to tissue mast cells. On the mast cell it serves as a sentinel to detect and respond to specific antigens by causing the mast cell to release granules that contain potent vasoactive mediators. IgE is optimized to control invasion by parasites such as helminths or arthropods. However, it also mediates a rapid acute inflammation in allergic states and can trigger life-threatening anaphylaxis. The function of IgD is unclear, but it is believed to play a role in the response to the normal microbiota.

T Cell Help in Animals

As discussed earlier, antibody responses are regulated by the need to receive prior approval from helper T cells. The helper T cells in turn can only be activated when they bind antigen fragments presented by specialized antigen-presenting cells called dendritic cells.

Dendritic cells are macrophage-like cells whose role is to capture and process foreign antigens. Their name derives from their many long, thin filamentous processes or dendrites that extend through tissues to form an antigen-trapping web. For example, a subpopulation of dendritic cells called Langerhans' cells are found in the dermis, where they trap organisms seeking to enter the body through damaged skin. Dendritic cells capture and phagocytize invading microorganisms. Fragments of these foreign antigens persist within the dendritic cells, where they become attached to receptor molecules called MHC molecules. Once formed, these antigen-receptor complexes move to the dendritic cell surface, where they can be recognized by helper T cells.

The receptors in dendritic cells that present antigen fragments are specialized proteins encoded by genes clustered together in the Major Histocompatibility Complex (MHC) (originally identified as the antigens that cause graft rejection, hence their unusual name). There are many thousands of different MHC molecules expressed within an animal population, but relatively few are expressed in any individual animal. Because they play a critical role in binding antigen fragments and activating T cells, MHC molecules effectively determine whether an individual can respond to a foreign antigen. An individual animal possesses MHC molecules that can bind many, perhaps most, foreign antigens, but not all of them. If an animal lacks MHC molecules that can bind an antigen, it will be unable to respond to that specific antigen.

Like B cells, helper T cells possess specific antigen receptors on their surface that are generated randomly when the cells are first produced. When helper T cells mature within the thymus, any cells with receptors that can bind normal body components are killed. As a result, the surviving T cells can respond only to foreign antigens. The antigen receptors on T cells, like those on B cells, are identical on any single cell. Unlike those on B cells, however, the receptors can recognize antigen only when it is bound to an MHC molecule. Thus, when a dendritic cell presents

MHC-associated antigen to T cells, only those T cells with appropriate receptors will bind to the dendritic cell. Once in contact, the cells exchange signals that confirm that the T cell is responding to a correctly processed antigen. After T cells receive all the necessary signals, they secrete cytokines that permit their attached B cells to respond to antigens and allow antibody production to proceed.

Antibodies are produced in response to, and directed against, extracellular bacteria. Cell-mediated responses, in contrast, are directed against viruses and intracellular bacteria. The selection of the appropriate form of the immune response is made at an early stage in the immune response. Thus, there are two populations of dendritic cells that can trap and process antigens. One population (DC1 cells) triggers cell-mediated immunity, whereas the other (DC2 cells) triggers antibody formation. These dendritic cell populations send different messages to T cells because they use different cytokines for signaling; for example, DC1 cells secrete IL-12, whereas DC2 cells secrete IL-1. In turn, these different cytokines stimulate two different helper T cell populations: Th1, which promotes cell-mediated immunity, and Th2, which promotes B cell responses and antibody production. Th1 cells secrete a mixture of cytokines typified by interferon-gamma (IFN-gamma). Th2 cells secrete a mixture of cytokines typified by IL-4. B cells will usually respond optimally to a foreign antigen only if they are stimulated by the presence of IL-4 from Th2 cells.

Cell-mediated Immunity

As described above, cell-mediated immune responses are needed to combat intracellular invaders such as viruses and some bacteria. The immune system combats viral infections simply by killing virus-infected cells. The cells responsible for this killing are called effector or cytotoxic T cells. These are also known as CD8+ cells, based on proteins they express on their surface. Cytotoxic T cells also undergo development and selection within the thymus so that any cells capable of killing normal, healthy cells are eliminated. The surviving cytotoxic T cells are released into the body, where they circulate continuously through the tissues, seeking out abnormal cells to kill.

All nucleated cells produce many different proteins. Virus-infected cells, however, are forced by the virus to produce viral proteins. The body, therefore, requires that all nucleated cells send a sample of their newly synthesized proteins to the cell surface. Thus, the cell diverts a small amount of each new protein into a complex enzyme system called a proteasome. The resulting protein fragments are then attached to MHC molecules and carried to the cell surface, where they are available for inspection by effector T cells. If the T cell's receptors do not bind the complex, then it will be left alone. If, however, their antigen receptors bind to a foreign antigen fragment in an MHC-protein complex, then the T cell will kill the cell it is attached to. Like B cells, cytotoxic T cells only function if they receive costimulation from a helper T cell, specifically a Th1 cell. These cells are also called CD4+ helper T cells based on their surface proteins. The cytokines from Th1 cells, especially IFN-gamma, must be present if a cytotoxic T cell is to kill its target.

Cytotoxic T cells bind tightly to any cells expressing foreign antigens and then signal them to commit suicide through apoptosis. The T cells inject their targets with enzymes called granzymes that trigger this process. As a result, cytotoxic T cells eliminate virus-infected cells but not normal, healthy cells. Most cytotoxic T cells die within a few days once they are no longer needed, but a few survive to become long-lived memory cells that respond rapidly should the animal encounter the virus a second time.

Cytotoxic T cells are especially effective at killing target cells producing foreign antigens. However some intracellular organisms, especially intracellular bacteria, are more effectively destroyed by other cell-mediated mechanisms. In these cases, IFN-gamma from Th1 cells activates M1 macrophages. As a result, bacteria that can survive within normal macrophages are rapidly destroyed by activated macrophages.

IMMUNOLOGIC MEMORY

The effectiveness of adaptive immunity is largely a result of its ability to recognize invading microbes encountered previously and to mount an enhanced and accelerated response against them. The more an animal encounters an antigen, the greater will be its immune response. Immunologic memory depends on the presence of persistent populations of memory cells that accumulate as an animal ages. These memory cells may be very long-lived or, more likely, turn over very slowly. As a result, animals may make small amounts of antibodies to vaccine antigens for many years after vaccination. Cell-mediated memory is also due to the development of very long-lived populations of memory T cells. The effectiveness of vaccines in inducing long-lasting immunity depends in large part on their ability to induce memory cell populations.

Cytokines

The cells of the adaptive immune system communicate in many ways. They can come into physical contact and exchange signals through receptors within the contact area or immunologic synapse. Examples include the contact between T cells and dendritic cells or between effector T cells and their targets. Immune cells can also signal nearby cells by secreting signaling proteins called cytokines. Several hundred different cytokines have been identified. Signaling cells secrete a mixture of cytokines that then bind to receptors on nearby cells. The target cell receives multiple signals that it must integrate to respond appropriately. Cytokines, acting through their specific receptors, can turn the synthesis of specific proteins on or off. They can cause the target cell to divide or differentiate, and they may trigger apoptosis. With hundreds of different cytokines acting in complex mixtures it is sometimes difficult to predict exactly how a specific target cell will respond. Major families of cytokines include the interleukins that mediate signaling between leukocytes, interferons that mediate interactions between cells and have significant antiviral activity, growth factors that regulate growth and differentiation of many different cell types, and tumor necrosis factors that modulate inflammatory responses.

Regulatory Cells

The adaptive immune system is carefully regulated by several different cell populations. Helper T cells that promote immune responses are described earlier. Other T cells are called regulatory T cells (T_{reg} cells). These secrete a mixture of cytokines that inhibit conventional immune responses. They serve to turn off an immune response once it has completed its task and the invading microorganism is eliminated. T_{reg} cells also play a central role in preventing the development of autoimmunity.

IMMUNE DYSFUNCTION AND CLINICAL IMMUNOLOGY

The immune system is a highly regulated and balanced system and when the balance is disturbed, disease can result. Research in this area involves studying disease that is caused by immune system dysfunction.

Much of this work has significance in the development of new therapies and treatments that can manage or cure the condition by altering the way the immune system is working or, in the case of vaccines, priming the immune system and boosting the immune reaction to specific pathogens.

Immuno-deficiency disorders involve problems with the immune system that impair its ability to mount an appropriate defence. As a result, these are almost always associated with severe infections that persist, recur and/or lead to complications, making these disorders severely debilitating and even fatal. There are two types of immunodeficiency disorders: primary immunodeficiencies are typically present from birth, are generally hereditary and are relatively rare. Such an example is common variable immunodeficiency (CVID). Secondary immunodeficiencies generally develop later in life and may result following an infection, as is the case with AIDS following HIV infection.

The development of novel tools and technologies has been fundamental to the advancement of basic and applied immunology across species. The rate of progress of immunological reagent development for veterinary species has been much slower than that for humans and small rodent biomedical model species, and has impacted research capability in those species.

Historically, however, innovations in surgical procedures in veterinary species have resulted in major step-changes in our understanding of the ontogeny, compartmentalization and function of the immune system. For example, bursectomy in chickens shed new light on mechanisms of B cell development and immunoglobulin production, in utero thymectomy of lambs revealed the importance of the thymus for lymphocyte development and lymphatic cannulation of sheep revealed that lymphocyte subsets differ between blood, afferent and efferent lymph. These ground-breaking experiments were feasible, in part, due to the size of the species under investigation, particularly for the technique of lymphatic cannulation due to the diameter of lymphatic vessels in ruminants.

However, this momentum in veterinary immunological studies was not maintained; the vast majority of technological innovations and discoveries in immunology in the past 50 years have been made in mice. The development of congenic mice, differing at a single histocompatibility locus, was a fundamental technological innovation in immunology that led to mice being the primary species of choice for research.

That pioneering work of George Snell and the later capability of genetically manipulating congenic mice has allowed immunologists to ascribe functions to genes, molecules and cells with high precision. The development of monoclonal antibody (mAb) technology using congenic mice subsequently created almost boundless opportunities for research in basic and translational immunology.

The availability of mAbs that could phenotype cells and detect cytokines by ELISA underpinned the discovery of two distinct $CD4^{+ve}$ T-cell subsets in congenic mice . The subsequent Th1/Th2 paradigm provided a fundamental framework for investigating immune activation and regulation that has expanded far beyond those original two subsets. Current capability now extends to multi-parametric analyses such as simultaneous fourteen-color flow cytometry that can identify 89 functionally-relevant $CD4^{+ve}$ T-cell subsets in human blood. Mass cytometry (CyTOF) methods using panels of well over 40 conjugated antibodies are now allowing for even deeper analysis of single cell expression, offering new insights into cellular subsets and their differentiation.

Such technologies cannot usually be applied directly to different species since molecular differences in immunological orthologs result in low cross-reactivity of reagents across species as affirmed by a recent comparison of reactivity of immune protein reagents for other species with swine orthologs. Thus, reagent development needs to be evaluated on a case-by-case basis. Gaps in capability for veterinary species are often prioritized based on the extensive mouse and human immunological toolboxes. The expansion of the toolboxes has revealed substantial differences in the ways that humans, mice and veterinary species respond to disease and highlighted to need for studying different species in their own right. There have been coordinated efforts to evaluate species cross-reactivity of anti-human CD antigen mAbs through the animal homologs section of the human leukocyte differentiation antigen (HLDA) workshops: for horses, dogs, pigs, and ruminants.

In an effort to generate greater international co-ordination for immune reagent characterization activities, the International Union of Immunological Societies (IUIS) Veterinary Immunology Committee (VIC) supported a Toolkit Workshop at the 6th International Veterinary Immunology Symposium (IVIS) in Upsala, Sweden in 2001. This set the scene for a series of VIC Toolkit Workshops. It is almost 10 years since the last published review of the veterinary immunology toolbox from the IUIS VIC Toolkit Workshop at the 9th IVIS in Tokyo, Japan. Here, we review progress over the past decade by reporting on the IUIS VIC Toolkit Workshop at the 12th IVIS in Seattle, USA in 2019 and take a forward look to the future of the veterinary immunology toolbox.

The Past

The success of the HLDA workshops was based on good co-ordination, high-quality work and collective effort by the veterinary immunology community, as well as results from past species-specific CD workshops supported by IUIS VIC. Common standards were applied to the distribution and evaluation of anti-human CD reagents being assessed in different laboratories and the collective generated data being reviewed centrally. The outcome was an evidence-based assessment for the activity of species cross-reactive mAbs, with affirmation that only a limited number of mAb directed against human CD antigens actually cross-react with other animal species. These results instilled confidence in the performance of those reagents and promoted their uptake by the research community and industry, including companies that market and sell veterinary immunological reagents.

Although the HLDA workshops were primarily focused on evaluation of species cross-reactive antibodies, they played an important role in informing of capability gaps and therefore the prioritization of reagents for future development. A major step-change in the way veterinary immunological reagent development was supported came with the inception of a UK Immunological Toolbox funded by the Biotechnology and Biological Sciences Research Council (BBSRC) and the Scottish Executive Environment and Rural Affairs Department (SEERAD) in 2003.

This was unique as it united several laboratories within a single project to take a collective multi-species approach to immunological reagent development. This was followed by the Veterinary Immune Reagent Network (VIRN) funded by United States Department of Agriculture (USDA)/National Institute of Food and Agriculture (NIFA) in the US in 2005. Both projects included the creation of databases listing available veterinary immunological reagents, which will be discussed later. They also expanded the emphasis from mAb anti-CD antigens to expression of immune proteins (cytokines and chemokines) and protein reactive mAbs. The US project included direct collaboration with commercial partners to express these immune proteins.

The US and UK projects worked together under a Memorandum of Understanding (MOU) to avoid duplication of effort. This MOU was created in the absence of a mechanism for joint international funding by the respective national agencies. The structure, priorities and achievements of these projects has been published previously. A key output from these initiatives was an increased recognition of the importance of coordinated, complementary approaches to reagent prioritization and development. Their success has also been reflected by continued support for reagent development initiatives by funders seeking to build on the significant benefits from their original investments, with the assertion that long-term sustainability is essential.

The funding for veterinary immunology reagent development has changed over the past 10 years, moving from the multi-species models of the UK Immunological Toolbox and US VIRN, to single-species projects. With the exception of ruminants, there is very little species cross-reactivity of veterinary reagents, highlighting that the genes involved in immune responses are amongst the most rapidly evolving in vertebrate genomes.

However, this does not diminish their potential as disease models. BBSRC and USDA/NIFA have supported reagent development projects for ruminants, swine, horses, aquaculture species and poultry in the past 10 years. A barrier to formal international collaboration was lifted in 2013 when USDA/NIFA and BBSRC launched a pilot call to support animal disease research of strategic importance to both the US and UK which included the development of veterinary immunological reagents for agriculturally-relevant animal species. The swine toolkit was a landmark first transatlantic veterinary immunology reagent project funded under this initiative in 2015.

Although we have focused here on projects funded specifically to develop reagents and supporting technologies, this is not intended to ignore the veterinary immunological reagent development that is conducted within disease-driven projects, networks and within strategic programmes of government research institutes across the globe. The challenge is in capturing the outputs of these diverse activities. The websites of commercial reagent suppliers and peer-reviewed publications are sources of validated information on reagent activity.

However, they do not capture everything, a particular gap being the paucity of "negative" data when reagents are found to be non-functional or where repeated attempts fail to generate specific antibodies. These are very valuable data as they can potentially prevent the duplication of wasted effort. The solution lies in community engagement for the sharing of knowledge on reagent availability and performance.

Workshops such as those hosted by IUIS VIC Toolkit are a focal point for international information exchange, but they do not have the facility to capture, store and disseminate information at a detailed level. It has been recognized for many years that a major unmet need in veterinary immunology is the lack of centralized, non-commercial, searchable reagent databases.

The Present

The current landscape of the veterinary immunology toolbox has been shaped by new funding approaches to facilitate reagent development while also addressing the complex issues of database construction, collection and validation of data, and sustainability of the database and biobanks of the reagents listed therein. This report summarizes the outcomes of several international workshops where these various elements have been considered.

Before summarizing those outcomes, it is worth reviewing the scope of the toolbox in terms of species coverage and knowledge of immunological capability within those species. In the broadest sense, the concept of a veterinary immunological toolbox encompasses a broad range of livestock, companion animal, biomedical model and wildlife species. There has been progress in reagent development across all of those species in the past 10 years which has been presented at various meetings and workshops. We have identified a number of published articles where reagent availability for different species have been reviewed. For the purposes of the toolbox, livestock species can largely be regarded as belonging to one of four major groupings, namely swine, ruminants, poultry, and aquaculture. Companion animals include horses, cats, and dogs.

The mice are the most common small-animal biomedical model for human. However, rabbitsand ferretsare also popular small-animal biomedical models for human disease. There is interest in expanding the immunological toolboxes for wildlife species, for example buffaloand badgersdue to their potential to act as reservoirs for economically-important livestock diseases. There is also interest in developing immunological reagents for marine mammals such as dolphins. In addition, although camelid species are not often regarded as a major target host species for disease studies, they have come to the fore with heightened awareness of MERS-CoV and the potential to reduce zoonotic transmission by investigating vaccine-induced responses in camels. Importantly, camels make a unique technological contribution to the immunological toolbox via the production of nanobodies.

HISTORY OF IMMUNOLOGY

In Western society, it was not until the late eighteenth century that a rational approach to the origin of disease developed. Prior to the discovery that disease was the result of pathogenic organisms, it was commonly accepted that disease was a punishment from God (or the Gods), or even a witches curse. Eastern cultures perceived disease as an imbalance in the energy channels within the body. Later, the great plagues of Europe were assumed the result of virulent or noxious vapors. Nevertheless, there were intimations as early as 430 B.C. that if one survived a disease, the person thereafter became "immune" to any subsequent exposures. However, this was never recognized as evidence of some type of internal defense system until the later part of the seventeenth century.

Although most historical accounts credit Edward Jenner for the development of the first immunization process, a previous similar procedure had become established in China by 1700. The technique was called variolation. This was derived from the name of the infective agent—the variola virus . The basic principal of variolation was to deliberately cause a mild infection with unmodified pathogen. The risk of death from variolation was around two to three percent. Although still a risk, variolation was a considerable improvement on the death rate for uncontrolled infection. Immunity to smallpox was conferred by inserting the dried exudate of smallpox pustules into the nose. This technique for the transfer of smallpox, as a form of limited infection, traveled to the west from China along the traditional trade routes to Constantinople where it spread throughout Europe. Hearing of this practice, the Royal family of England had their children inoculated against the disease in 1721, but the practice aroused severe opposition as physicians felt it was far too risky.

In 1798, Edward Jenner, noticed that milkmaids were protected from smallpox if they had been first infected with cowpox . It was not his intention to make medical history, as his interests were mostly scholarly and involved the transfer of infections from one species to another, especially from animals to humans. However, Jenner's work led him to the conclusion, that inoculation with cowpox (a bovine analogue of smallpox) could confer immunity to smallpox. Thus, the concept of vaccination was initiated. (Incidentally, the Latin word for cow is *vacca*). Jenner's ideas first made him a medical as well as a social pariah, as they were in opposition to both the church and popular beliefs. Because his method was much safer then variolation, however, the use of vaccinations gradually became widely accepted and most European countries had some form of compulsory program within fifty years of Jenner's discovery.

The idea that a pathogenic organism caused disease was not fully realized until certain technological advances had occurred. Initially, Antoni van Leeuwenhoek 's development of the microscope and the subsequent realization that entities existed that were not visible to the human eye, allowed the concept of germs to be appreciated.

That these organisms were the causative agent of disease was not recognized until Louis Pasteur developed his germ theory of disease . His original interests were in fermentation in wine and beer, and he was the first to isolate the organisms that caused the fermentation process. Pasteur's work eventually led him to the development of pasteurization (heating) as a means of halting fermentation. While working with silk worms and anthrax , he was able to demonstrate that the same method for transferring the fermentation process also worked in transmitting disease from infected animals to unaffected animals.

Finally, in 1878, Pasteur accidentally used an attenuated (weakened) chicken cholera culture and realized, when he repeated the experiment using a fresh culture, that the weakened form protected the chickens from the virulent form of the disease. Pasteur went on to develop an attenuated vaccine against rabies and swine erysipelas.

Pasteur was not the only proponent of the germ theory of disease. His chief competitor was Robert Koch. Koch was the first to isolate the anthrax microbe and, unaware of Pasteur's work, he was able to show that it caused the disease. Then in 1882, Koch was able to demonstrate that the germ theory of disease applied to human ailments as well as animals, when he isolated the microbe that caused tuberculosis . His "Koch's postulates" are still used to identify infective organisms.

Much of the basis for modern medicine, as well as the field of immunology , can be traced back to these two scientists, but the two major questions still to be answered were how did infection cause the degradation of tissue, and how did vaccines work? The first question was addressed in 1881 by Emile Roux and Alexander Yersin when they isolated a soluble toxin from diphtheria cultures. Later, Emil von Behring and Shibasaburo Kitasato were able to demonstrate passive immunity when they took serum from animals infected with diphtheria and injected into healthy animals.

These same animals were found to be resistant to the disease. Eventually these serum factors were recognized in 1930 as antibodies. However, thirty years before antibodies were finally isolated and identified, Paul Ehrlich and others, recognized that a specific antigen elicited the production of a specific antibody . Ehrlich hypothesized that these antibodies were specialized molecular structures with specific receptor sites that fit each pathogen like a lock and key.

Thus, the first realization that the body had a specific defense system was introduced. In addition, sometime later, he realized that this powerful effector mechanism, used in host defense would, if turned against the host, cause severe tissue damage. Ehrlich termed this *horror autotoxicus.* Although extremely valuable, his work still left a large gap in understanding how the immune system fights a pathogenic challenge. The idea that specific cells could be directly involved with defending the body was first suggested in 1884 by Élie Metchnikoff . His field was zoology and he studied phagocytosis in single cell organisms.

Metchnikoff postulated that vertebrates could operate in a similar manner to remove pathogens. However, it was not until the 1940s that his theories were accepted and the cell mediated, as opposed to the humoral, immune response was recognized.

The clarification of the immune response and the science of immunology did not progress in a systematic or chronological order. Nonetheless, once scientists had a basic understanding of the cellular and humoral branches of the immune system, what remained was the identification of the various components of this intricate system, and the mechanisms of their interactions. This could not have been accomplished without the concomitant development of molecular biology and genetics.

Milestones in the history of immunology include:

- 1798 Edward Jenner initiates smallpox vaccination.
- 1877 Paul Erlich recognizes mast cells.
- 1879 Louis Pasteur develops an attenuated chicken cholera vaccine.
- 1883 Elie Metchnikoff develops cellular theory of vaccination.
- 1885 Louis Pasteur develops rabies vaccine.
- 1891 Robert Koch explored delayed type hypersensitivity.
- 1900 Paul Erlich theorizes specific antibody formation.
- 1906 Clemens von Pirquet coined the word allergy.
- 1938 John Marrack formulates antigen-antibody binding hypothesis.
- 1942 Jules Freund and Katherine McDermott research adjuvants.
- 1949 Macfarlane Burnet & Frank Fenner formulate immunological tolerance hypothesis.
- 1959 Niels Jerne, David Talmage, Macfarlane Burnet develop clonal selection theory.
- 1957 Alick Isaacs & Jean Lindemann discover interferon (cytokine).
- 1962 Rodney Porter and team discovery the structure of antibodies.
- 1962 Jaques Miller and team discover thymus involvement in cellular immunity.
- 1962 Noel Warner and team distinguish between cellular and humoral immune responses.
- 1968 Anthony Davis and team discover T cell and B cell cooperation in immune response.
- 1974 Rolf Zinkernagel and Peter Doherty explore major histocompatibility complex restriction.

- 1985 Susumu Tonegawa, Leroy Hood, and team identify immunoglobulin genes.
- 1987 Leroy Hood and team identify genes for the T cell receptor.
- 1985 Scientists begin the rapid identification of genes for immune cells that continues to the present.

IMMUNE SYSTEM

The immune system protects your child's body from outside invaders. These include germs such as bacteria, viruses, and fungi, and toxins (chemicals made by microbes). The immune system is made up of different organs, cells, and proteins that work together.

The innate immune system

This is your child's rapid response system. It is the first to respond when it finds an invader. It is made up of the skin, the eye's cornea, and the mucous membrane that lines the respiratory, gastrointestinal, and genitourinary tracts. These all create physical barriers to help protect your child's body.

They protect against harmful germs, parasites (such as worms), or cells (such as cancer). The innate immune system is inherited. It is active from the moment your child is born. When this system recognizes an invader, it goes into action right away. The cells of this immune system surround and cover the invader. The invader is killed inside the immune system cells (called phagocytes).

The acquired immune system

The acquired immune system, with help from the innate system, makes special proteins (called antibodies) to protect your body from a specific invader. These antibodies are developed by cells called B lymphocytes after the body has been exposed to the invader. The antibodies stay in your child's body. It can take several days for antibodies to form. But after the first exposure, the immune system will recognize the invader and defend against it. The acquired immune system changes during your child's life. Immunizations train your child's immune system to make antibodies to protect them from harmful diseases.

The cells of both parts of the immune system are made in different organs of the body, including:

- Adenoids. Two glands located at the back of the nasal passage.
- Bone marrow. The soft, spongy tissue found in bone cavities.
- Lymph nodes. Small organs shaped like beans, which are located all over the body and connect via the lymphatic vessels.

- Lymphatic vessels. A network of channels all over the body that carries lymphocytes to the lymphoid organs and bloodstream.
- Peyer patches. Lymphoid tissue in the small intestine.
- Spleen. A fist-sized organ located in the belly (abdominal) cavity.
- Thymus. Two lobes that join in front of the windpipe (trachea) behind the breastbone.
- Tonsils. Two oval masses in the back of the throat.

IMMUNE SYSTEM RESPONSES IN DOGS

The primary role of the immune system is to defend the body against foreign invaders or abnormal cells that invade or attack it. In order to do this, the immune system must distinguish between "self" and "non-self."

By recognizing invading microorganisms (such as viruses), chemical agents, or other foreign substances that are "non-self," a body can protect itself from attack. Substances that stimulate an immune response in the body are called antigens. Antigens may be contained within or on bacteria, viruses, other microorganisms, or cancer cells. Antigens may also exist on their own—for example, as pollen or food molecules. A normal immune response consists of recognizing a foreign antigen, mobilizing forces to defend against it, and attacking it. There are 3 lines of defense against invaders: physical barriers, nonspecific (or innate) immunity, and specific (or adaptive) immunity. Nonspecific and specific immunity involve various white blood cells.

Physical Barriers

The first lines of defense against invaders are mechanical or physical barriers. These include the skin, the cornea of the eye, and the membranes lining the respiratory, digestive, urinary, and reproductive tracts. As long as these barriers remain unbroken, many invaders cannot penetrate them. However, if a barrier is broken (for example, if the skin is broken by a wound), the risk of infection is increased.

In addition, the physical barriers are defended by "good" bacteria that live in the area and by secretions containing enzymes that can destroy harmful bacteria. Examples are tears in the eyes, secretions in the digestive tract, and normal "gut flora" (bacteria) that live in the digestive tract.

Nonspecific Immunity

Nonspecific (innate) immunity is present at birth. It is so named because its components treat all foreign substances in much the same way. Acute inflammation is the most important process involved in nonspecific immunity. During inflammation, white blood cells (such as neutrophils and macrophages) rapidly travel from the blood into the tissues to kill invading organisms and remove injured cells. Other white blood cells involved in nonspecific immunity are monocytes (which develop into macrophages), eosinophils, basophils, and natural killer cells (see also White Blood Cells of Dogs). These nonspecific types of white blood cells usually act on their own to destroy invaders. The complement system and cytokines are molecules produced by the immune system that also participate in nonspecific immunity.

Specific Immunity

Specific (adaptive) immunity is not present at birth; it is acquired. As the immune system encounters different antigens, it learns the best way to attack each antigen, and it begins to develop a memory for that antigen. Specific immunity is so named because it tailors its attack to a specific antigen previously encountered. It takes time to develop specific immunity after initial exposure to a new antigen; however, when the antigen is encountered in the future, the response is more rapid and more effective than that generated by nonspecific immunity. Specific immunity involves the action of lymphocytes (B cells and T cells), antibodies, antigen-presenting cells, and cytokines. Most vaccines work by stimulating the development of specific immunity. Vaccinations have been developed for many diseases in animals and are an effective way of enhancing the immune response.

Mounting an Immune Response

To destroy invaders, the immune system must first recognize them. It can make this distinction because all cells have unique markers on their surface that identify them. A cell with markers on its surface that are not identical to those on the body's own cells is identified as being foreign. The immune system then attacks that cell.

Some white blood cells (B cells) recognize invaders, or antigens, directly. When a B cell recognizes and attaches to the antigen, it produces antibodies, which coat the surface of the virus or bacteria to stop it from multiplying or infecting other cells. This process is called neutralization. Antibodies also label the foreign invaders so that other immune defenses can find and attack them. To prevent inappropriate immune responses, B cells usually require "permission" from helper T cells to produce antibodies.

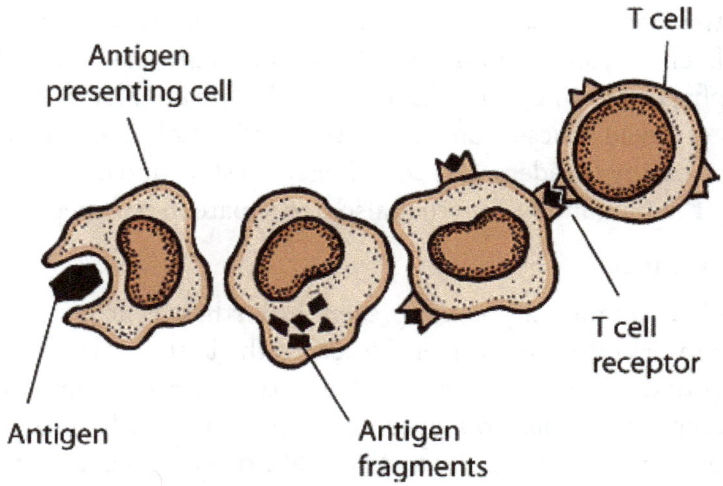

Fig. 8. Antigens and T cells

T-cells are white blood cells that also need help from cells that first ingest the invader and break it into fragments. The fragments are then presented to the T cells so that they can recognize and destroy them. These helper cells are called antigen presenting cells.

After an infectious organism has been eliminated, most of the immune cells and antibodies that fought the infection disappear. However, a small group of "memory" immune cells remain in the body. If the memory cells are later exposed to an antigen that they remember, they help the body respond much faster and with a stronger response. This is the reason why vaccinations are successful in preventing many diseases. Vaccinations prime the immune system to respond quickly by exposing the T and B cells to antigens present on the infectious organism.

TYPES OF IMMUNE SYSTEM DISORDERS

The immune system does not always function properly. Immune system disorders, called immune-mediated disorders, occur when the immune system is overactive or underactive. Disorders resulting from an underactive immune system, called immunodeficiencies, put animals at an increased risk for infections. Alternatively, an overactive immune system can attack parts of its own body that it misidentifies as foreign, causing what is known as an autoimmune disorder. At other times, the immune system overreacts to foreign invaders by producing too many antibodies or other chemicals (known as hypersensitivity or allergic reactions). There are 4 general classifications or types of these disorders.

Type I Reactions (Anaphylaxis)

Type I reactions are excessive immune responses triggered by antibodies, mast cells, and eosinophils. It includes allergic reactions, the most serious of which is anaphylaxis. Anaphylaxis is a rare, life-threatening, immediate allergic reaction to something that has entered the body (for example, eaten or injected). In a normal immune system, the binding of an antigen to an antibody activates various cells, which produce chemicals such as histamines. In anaphylaxis, the body activates an excessive number of cells, resulting in the production of very large numbers of histamines and other chemicals. These chemicals can affect various organs such as the blood vessels and muscles. The severity of the reaction depends on the type and amount of antigen, the amount of antibodies produced, and the route of exposure. Agents that can cause anaphylactic and allergic reactions include biting insects, vaccines, drugs, food, and blood products. The most common signs include restlessness, excitement, swelling of the face, drooling, vomiting, abdominal pain, diarrhea, difficulty breathing, shock, collapse, convulsions, and death.

Type II Reactions (Antibody-mediated Cytotoxic Reactions)

Type II reactions occur when an antibody binds to an antigen present at the surface of its own cells. This antibody–antigen complex then activates a cell-killing series of proteins called complement, resulting in cell death and tissue damage. An infection can trigger this reaction, or "cross-reactive" antibodies can target normal cells. Some animals appear to be born with a higher risk of this disorder.

Signs of Type II hypersensitivity vary, and they depend on the organ in which the reaction is occurring. Immune-mediated destruction of red blood cells and platelets are the most common Type II reactions. The skin and muscles are other potential targets. The method of diagnosis also varies depending on the affected organ. Supportive treatment consists of elimination of the infectious agent (if determined) and anti-inflammatory or immunosuppressive drug treatment.

Type III Reactions (Immune Complex Disease)

Type III reactions occur when a large number of antigen–antibody complexes lodge in certain organs, causing damage to blood vessels. There are many possible reasons for the continuous presence of antigens, including persistent infections, cancer, and longterm exposure to inhaled antigens. In addition, antibody responses to certain drugs can occur, particularly in the case of long-acting drugs or drugs that are given continually over a long period of time. Some animals can react and produce antibodies against self antigens. However, in many cases, the cause of the disease is unidentifiable.

The most commonly affected sites include the joints, skin, kidneys, lungs, and brain. Signs vary and may include fever, skin lesions, lameness that shifts from leg to leg, painful or swollen joints, behavioral changes, vomiting, diarrhea, and abdominal pain. An immune complex disease is usually diagnosed with blood tests, biopsies, and by ruling out other causes of disease. Treatment generally includes supportive treatment for the affected organ, removal of the causative agent, or treatment of the infection (such as appropriate antibiotic treatment for bacterial infection). Anti-inflammatory drugs may be needed to stop the continued formation of immune complexes and to decrease the inflammation associated with these reactions.

Type IV Reactions (Cell-mediated Reactions)

Type IV or delayed hypersensitivity occurs more than 24 hours after the body was exposed to an antigen. Unlike the other types of reactions that involve antibodies, Type IV reactions involve immune cells, such as T cells and macrophages. The antigens responsible for the development of Type IV reactions can come from bacteria, parasites, viruses, chemicals, and certain cells. This type of reaction can occur in any organ. For this reason the signs will vary. The reaction is diagnosed based on excluding other causes for organ-specific diseases and by laboratory tests on the tissue. The goals of treatment are to provide supportive treatment based on the organ-specific disease process, to identify (if possible) and eliminate the source of the antigen causing the reaction, and to control inflammation and immune suppression.

THE IMMUNE SYSTEM OF HORSES

The immune system consists of a network of white blood cells, antibodies, and other substances that fight off infections and reject foreign proteins. In addition, the immune system includes several organs. Some, such as the thymus gland and the bone marrow, are the sites where white blood cells are produced. Others, including the spleen, lymph nodes, and liver, trap microorganisms and foreign substances and provide a place for immune system cells to collect, interact with each other and with foreign substances, and generate an immune response.

The primary role of the immune system is to defend the body against foreign invaders or abnormal cells that invade or attack it. To do this, the immune system must distinguish between "self" and "non-self." By recognizing invading microorganisms (such as viruses), chemical agents, or other foreign substances that are "non-self," a body can protect itself from attack. Substances that stimulate an immune response in the body are called antigens. Antigens may be contained within or on bacteria, viruses, other microorganisms, or cancer cells. Antigens may also exist on their own—for example, as pollen or food molecules. A normal immune response consists of recognizing a foreign antigen, mobilizing forces to defend against it, and attacking it. There are three lines of defense against invaders: physical barriers, nonspecific (or innate) immunity, and specific (or adaptive) immunity. Nonspecific and specific immunity involve various white blood cells.

The immune system of the horse is a fascinating and complex, yet typically effective physiological means of fighting off disease causing agents such as bacteria, viruses and other pathogens. The three main factors that influence immune system function in the horse include: stress, nutrition and age. If a horse is young or very old, when they are not receiving an appropriate level of nutrition, or when they are otherwise stressed, their immune system may fail to protect them effectively, therefore increasing the risk of disease. At this time of year, cold stress combined with age, low body condition, or some combination of the three may create a situation where horses are more susceptible to illness.

When considering the many factors of stress causing agents, maintaining proper immune system function is a primary concern. When horses are transported to events where large numbers of unfamiliar horses congregate, such as a horse show, rodeo or organized trail ride, there is the potential for them to be exposed to pathogens. It is imperative to realize that their immune system may be compromised by the stress of travel or a change in routine.

The role of antibodies

One of the ways in which the acquired immune system works is to create and maintain enough antibodies (a type of protein) in the blood that can identify and neutralise foreign objects within the body such as bacteria and viruses. Another important role is 'cell-mediated immunity', which involves the production of white blood cells that specifically fight infections without the production of antibodies. All these components work together to provide protection for your horse.

What can compromise the immune system?

The immune system can be compromised by many things such as the amount and type of pathogen (bug) it has to fight off as well as the horse's natural ability to fight disease. Youngsters, older horses and those that have other disease challenges, for example Cushing's, will often have compromised immunity.

What do vaccinations do?

Prevention is key to the control of equine disease. The intention is to reduce the level of challenge whilst maximising the horse's immunity and vaccination is one of the most important ways to help achieve this. Vaccinations have two main functions, depending on the type of disease. The first is to provide protective immunity against diseases such as tetanus. The second is to reduce the spread of contagious diseases such as equine influenza.

How do vaccines work?

Simplistically a vaccine imitates a specific disease in order to stimulate the acquired immune response more quickly and with greater magnitude than in an unvaccinated horse. The immune system then communicates with the other body systems to regulate and destroy this foreign material or 'pathogen'. Vaccination helps to provide protective immunity, priming the animal's own immune system to allow it to remember specific diseases. This enables it to mount an improved immune response more quickly and with a greater magnitude when challenged in the future.

To work successfully an effective vaccine must be used and the horse must have a healthy immune system, both at time of vaccination and at time of challenge. However, because each horse is an individual, some may respond differently to others to exactly the same vaccination protocol.

EVOLUTION OF THE IMMUNE SYSTEM

Evolution of immunity happens at many timescales, from the deep time evolution of whole systems, to the evolution of variants of pathogens and individuals over the lifetime of a host species, to the changes in frequency of lymphocyte clones within an individual during an infection. It would have been impossible to do justice to even one of these vast subjects in a single day, so a few speakers were invited to touch on some of the highlights. The talks were held in the beautiful auditorium at Peterhouse, followed by a reception at the Fitzwilliam Museum during which the participants could enjoy the ongoing exhibition *Endless Forms: Charles Darwin, Natural Science and the Visual Arts*, followed by the conference dinner in the great hall of Christ's College, where Darwin was a student.

It was long thought that adaptive immunity was a property of jawed vertebrates alone, so it has been a major revolution to find that some invertebrates have their own adaptive immune systems, based on molecules other than antibodies (Abs), T-cell receptors (TCRs) and major histocompatibility complex (MHC) molecules. The first glimpse of this reality was provided by work on snails,[2,3] which failed to shatter the old paradigm. Among other indications, the inability to find a multigene family of immunoglobulin variable (V) receptors in the genome sequence of the fruit fly *Drosophila melanogaster* confirmed the prevailing view that invertebrates relied only on innate immunity.

Therefore, it was particularly apt for Dietmar Schmucker (Harvard University, Boston, USA) to describe the properties of Down's syndrome cell-associated molecule (DSCAM) in insects and crustaceans, in which a single gene generates thousands of variant isoforms by alternative splicing.[4–6] DSCAM in humans is expressed in the nervous system, and in fruit flies many variants are involved in development of the nervous system, including specifying axonal connections between neurons.

However, insect and crustacean DSCAM variants are also expressed in cells involved in immunity, including haemocytes and the fat body, and are secreted into the haemolymph. Knockdown of fruit fly DSCAM in haemocytes decreases phagocytosis, and transient silencing in the mosquito *Anopheles gambiae* leads to decreased resistance to bacterial pathogens and malarial parasites. The DSCAM molecule contains eight immunoglobulin V domains arranged in an S-shape, and the variability clusters into two sites in the structure, one that specifies homophilic (and limited heterodimeric) pairing and one that may contribute to specific antigen binding. In the nervous system, homophilic interaction of DSCAM expressed on some neurons leads to repulsion.

At the base of the vertebrates are the jawless fish, lampreys and hagfish, which have yet another adaptive immune system, described by Max Cooper (Emory University, Atlanta, USA). Lamprey lymphocytes could be identified by flow cytometry, and immunization with bacteria, foreign erythrocytes or plant mitogens led to the appearance of lymphoblasts. Large-scale sequencing of cDNAs from such lymphocytes resulted in no obvious Ab, TCR or MHC sequences, but many different leucine-rich repeats [LRRs, as are found in Toll-like receptors (TLRs)] were discovered and named variable lymphocyte receptors (VLRs). Analysis of genomic DNA revealed a few VLR genes in the haploid genome to which LRR sequences are added by a copy choice mechanism from LRR pseudogenes, resulting in upwards of 10^{14} different sequences with evidence for both allelic exclusion and clonal expression. The resulting proteins can be anchored in the cell membrane by glycolipid linkage, or may be secreted as pentamers of dimers. These pentamers have low affinity but high avidity for antigen, and X-ray structural analysis shows antigen bound 'as in the palm of a cupped hand'.

Two kinds of VLR genes were found, VLR-A and VLR-B, for which monoclonal antibodies (mAbs) defined two kinds of lymphocytes with different distributions in lamprey tissues. Both kinds of lymphocytes respond to antigens; VLR-B cells bind antigen and secrete VLRs, while VLR-A cells do not but instead respond to a phytohaemagglutinin, a T-cell mitogen. Gene expression analysis showed many differences between these two kinds of lymphocytes, including cytidine deaminases, transcription factors, kinases, cell surface proteins, cytokines, chemokines and TLRs. Overall, the data suggest that the VLR-A lymphocytes may be like T cells and the VLR-B lymphocytes like B cells, leading immediately to the question of whether lymphocytes specialized into functionally different subsets independently in jawless fish and jawed vertebrates, or only once, after which different receptor molecules evolved (or persisted) in jawless fish and in the jawed vertebrates.

Coming to the adaptive immune system of jawed vertebrates, Jim Kaufman (University of Cambridge, UK) reviewed some of the data and speculations concerning the emergence of the key molecular components: Ab, TCR and MHC molecules.[10,11] It is generally accepted that the key event occurred at the base of the jawed vertebrates some 500 million years ago: the creation of the first split V gene from the insertion of a transposon into the immunoglobulin V exon of what is presumed to have been a membrane-bound receptor, which used recombination-activating genes (RAGs) to specify imprecise joining of the different parts of the split V gene.

It has been argued that this first receptor was a TCR-like molecule, based on the fact that diversity is generated by recombinational joining only at complementarity-determining region 3 (CDR3), which is the major contact with peptide in MHC molecules. In this view, $\alpha\beta$ T cells emerged first, followed by $\gamma\delta$ T cells and then by B cells. The first MHC molecule was probably a class II-like homodimer, the gene for which duplicated and diverged to create a heterodimer, from which the first class I heavy chain and β_2-microglobulin genes could be generated by an inversion.

Many if not most non-mammalian vertebrates share the salient features first found in the chicken MHC, with MHC genes located close to polymorphic antigen-processing genes to allow co-evolution as stable haplotypes. The familiar organization of the human MHC probably arose from an inversion which put the class III region in between the class I and class II regions, leaving the tapasin, transporter associated with antigen presentation and inducible proteasome genes in the class II region. The organization of the primordial MHC allowed the ancestors of the MHC and antigen-processing genes to co-evolve from their original functions an antigen presentation pathway.

Two rounds of genome-wide duplication at the base of the vertebrates led to MHC paralogous regions, including the CD1 region and arguably the regions containing natural killer (NK) receptor genes in humans. The discovery of NK receptor and CD1 genes in the chicken MHC was the first of many examples, including a TCR-like gene in the frog MHC, which suggest that the primordial MHC contained the genes that co-evolved into receptor–ligand pairs. In this view, the primordial MHC was the birthplace of the adaptive immune system, which has been breaking apart ever since.

A crucial property for an adaptive immune system with variable antigen-specific receptors is self-tolerance, part of which occurs in the thymus during development of T cells. Thomas Boehm (Max-Planck-Institute for Immunobiology, Freiburg, Germany) described the minimal gene networks which may have been necessary for the appearance of the T cells developing through the thymus. Taking advantage of the transparency of zebrafish (*Danio rerio*) embryos and the ease of knock-downs, a chemokine system was identified for homing of thymic lymphoid precursors: zebrafish chemokine (C-C motif) ligand 25 (CCL25) (equivalent to human tyrosine kinase expressed in hepatocellular carcinoma) and zebrafish chemokine (C-X-C motif) ligand 12 (CXCL12) (equivalent to human CXCR12, or stromal cell derived factor 1).

Both these genes were found throughout the jawed vertebrates, but only the equivalent of CCL25 was found in the jawless fish lamprey (*Lampetra planeri*), which lacks an obvious thymus, and neither was found in the protochordate amphioxis (*Branchiostoma floridae*), which lacks lymphocytes altogether. Using FoxN1 knock-out mice with adoptive transfer of transgenic cells, reconstitution of the thymic niche was shown to depend on Notch, delta-like ligand 4, kit ligand, CCL25 and CXCL12 under the control of the FoxN1 gene.

Of these five genes, only the delta-like ligand gene is present in lamprey and amphioxis but still under control of the equivalent of FoxN1, suggesting that the stroma began to evolve the regulatory gene network for the formation of the thymus prior to the emergence of T cells.

On a shorter timescale, host species evolve adaptations to their pathogens, and different individuals may respond appropriately for protection, under-respond allowing infection, or over-respond leading to pathogenesis. Rick Maizels (Edinburgh University, UK) discussed the precarious balance between protective responses to multicellular parasites and pathogenic responses to harmless allergens or to self antigens. Although at least 2·3 billion people (of approximately 6·9 billion) are infected with just five species of helminth worms, the majority escape severe pathology, with the parasites regulated by T helper type 2 (Th2) and regulatory T (Treg) cells.

Many studies show an inverse correlation between the level of such parasites in a population and the prevalence of allergy, asthma and autoimmune diseases such as multiple sclerosis, a concept called the 'hygiene hypothesis'. One example of how this can work is the reduction of lung allergy and autoimmunity in experimental allergic encephalitis (EAE) produced by infection of the mouse intestine with the nematode worm *Heligmosomoides polygyrus*, apparently through the parasite secreting a molecule(s) that expands Treg (FoxP3-positive) cells through binding the transforming growth factor (TGF)-β receptor. Overall, the evidence suggests that hosts evolved with strong selective pressure from parasites, leading to some individuals with an immune response that protects from parasites but leads to pathological responses in the absence of parasites.

This theme was continued by Ken Smith (University of Cambridge, UK) who described the importance of an antibody receptor called FcãRIIB in the balance between susceptibility to systemic lupus erythromatosis (SLE) and protection from malaria.[16,17] The FcãRIIB locus is one of the stronger susceptibility loci among the 40 found by genome-wide association (GWA) studies, which overall explain %25 of the genetic variation of SLE. Copy number variation (CNV) of the FcãRIIB gene is important, with knock-outs in mice leading to autoimmunity and with three or more copies leading to a reduction in SLE but also a reduction in the response to pathogens such as bacteria.

Single nucleotide polymorphisms (SNPs) in FcãRIIB genes can also be important, with the I232T mutation in the transmembrane region abolishing function, apparently by blocking entry into lipid rafts in the cell membrane. The population distribution of T232 world-wide correlates both with susceptibility to SLE and with the geographic distribution of malaria, and the frequency of severe malaria in T232 homozygotes is half that of heterozygotes or I232 homozygotes. The balance between the inhibitory FcãRIIB molecule and the activatory FcãRIIIB molecule determines, at least in part, the immune response, with less inhibition apparently driven by the advantage of increased survival from malaria.

Like hosts, pathogens also evolve on several timescales, and Gordon Dougan (Sanger Institute, Hinxton, UK) described the evolution of some bacterial pathogens. An emerging theme is the existence of groups of 'promiscuous species' infecting a variety of different host species using generalist strategies and differing in 1–2% of their DNA, which occasionally give rise to single species, clades or serovars adapted to a particular host with a specialist strategy and differing only in SNPs or indels. Examples include *Salmonella, Pertussis, Yersinia, Mycobacteria* and many others. For instance, *Salmonella enteritidis* infects the intestines of many hosts, resulting in inflammation and eventual clearance, but gave rise to *Salmonella typhi*, which infects only humans using a stealth approach which allows systemic infection, leading in some cases to eventual death. Complete genomic sequences of thousands of *S. typhi* isolates revealed only 2000 SNPs, a similar level of diversity as in humans, consonant with a jump to infecting humans about 30,000 years ago. New haplotypes can be formed by loss of genes, and there are examples of replacement of local haplotypes by 'superfit' strains, but now the major epidemics in South Africa are 'non-typhoidal Salmonella' (NTS) as a result of replacement by *Salmonella typhimurium*. Another kind of adaptation is illustrated by *Clostridium difficile*, different isolates of which have 2–4% difference in DNA sequence, apparently having crossed into human populations from several sources. In comparison, the 'super-fit' 027 ribotype has only 30 SNPs across the world. The emergence of this medical problem is presumably a result of the use of antibiotics, as *C. difficile* colonizes the intestine of humans after antibiotic treatment has changed the normal spectrum of microbiota, allowing such people to become highly infectious 'super-shedders'.

Many pathogens can evolve over very short timescales, and Andrew McMichael discussed the evolution of human immunodeficiency virus (HIV) within individuals.[21–23] An HIV inoculum is generally very complex (10^4–10^6 viral sequences), but most individuals are initially infected by only a single virus (at least by the early peak of viraemia). The characteristics of this virus and the individual can determine the course of the infection, in particular the viral set point, the level of viraemia after the early peak. Many host genes contribute to resistance and susceptibility, and the virus evolves in response. As just one example of many, MHC class I genes present viral peptides to CD-8bearing cytotoxic T lymphocytes (CTLs) which can kill infected cells, with particular class I alleles [such as human leucocyte antigen (HLA)-B57] leading to low set points and greatly enhanced survival. As one example of the counter-response, the viral protein Nef down-regulates class I molecules. Whatever the class I molecule, the T-cell response destroys the infected cells, with selection eventually resulting in a viral sequence that has lost the relevant T-cell epitope. Viruses even escape highly protective MHC alleles like HLA-B57, but more slowly and with a clear fitness cost to the virus. The new viral sequence will in turn select for new CTLs while the old CTLs disappear, an evolutionary process inside a single individual that continues until the immune response is apparently exhausted.

Such evolution occurs constantly inside each individual of the jawed vertebrates, as clones of lymphocytes with different antigen-specific variable receptors wax and wane.

In mammals, the transition from high-avidity immunoglobulin M (IgM) to high-affinity IgG is accomplished by cycles of mutation and selection within germinal centres (GC) of lymph nodes. In the process, diversity is spread to the periphery of the CDRs, aided by the presence of somatic hypermutation (SHM) hotspots. The SHM process is triggered by a member of the apolipoprotein B mRNA editing enzyme, catalytic polypeptide-like (APOBEC) family called activation-induced deaminase (AID), which is a B-cell-specific enzyme and thereby drives somatic mutation of Abs but not TCRs. AID is also the critical trigger of Ab diversity produced by gene conversion in birds, Ab class switching (first apparent in amphibians), somatic mutation (first apparent in jawed fish) and, quite probably, segmental recombination of LRR sequences in VLRs of jawless fish. The presence of such genes in jawless fish, cytidine deaminase (CDA) 1 in VLR-A cells and CDA2 in VLR-B cells, highlights the age of this gene family. Other members of the APOBEC family have appeared subsequently, but are involved in RNA editing and resistance to retroviruses, including HIV. The similarity of the structure of AID/APOBEC proteins to bacterial enzymes involved in nucleotide metabolism and in transfer RNA (tRNA) editing suggests a very ancient origin indeed.

Having touched in this meeting on some highlights of the importance of evolution to every level of immunity, Chris Howe (University of Cambridge, UK) reminded the audience that the only figure in *The Origin of Species* was a phylogenetic tree, a method that became a powerful workhorse of evolutionary analysis. This approach can be extended beyond the investigation of life to the analysis of manuscripts, language and even carpet designs.[27] We can only imagine what Darwin would have thought of the day's presentations, but hopefully he would have appreciated how far we have come since his day and understood how far we have yet to go.

All living organisms are continuously exposed to substances that are capable of causing them harm. Most organisms protect themselves against such substances in more than one way - with physical barriers, for example, or with chemicals that repel or kill invaders. Animals with backbones, called vertebrates, have these types of general protective mechanisms, but they also have a more advanced protective system called the immune system. The immune system is a complex network of organs containing cells that recognize foreign substances in the body and destroy them. It protects vertebrates against pathogens, or infectious agents, such as viruses, bacteria, fungi, and other parasites. The human immune system is the most complex.

Although there are many potentially harmful pathogens, no pathogen can invade or attack all organisms because a pathogen's ability to cause harm requires a susceptible victim, and not all organisms are susceptible to the same pathogens. For instance, the virus that causes AIDS in humans does not infect animals such as dogs, cats, and mice. Similarly, humans are not susceptible to the viruses that cause canine distemper, feline leukemia, and mouse pox.

TWO KINDS OF IMMUNITY

All animals possess a primitive system of defense against the pathogens to which they are susceptible. This defense is called innate, or natural, immunity and includes two parts. One part, called humoral innate immunity, involves a variety of substances found in the humors, or body fluids. These substances interfere with the growth of pathogens or clump them together so that they can be eliminated from the body. The other part, called cellular innate immunity, is carried out by cells called phagocytes that ingest and degrade, or "eat" pathogens and by so-called natural killer cells that destroy certain cancerous cells. Innate immunity is nonspecific - that is, it is not directed against specific invaders but against any pathogens that enter the body.

Only vertebrates have an additional and more sophisticated system of defense mechanisms, called adaptive immunity, that can recognize and destroy specific substances. The defensive reaction of the adaptive immune system is called the immune response. Any substance capable of generating such a response is called an antigen, or immunogen. Antigens are not the foreign microorganisms and tissues themselves; they are substances - such as toxins or enzymes - in the microorganisms or tissues that the immune system considers foreign. Immune responses are normally directed against the antigen that provoked them and are said to be antigen-specific. Specificity is one of the two properties that distinguish adaptive immunity from innate immunity. The other is called immunologic memory. Immunologic memory is the ability of the adaptive immune system to mount a stronger and more effective immune response against an antigen after its first encounter with that antigen, leaving the organism better able to resist it in the future. Adaptive immunity works with innate immunity to provide vertebrates with a heightened resistance to microorganisms, parasites, and other intruders that could harm them. However, adaptive immunity is also responsible for allergic reactions and for the rejection of transplanted tissue, which it may mistake for a harmful foreign invader.

Lymphocytes - Heart of the Immune System

Lymphocytes - a class of white blood cells - are the principal active components of the adaptive immune system. The other components are antigen-presenting cells, which trap antigens and bring them to the attention of lymphocytes so that thev can mount their attack.

How lymphocytes recognize antigens

A lymphocyte is different from all other cells in the body because it has about 100,000 identical receptors on its cellular membrane that enable it to recognize one specific antigen. The receptors are proteins containing grooves that fit into patterns forrned by the atoms of the antigen molecule - somewhat like a key fitting into a lock - so that the lymphocyte can bind to the antigen. There are more than 10 million different types of grooves in the lymphocytes of the human immune system.

When an antigen invades the body, normally only those lymphocytes with receptors that fit the contours of that particular antigen take part in the immune response. When they do, so-called daughter cells are generated that have receptors identical to those found on the original lymphocytes. The result is a family of lymphocytes, called a lymphocyte clone. with identical antigen-specific receptors.

A clone continues to grow after lymphocytes first encounter an antigen so that, if the same type of antigen invades the body a second time, there will be many more lymphocytes specific for that antigen ready to meet the invader This is a crucial component of immunologic memory.

How lymphocytes are made

Like all blood cells, lymphocytes are made from stem cells in the bone marrow. (In fetuses, or unborn offspring, lymphocytes are made in the liver.) Lymphocytes then undergo a second stage of development, or processing, in which they acquire their antigen-specific receptors. By chance, some lymphocytes are created with receptors that happen to be specific to normal, healthy components of the body. Fortunately, a healthy immune system purges itself of these lymphocytes, leaving only lymphocytes that ignore normal body components but react to foreign intruders. If this purging process is not completely successful, the result is an autoimmune (literally "self-immune") disease in which the immune system attacks normal components of the body as though they were foreign antigens, destroying healthy molecules, cells, or tissues.

Some lymphocytes are processed in the bone marrow and then migrate to other areas of the body - specifically the lymphoid organs. These lymphocytes are called B lymphocytes, or B cells (for bone-marrow-derived cells). Other lymphocytes move from the bone marrow and are processed in the thymus, a pyramid-shaped lymphoid organ located immediately beneath the breastbone at the level of the heart. These lymphocytes are called T lymphocytes, or T cells (for thymus-derived cells).

These two types of lymphocytes - cells and T cells - play different roles in the immune response, though they may act together and influence one another's functions. The part of the immune response that involves B cells is often called humoral immunity because it takes place in the body fluids. The part involving T cells is called cellular immunity because it takes place directly between the T cells and the antigens. This distinction is misleading, however, because, strictly speaking, all adaptive immune responses are cellular - that is, they are all initiated by cells (the lymphocytes) reacting to antigens. B cells may initiate an immune response, but the triggering antigens are actually eliminated by soluble products that the B cells release into the blood and other body fluids. These products are called antibodies and belong to a special group of blood proteins called immunoglobulins When a B cell is stimulated by an antigen that it encounters in the body fluids, it transforms, with the aid of a type of T cell called a helper T cell (see "T cells"), into a larger cell called a blast cell. The blast cell begins to divide rapidly, forming a clone of identical cells. Some of these transform further into plasma cells - in essence, antibody-producing factones. These plasma cells produce a single type of antigen-specific antibody at a rate of about 2,000 antibodies per second. The antibodies then circulate through the body fluids, attacking the triggering antigen.

Antibodies attack antigens by binding to them. Some antibodies attach themselves to invading microorganisms and render them immobile or prevent them from penetrating body cells. In other cases, the antibodies act together with a group of blood proteins, collectively called the complement system, that consists of at least 30 different components. In such cases, antibodies coat the antigen and make it subject to a chemical chain reaction with the complement proteins. The complement reaction either can cause the invader to burst or can attract scavenger cells that "eat" the invader.

Not all of the cells from the clone formed from the original B cell transform into antibody-producing plasma cells; some serve as so-called memory cells. These closely resemble the original B cell, but they can respond more quickly to a second invasion by the same antigen than can the original cell. T cells. There are two major classes of T cells produced in the thymus: helper T cells and cytotoxic, or killer, T cells. Helper T cells secrete molecules called interleukins (abbreviated IL) that promote the growth of both B and T cells. The interleukins that are secreted by lymphocytes are also called lymphokines. The interleukins that are secreted by other kinds of blood cells called monocytes and macrophages are called monokines. Some ten different interleukins are known: IL-1, IL-2, IL-3, IL-4, IL-5, IL-6, IL-7, interferon, lymphotoxin, and tumor necrosis factor. Each interleukin has complex biological effects.

Cytotoxic T cells destroy cells infected with viruses and other pathogens and may also destroy cancerous cells. Cytotoxic T cells are also called suppressor lymphocytes because they regulate immune responses by suppressing the function of helper cells so that the immune svstem is active onlv when necessary.

The receptors of T cells are different from those of B cells because they are "trained" to recognize fragments of antigens that have been combined with a set of molecules found on the surfaces of all the body's cells. These molecules are called MHC molecules (for major histocompatibility complex). As T cells circulate through the body, they scan the surfaces of body cells for the presence of foreign antigens that have been picked up by the MHC molecules. This function is sometimes called immune surveillance.

IMMUNE RESPONSE

When an antigen enters the body, it may be partly neutralized by components of the innate immune system. It may be attacked by phagocytes or by preformed antibodies that act together with the complement system. Often, however, the lymphocytes of the adaptive immune system are brought into play.

The human immune system contains approximately l trillion T cells and l trillion B cells, located in the lymphoid organs and in the blood, plus approximately 10 billion antigen-presenting cells located in the lymphoid organs.

To maximize the chances of encountering antigens wherever they may invade the body, lymphocytes continually circulate between the blood and certain lymphoid tissues. A given lymphocyte spends an average of 30 minutes per day in the blood and recirculates about 50 times per day between the blood and lymphoid tissues.

If lymphocytes encounter an antigen trapped by the antigen-presenting cells of the lymphoid organs, lymphocytes with receptors specific to that antigen stop their migration and settle to mount an immune response locally. As these lymphocytes accumulate in the affected lymphoid tissue, the tissue often becomes enlarged - for example, the lymph nodes in the groin become enlarged if there is an infection in the thigh area.

Antigen-presenting cells degrade antigens and often eliminate them without the help of lymphocytes. If there are too many antigens for them to handle alone, however, the antigen-presenting cells secrete IL- 1 and display fragments of the antigens (combined with MHC molecules) to alert the helper T cells.

The IL-1 facilitates the responsiveness of T and B cells to antigens and, if released in large amounts (as it is in the course of infections), can also cause fever and drowsiness. Helper T cells that encounter IL- 1 and fragments of antigens transform into cells called lymphoblasts, which then secrete a variety of interleukins that are essential to the success of the immune response.

The IL-2 produced by helper T cells promotes the growth of cytotoxic T cells, which may be necessary to destroy tumorous cells or cells infected with viruses. The IL-3 increases the production of blood cells in the bone marrow and thus helps to maintain an adequate supply of the lymphocytes and lymphocyte products necessary to fight infections.

Helper T cells also secrete interleukins that act on B cells, stimulating them to divide and to transform into antibody-secreting plasma cells. The antibodies then perform their part of the immune function.

The process of inducing an immune response is called immunization. It may be either natural - through infection by a pathogen - or artificial - through the use of serums or vaccines. The heightened resistance acquired when the body responds to infection is called active immunity.

Passive immunity results when the antibodies from an actively immunized individual are transferred to a second, nonimmune subject. Active immunization, whether natural or artificial, is longer-lasting than is passive immunization because it takes advantage of immunologic memory.

Monoclonal Antibodies

Scientists can now produce antibody-secreting cells in the laboratorv by a method known as the hybridoma technique. Hybridomas are hybrid cells made by fusing a cancerous, or rapidly reproducing, plasma cell and a normal antibody-producing plasma cell obtained from an animal immunized with a particular antigen. The hybridoma cell can produce large amounts of identical antibodies — called monoclonal, or hybridoma, antibodies — which have widespread applications in medicine and biology.

CHAPTER

DISEASES OF IMMUNITY 2

IMMUNE SYSTEM: AN INTRODUCTION

The immune system is a defensive system whose primary functions are to protect against infectious organisms, such as bacteria, viruses, fungi, and parasites, and the development of cancer. The complexity by which these functions occur is evidenced not only by the cell types, recognition molecules, and soluble factors involved and interactions with other systems (e.g., endocrine, nervous) but also by the ability to recognize virtually any foreign antigen. Immunologic responses result in pathologic processes, primarily inflammatory responses, as a result of either normal immune responses to foreign antigens (e.g., microbial pathogens) or from aberrations of the immune system as in the case of hypersensitivity reactions and autoimmune diseases. Finally, the importance of a normal functional immune system cannot be more evident than in instances in which it is deficient as the result of a genetic defect or as the result of an acquired immunodeficiency disease.

Immunity is the result of nonspecific (innate) and specific (adaptive) responses that together provide effective protection. The immune system's recognition and response functional capabilities are key components of both innate and adaptive immune responses. The recognition capabilities are highly specific and allow immune responses to develop against a diverse group of foreign (nonself) antigens and prevent the development of immune responses to self-antigens. Innate and adaptive immune responses feature effector mechanisms for eliminating or neutralizing the antigen, whereas adaptive immunity has the additional feature of memory.

The emphasis of this chapter is on diseases that are the result of inadequate or inappropriate immune responses. Before one can understand the pathogenic mechanisms of these diseases, one must first have an understanding of the basic elements of the immune system. The chapter begins with an overview of our current understanding of innate and adaptive immunity, cells of the immune system, cytokines, and major histocompatibility complex (MHC) molecules.

This overview facilitates the discussion of disorders of the immune system that includes hypersensitivity reactions, autoimmunity, and immunodeficiency. This chapter concludes with a discussion of amyloidosis, a diverse group of conditions characterized by the deposition of a pathologic extracellular protein. One of the conditions is associated with the deposition of immunoglobulin components. Although the focus of this text is on the pathologic basis of veterinary diseases, with an emphasis on domestic species, in this chapter we use the vast knowledge base regarding human and rodent immunology as our basis and interject major known relevant species differences as appropriate.

INNATE IMMUNITY (NONSPECIFIC IMMUNITY)

As stated previously, the function of the immune system is to protect against infectious pathogens and the development of cancer. There are two categories of immune responses that are based in part on their specificity for the antigen: (1) innate immunity and (2) adaptive immunity (Fig. 1). Innate immune responses are considered the first-line defense mechanisms, are not specific to the antigen, and lack memory. These defense mechanisms are the result of anatomic (e.g., skin, mucosal epithelia, cilia) and physiologic (e.g., stomach pH, body temperature) properties, and phagocytic and inflammatory responses. Major components of innate immunity are intact epithelial barriers, phagocytic cells, natural killer (NK) cells, and a number of plasma proteins, the most important of which are the proteins of the complement system.

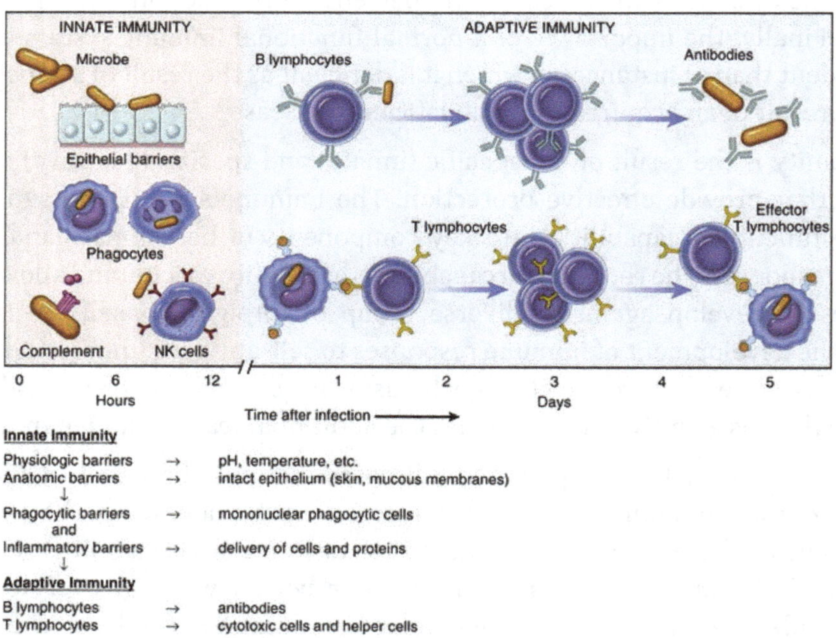

Fig 1. Innate (nonspecific) and adaptive (specific) immunity are depicted in relation to the time course of an infection.

Phagocytic cells are recruited to sites of infection during an inflammatory response where they have a number of functions, two of which are to ingest and destroy pathogenic organisms and neutralize toxins. Neutrophils, monocytes, and tissue macrophages are the major cells involved in phagocytosis. These cells recognize components of microbial pathogens through the expression of several membrane receptors, including receptors for mannose residues and *N*-formyl-methionine containing peptides and a family of pattern recognition receptors (PRRs) that, when activated by microbial components, signal the activation of transcription factors that facilitate the microbicidal mechanisms of the phagocytic cell and are discussed later. NK cells are the cytotoxic cells of innate immunity and are also discussed later.

The complement system can be activated by either the innate immune system (alternative and mannose/lectin pathways) or the adaptive immune system (classical pathway). Other important plasma proteins of the innate immune system include mannose-binding protein and C-reactive protein; two of the functions of these proteins are to facilitate phagocytosis through opsonization of pathogens and complement activation. Inflammatory responses comprise vascular, permeability, and cellular phases that act in response to damage to vascularized tissue.

RECOGNITION MOLECULES OF INNATE IMMUNITY

The recognition molecules of innate immunity provide an opportunity to recognize pathogens by cells other than lymphocytes. These germline-encoded molecules function to sense molecular structures shared by microbes and endogenous molecules associated with inflammation. The recognition molecules associated with microbes are generally referred to as pathogen-associated molecular patterns (PAMPs). The function of the innate immune system extends beyond microbial pathogen recognition to include endogenous molecules associated with cell damage and inflammation which are generally referred to as danger or damage associated molecular patterns (DAMPs).

The activation of the innate immune system through these invariant PRRs not only precedes lymphocyte activation but also is required to initiate the adaptive immune responses. PRRs molecular patterns are associated with microbial pathogens and classified as secreted, transmembrane, and cytosolic forms. Collectins and pentraxin are examples of secreted PRRs that largely function to bind to microbial surfaces and activate the complement system. Collectins, having properties of collagen and lectins, include mannose binding lectins and pulmonary surfactants A and D.

Pentraxin is comprised of five identical subunits to form a pentamer and include C-reactive protein, an activator of the classical pathway of complement. Toll-like receptors (TLRs) and C-type lectins are examples of the transmembrane PRRs, and they have limited cellular distribution, including macrophages, NK cells, and dendritic cells. TLRs are expressed on the plasma membrane or in endosomal/

lysosomal organelles. The cytosolic PRRs are more widely distributed, including all nucleated cells, and include retinoic acid–inducible gene (RIG)-1–like receptors (RLRs) and nucleotide-binding domain (NOD) and leucine-rich repeat–containing receptors (NLRs).

These recognition molecules provide the host with the ability to sense "danger" either through PAMPs in the case of microbial infections or through DAMPs in the presence of cellular damage or stress. This allows the innate immune system to detect and initiate immune responses in response to infectious and noninfectious causes. NLR molecules as immune sensors are not unique to mammals because they have been found in plants and urchins. The molecules are designated based on the structure of the molecule NLR with a suffix of P (pyrin domain) or C (caspase activation and recruitment domains [CARD]), referring to the N-terminal moiety followed by a number (e.g., NLRP1, NLRP2, or NLRP3).

The function of these pattern recognition molecules is also extended beyond the initiation of adaptive immunity to also include regulation of cell death (apoptosis). As is often the case in immunology, our understanding of immune responses is greatly enhanced through the identification of genetic immunologic disorders. Deficiencies in components of the NLRs have been described in humans and are most frequently associated with inflammatory disorders (e.g., Crohn's disease and inflammatory bowel disease).

Analogous to the adaptive immune response, which has developed the ability to defend the host against a diverse array of microbial pathogens (humoral versus cell-mediated responses), the innate immune system is now seen as also having an ability to distinguish specific types of pathogens. Intracellular (e.g., viruses) and extracellular (extracellular bacteria) pathogens require different types of immune responses to control them. The innate immune system has developed cell-intrinsic and cell-extrinsic recognition mechanisms dependent on if it is mediated by an infected cell or an uninfected cell.

Cell-extrinsic recognition mechanisms are a way in which an uninfected cell can participate in the immune response and are mediated through transmembrane receptors (e.g., TLRs) on specialized cells of the innate immune system such as macrophages and dendritic cells. Cell-intrinsic recognition mechanisms are essential for recognizing intracellular pathogens and involve type I interferon (IFN) gene transcription signaling by members of the RLRs.

Three members of the RLR family are RIG-1, melanoma differentiation-associated gene-5 (MDA-5), and laboratory of genetics and physiology gene 2 (LPG-2). In viral sensing, the RLRs are highly discriminating with regards to the cytoplasmic localization and sensing of specific RNAs. They specifically detect RNA molecular patterns not normally present in the cytoplasm. Abnormal RNA patterns include chemical modifications, secondary or tertiary RNA conformations, specific RNA sequences, or double-stranded RNA. While much of what is currently known about RLRs is centered around the sensing of RNA viruses, there is preliminary evidence that similar intracellular mechanisms may exist for sensing DNA viruses and some intracellular bacteria.

Members of the NLR are central regulators of immunity and inflammation largely through activation of transcription factors like nuclear factor (NF) kappa B, interferon regulatory factor (IRF), or nuclear factor of activated T lymphocytes (NFAT). Some members of the NLR family form multiprotein complexes with the cysteine protease pro-caspase-1 and the adapter molecule ASC (apoptosis-associated speck-like protein containing a CARD) referred to as inflammasomes. The inflammasome is a multiprotein complex that activates caspase-1. PAMPs and DAMPs are sensed through activation of the inflammasome complex, resulting in activation of caspase-1, which elicits effector functions through proteolytic cleavage of cytosolic proinflammatory cytokines (e.g., pro-interleukin [IL]-1b and pro-IL-18), which are then secreted in their active form.

The inflammasome model is analogous to the model for the activation of the apoptotic caspases by CD95/Fas death–inducing signaling complex (DISC) and the Apaf-1 apoptosome. IL-1β functions in localized and systemic responses to infections and injury, to cause fever, activation of lymphocytes, and the extravasation of leukocytes at sites of injury or infection. IL-18 functions to induce IFN-g by activated T lymphocytes and NK cells during a TH1 response and to induce secondary inflammatory cytokines, chemokines, cell adhesion molecules, and nitric oxide (NO) synthesis. Other members of the NLR family are involved in inflammasome-independent (non-inflammasome) innate immune responses and signal through different multicomponent signalosomes such as nodosomes, transcriptosomes, mito-signalosomes. Noninflammasome-mediated innate immune responses occur through NF kappa B activation, mitogen-activated protein kinase (MAPK) activation, cytokine and chemokine production, antimicrobial reactive oxygen species production, type I interferon (IFN-a and IFN-b) production, and ribonuclease L activity.

Toll-Like Receptors

TLRs are the mammalian homologue of the Toll receptor originally identified in Drosophila. It has not only an embryologic function but also an immunologic function. In mammals, TLRs are membrane molecules that function in cellular activation by a wide range of microbial pathogens. TLRs are classified as PRRs because they recognize PAMPs and signal to the host the presence of an infection. Pathogen associated molecules include lipopolysaccharide (LPS) from Gram-negative bacteria, peptidoglycan from Gram-positive bacteria, double-stranded RNA from viruses, or a-glucans from fungi.

In general, TLRs 1, 2, 4, and 6 recognize unique bacterial products that are found on the cell surface, and TLRs 3, 7, 8, and 9 are involved in viral detection and nucleic acid recognition within endosomes. The specificity of TLRs for microbial products depends on interactions between TLRs and non-TLR adapter molecules. All TLRs contain an extracellular domain characterized by a leucine-rich repeat motif flanked by a cysteine-rich motif (Fig. 2). They also contain a conserved intracellular signaling domain, Toll/IL-1 receptor (TIR), that is identical to the cytoplasmic domain of the IL-1 and IL-18 receptors. Fig. 2 illustrates how TLRs function in the recognition of LPS. In the blood or extracellular fluid, the binding of LPS to LPS-binding protein (LBP) facilitates the binding of LPS to CD14, a plasma protein and glycophosphatidylinositol-linked membrane protein present on most cells. The binding of LPS to CD14 results in the dissociation of LBP and the association of the LPS-CD14 complex with TLR4. An accessory protein, MD2, complexes with the LPS-CD14-TLR4 molecule and results in LPS-induced cell signaling.

Briefly, TLR signaling through the binding of PAMP to a TLR leads to the activation of TIR, which forms a complex with the cytoplasmic adapter protein MyD88, an IL-1 receptor-associated kinase (IRAK), and tumor necrosis factor (TNF) receptor-associated factor 6 (TRAF6). Activated TRAF then activates the MAPK cascade leading to the activation of NF kappa B, a transcription factor. MyD88 is a universal signaling molecule for NF kappa B activation, and MyD88-deficient mice are incapable of activation by TLR, IL-1, and IL-18. Recent information suggests that there are also signaling mechanisms unique to individual TLRs.

TLRs and their pathogen-associated ligands are important recognition molecules for the innate immune system and trigger a number of antimicrobial and inflammatory responses. Up to 15 different TLR genes have been identified. The importance of these receptors in immunity is further supported by the observation of polymorphisms in the genes encoding them.

Although the individual TLRs exhibit ligand specificity, they differ in their cellular expression patterns and the signal pathways they activate, similar to that described for cytokines, which exhibit pleiotropy, redundancy, synergy, and antagonism. There are constitutively and inducibly expressed TLRs in different tissues. TLRs regulate cell recruitment to sites of infection through the upregulation of the expression of adhesion molecules, chemokines, and chemokine receptors during an inflammatory response. TLRs activate leukocytes (primarily neutrophils and NK cells of the innate immune system) and epithelial, endothelial, and hematopoietic cells. TLRs are also hypothesized to be essential for linking the innate immune response to the adaptive immune responses.

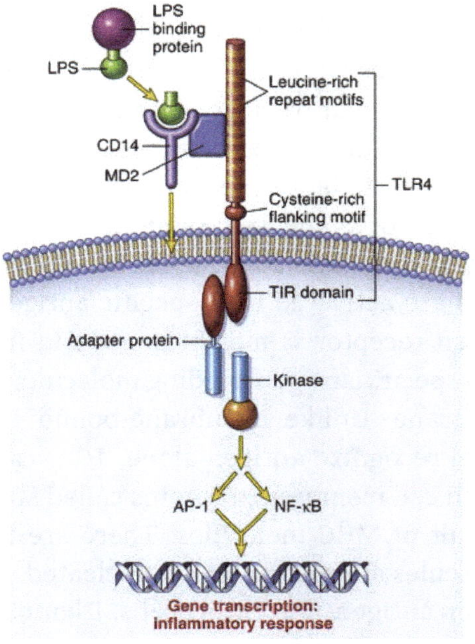

Fig. 2. Signaling pathway for Toll-like receptor 4 (TLR4) in response to bacterial lipopolysaccharide (LPS).The binding of LPS to TLR4 results in activation of a signal transduction pathway, leading to gene transcription and the elicitation of an inflammatory response. AP-1, Activating protein 1; NF-kB, nuclear factor-kappa B; TIR, Toll/interleukin-1 receptor.

Central to this hypothesis is the TLR-dependent dendritic cell-mediated control of T lymphocyte activation. Dendritic cells are important antigen-presenting cells for T lymphocyte activation. Dendritic cells uptake microbial antigens in the peripheral tissues and migrate to regional lymph nodes where they present peptide fragments, in the context of MHC molecules, to naïve T lymphocytes. In addition to the expression of the peptide-MHC signal, dendritic cells are also required to provide a second, co-stimulatory signal through the expression of B7, the ligand for the CD28 molecule on naïve T lymphocytes. The activation and maturation pathway related to the co-stimulatory signal occurs through TLR recognition of PAMPs.

There are species differences in the ligand specificity of TLRs and in the cellular responses elicited. Although sequences for canine, feline, and chicken TLR4 have been identified, no functional data have been published. With regard to domestic animals, a significant body of literature exists on TLRs of cattle.

Finally, TLRs have been implicated in "innate autoimmunity," with several reports of TLRs recognizing fibrinogen, heat-shock proteins, or DNA. There are also reports of TLR binding of DNA as a factor in directing antibody production by autoreactive B lymphocytes contributing to the pathogenesis of rheumatoid arthritis and systemic lupus erythematosus (SLE). Further studies are necessary to more fully understand these observations and the underlying immuno-pathogenesis.

ADAPTIVE IMMUNITY (SPECIFIC IMMUNITY)

Adaptive immunity in general consists of cell-mediated immunity, mediated by T lymphocytes against intracellular pathogens, and humoral immunity, mediated by B lymphocytes against extracellular pathogens and toxins (Fig. 3). The adaptive immune response is the second-line defense mechanism and is characterized by antigen specificity, diversity, memory, and self-/nonself-recognition. Antigen specificity and self-/nonself-recognition are the result of distinct membrane molecules. Mature B lymphocytes are activated by a specific antigen-binding molecule on its membrane. The antigen receptor is membrane-bound immunoglobulin. Mature T lymphocytes express a specific antigen-binding molecule, the T lymphocyte receptor (TCR), on their membrane. Unlike membrane-bound immunoglobulin on the B lymphocyte, which can recognize antigen alone, TCRs can recognize only antigens that are associated with cell membrane proteins called *MHC molecules.* Self-/nonself-recognition is the result of MHC molecules. There are two major classes of MHC molecules. Class I molecules are present on all nucleated cells, and class II molecules are present primarily on antigen-presenting cells. T lymphocytes and B lymphocytes are the major cells of adaptive immunity.

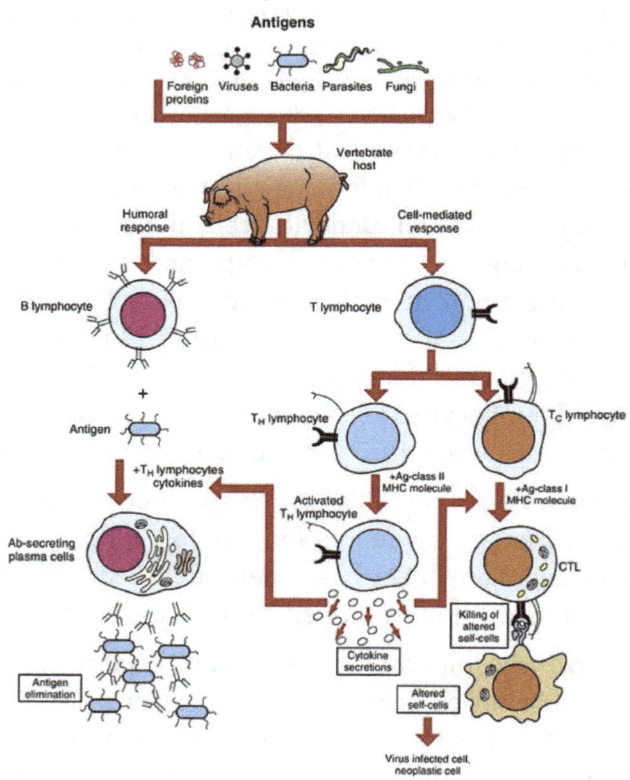

Fig. 3 Overview of humoral and cell-mediated arms of adaptive immunity. ***CTL,*** **Cytotoxic T lymphocyte**

CELLS AND TISSUES OF THE IMMUNE SYSTEM

T Lymphocytes

T lymphocytes are small nongranular cells that constitute 50% to 70% of the peripheral blood mononuclear cells. They originate in the bone marrow and migrate to the thymus (thus the "T" designation), where they undergo differentiation, selection, and maturation processes before exiting to the periphery as effector lymphocytes. In secondary lymphoid tissues, they are located primarily in the paracortical regions of lymph nodes and the periarteriolar sheaths (PALS) of the spleen. These specific anatomic sites elaborate chemoattractant cytokines (chemokines), for which the T lymphocytes express receptors. The definitive marker for T lymphocytes is the TCR, the polymorphic antigen-binding molecule. The antigen specificity of individual lymphocytes is attributed to their respective TCR, which is genetically determined. TCRs are classified as either αβ-TCR or γδ-TCR based on the composition of their disulfide-linked heterodimers. The individual polypeptide chains of the heterodimers contain variable (antigen-binding) and constant regions.

In mammals, most peripheral blood T lymphocytes express αβ-TCR; however, in ruminants and swine, these lymphocytes make up only 10% to 50%, and 10% of peripheral blood T lymphocytes, respectively. Both TCRs are associated with CD3, and together they form the TCR-CD3 complex. There are significant activation and functional differences between αβ-TCR– and γδ-TCR–expressing lymphocytes. Unlike membrane-bound immunoglobulin on B lymphocytes that can recognize soluble antigen, the αβ-TCR can only recognize antigen after it has been processed into peptide fragments and associated with MHC molecules. In most instances, the antigen is associated with the MHC on the surface of an antigen-presenting cell, a virally infected cell, a neoplastic cell, or a cell of a foreign tissue graft. Individual αβ-TCRs are covalently linked to a cluster of five polypeptide chains, three comprising the CD3 molecule and two comprising the β-chain.

The CD3 molecule and the β-chain are invariant, and although they do not bind antigen, they do function in the signal transduction after antigen binding by the TCR. Each T lymphocyte expresses a unique TCR with regard to structure and antigen specificity. The genes that encode α-, β-, γ-, and δ-chains of the TCR can undergo somatic rearrangements during their development in the thymus, resulting in tremendous diversity for antigen recognition. Not only are these rearrangements important for diversity, but also they can be used to molecularly phenotype proliferating populations of T lymphocytes as a diagnostic tool for the identification of clonal populations (neoplastic) and polyclonal populations (nonneoplastic).

In most species, a minority of T lymphocytes express γδ-TCR. The γδ-TCR lymphocytes develop in the thymus and migrate to the epithelium of the skin and intestine, mammary gland, and reproductive organs. Although these cells can be found within regional lymph nodes and the lamina propria, in these organs they primarily reside as intraepithelial lymphocytes (IELS). As stated, in some species, notably ruminants, γδ-TCR lymphocytes are the predominant circulating population of T lymphocytes. In contrast to the αβ-TCR lymphocytes, γδ-TCR lymphocytes can recognize native antigen in the absence of MHC binding and they do not rely exclusively on the δ-chain as a signal transducer. Most γδ-TCR lymphocytes use the γ-chain for signal transduction after activation. The diversity of antigens recognized by γδ-TCR is limited in most species except ruminants and swine, indicating their importance in these species. Some have suggested that they may provide early cell-mediated immune responses in neonates. The precise function of γδ-TCR lymphocytes remains unknown. Another small subset of T lymphocytes, called *NK-T lymphocytes,* expresses molecules found on NK cells in addition to a limited diversity of TCRs. NK-T lymphocytes primarily recognize glycolipids that are associated with an MHC-like molecule, CD1. The function of NK-T lymphocytes remains unknown.

Although all T lymphocytes express the TCR-CD3 complex, they are further classified according to accessory CD4 and CD8 molecules. These nonpolymorphic accessory molecules include CD4, CD8, CD2, integrins, and CD28. CD4 and CD8 functionally subdivide T lymphocytes into $CD8^+$ cytotoxic T lymphocytes (CTL [T_C]) and $CD4^+$ helper T lymphocytes (T_H). During antigen presentation, $CD4^+$ lymphocytes only recognize antigen bound to MHC class II molecules (Fig. 4), whereas CD^+8 lymphocytes only recognize antigen bound to MHC class I molecules. This coreceptor requirement is commonly referred to as *MHC class I and MHC class II restriction,* the basis for positive selection in the thymus. Although there have been reports in some species of CD4 lymphocytes that are functionally cytotoxic and CD8 lymphocytes that are functionally "helper"-like, these appear to be anomalies and for the purposes of this text are excluded. In most species, peripheral blood T lymphocytes express either CD4 or CD8. Except for ruminants and swine, lymphocytes negative for both CD4 and CD8—"double negative" lymphocytes—are rare in the peripheral blood. So-called "double positive" lymphocytes, positive for both CD4 and CD8, are rare, except in swine, where they can approach %25 of the T lymphocytes in the peripheral circulation. T lymphocytes require two signals for activation.

Signal 1 is provided by the TCR and the MHC-antigen complex and the CD4 or CD8 MHC complex. Signal 2 is provided by another accessory molecule expressed by T lymphocytes, the CD28 molecule. The ligands for CD28 are B7-1 (CD80) and B7-2 (CD81) expressed on activated dendritic cells, B lymphocytes, and macrophages (see Fig. 4). An inability to deliver the second signal results in an unresponsive T lymphocyte that either undergoes apoptosis or remains anergic. These molecules provide an important co-stimulatory signal for T lymphocyte activation.

When T lymphocytes are activated by antigen and receive the appropriate co-stimulatory signals, they clonally expand as a result of their secretion of IL-2. This clonally expanded population of T lymphocytes, of the same antigen specificity, differentiates into populations of effector lymphocytes and memory lymphocytes.

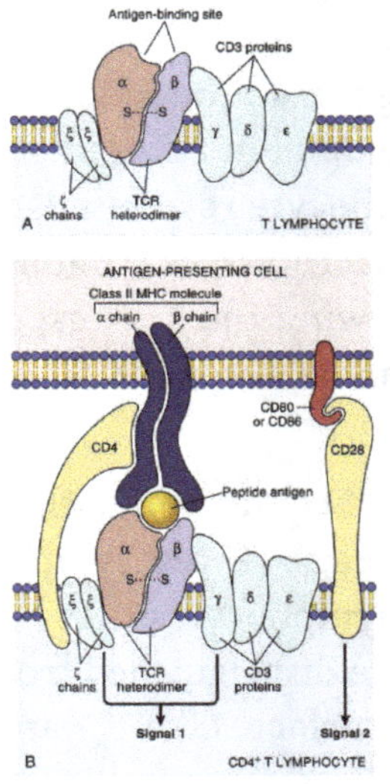

Fig. 4 The T lymphocyte receptor complex (T lymphocyte receptor [TCR]).A, TCR-a and TCRb chains complexed with CD3 g-, d-, and e-chains and the invariant, x-chains. B, Illustrating how the TCR recognizes antigen in the context of major histocompatibility complex on the antigen-presenting cell (top) and how the æ-chains and CD3 g-, d-, and x-chains deliver one of the two required signals for activation of the T lymphocyte. The second required signal is delivered by the co-stimulator molecules CD28 on the T lymphocyte and B7 on the antigen-presenting cell. MHC, Major histocompatibility complex.

TH lymphocytes can be classified based on their functional capacity and ability to elicit primarily an antibody response or a cell-mediated immune response. After activation of TH lymphocytes, by recognition of antigen bound to MHC class II molecules on the surface of an antigen-presenting cell, there is clonal expansion of TH lymphocytes of the same antigen specificity. These clonally expanded lymphocytes are important in directing the immune response as either primarily an antibody response or a cellular response. The type of response is dictated by a restricted cytokine profile that primarily activates B lymphocytes in the case of an antibody response or activates CTL (Tc) and macrophages in a cellular response. The restricted cytokine profile for TH lymphocytes allows for their classification as either TH1 or TH2 lymphocytes.

TH1 lymphocytes synthesize and secrete IL-2 and interferon-g (IFN-g), stimulating CTL (Tc) and macrophages, and induce a cell-mediated immune response. TH2 lymphocytes synthesize and secrete IL-4, IL-5, IL-6, and IL-13 that stimulate B lymphocytes to develop into antibody-secreting plasma cells and inhibit macrophage functions, and induce an antibody response. The type of immune response (antibody versus cell-mediated) can have a profound influence on the outcome of a disease. In the instance of an intracellular protozoal infection, a TH2 type response results in rapid proliferation of the organism and death of the host, whereas a TH1 type response results in elimination of the organism and survival of the host.

Similarly, a T_H2 response to an allergen results in the elaboration of immunoglobulin (Ig) E, through IL-4 production, stimulation of eosinophils, through IL-5 production, and the development of an allergic reaction. The exact regulation of the T_H1 versus the T_H2 lymphocyte response is unknown, but studies suggest that IL-12 produced by activated macrophages stimulates the T_H1 response, whereas IL-4 inhibits the T_H1 response, allowing the T_H2 response to dominate. T_H lymphocytes predominately drive the immune response to microbial pathogens by activating macrophages or B lymphocytes.

Another functionally distinct subpopulation of $CD4^+$ T lymphocytes is the regulatory T lymphocyte (T reg). T reg lymphocytes function to suppress the response of self-reactive CD4 lymphocytes that have escaped the negative selection process in the thymus. They are distinguished from other CD4 T lymphocytes by the expresson of CD25 on the cell surface. Like T_H1 and T_H2 lymphocytes (Table 1), T reg lymphocyte differentiation is driven by cytokine environments; however, where T_H1 and T_H2 lymphocyte activation occurs through transcripional activators T-bet and GATA-3, respectively, T reg lymphocytes are activated through the transcriptional repressor FoxP3 (Fig. 5).

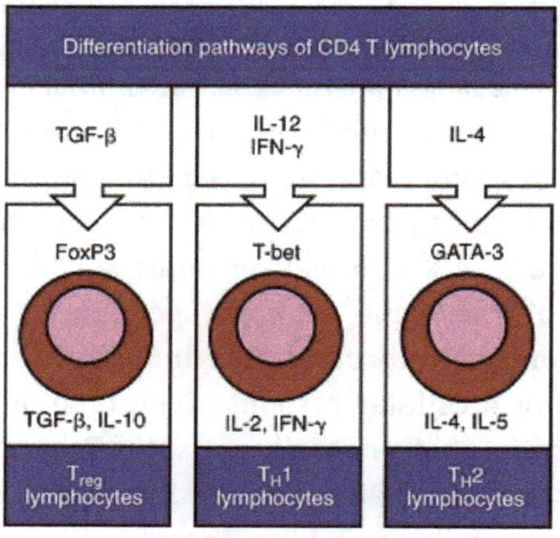

Fig. 5 Differentiation and expression of CD4 T lymphocytes. Cytokines in the extracellular tissue fluids direct the differentiation of CD4 T lymphocytes to specific secretory types, such that they secrete specific cytokines that have specific functions on other lymphocytes in the environment.

This subpopulation of T reg lymphocytes are often referred to as Fox3P lymphocytes and produce the immunosuppressive and antiinflammatory cytokines IL-4, IL-10 and TGF-β. FoxP3 lymphocytes are an intense area of investigation for their role as suppressor lymphocytes of immunity and inflammation. T reg lymphocytes have been shown to have a role in the prevention of organ-specific autoimmune diseases and in modulation of immune responses to microbial pathogens to prevent overwhelming inflammatory reactions.

Table 1. Basic Cytokine and Functional Profiles of TH_1 and TH_2 Lymphocytes

Cytokine	TH_1	TH_2
IL-2	+	
IFN-g	++	
TNF-b	++	
GM-CSF	++	+
IL-3	++	++
IL-4		++
IL-5		++
IL-13		++
Function		
Antibody	+	++
IgE		++
Eosinophils, mast cells		++
Macrophages	++	
Type IV hypersensitivity	++	
Cytotoxic T lymphocytes	++	

GM-CSF, Granulocyte-macrophage colony-stimulating factor; IFN-γ, interferon-γ; IgE, immunoglobulin E; IL, interleukin; TNF-β, tumor necrosis factor-β.

Finally, a subpopulation of CD4 lymphocytes characterized by the ability to produce IL-17 is designated as T_H17 lymphocytes. T_H17 lymphocyte differentiation is driven by TGF-β, IL-6, IL-1, and IL-23. T_H17 lymphocytes, through production of chemokines IL-17 and IL-22, induce the recruitment of monocytes and neutrophils to sites of inflammation. Again, one must recognize that this is an oversimplification of a complex regulatory mechanism and that as additional knowledge is gained about T_H1, T_H2, T reg, and T_H17 lymphocyte responses, we will be able to understand pathogenic mechanisms of diseases, which will lead to the development of more specific therapeutic targets.

B Lymphocytes

B lymphocytes constitute 5% to 20% of the peripheral blood mononuclear cells. B lymphocyte development occurs in two phases, an antigen-independent phase in the primary lymphoid tissues, followed by an antigen-dependent phase in secondary lymphoid tissues. B lymphocytes can be found in primary lymphoid tissues, such as the bone marrow and ileal Peyer's patches (a primary lymphoid tissue in some species because it is the site of B lymphocyte development, rather than the bone marrow), and in secondary lymphoid tissues, such as the spleen, lymph nodes, tonsils, and Peyer's patches. Within secondary lymphoid tissues, B lymphocytes are aggregated in the form of distinct lymphoid follicles, which on activation expand to form prominent pale regions called germinal centers (Fig. 6).

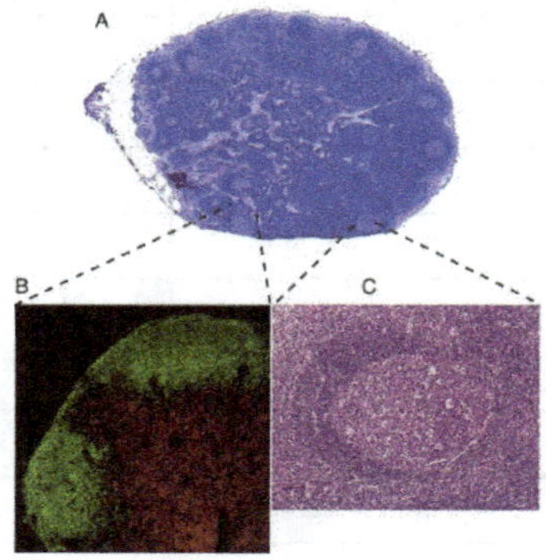

FIG. 6 Histology of a hyperplastic lymph node. A, Outer cortex, containing numerous secondary lymphoid follicles with characteristic pale centers, and inner medulla are easily identifiable. B, Localization of B lymphocytes (labeled with a B lymphocyte marker conjugated with a green fluorochrome) and T lymphocytes (labeled with a T lymphocyte marker conjugated with a red fluorochrome).

This anatomic localization, similar to T lymphocytes in the PALS and paracortex, is the result of elaboration of chemokines for which the B lymphocyte has receptors. The antigen receptor of the B lymphocyte is the membrane bound immunoglobulin. After the antigen-independent phase of development, B lymphocytes express IgM and IgD on their surface that signifies a mature B lymphocyte. In the antigen-dependent phase, antigen-activated mature B lymphocytes differentiate into IgM-secreting plasma cells or switch to another antibody isotype. Immunoglobulins can be generated against an almost unlimited number of antigenic determinants through the rearrangement of genes encoding the light chain and heavy chain components. As in the case of the TCR, an evaluation of the rearranged genes of a B lymphocyte can be used to molecularly phenotype B lymphocyte neoplasms.

Like the T lymphocyte, the B lymphocyte also has accessory molecules that function to form the antigen receptor complex (Fig. 7). These nonpolymorphic molecules are nonpolymorphic heterodimers composed of Ig-a (CD79a) and Ig-b (CD79b) that do not bind antigen but do interact with the transmembrane portion of surface immunoglobulin involved in cell activation.

B lymphocytes, unlike T lymphocytes, can recognize soluble antigens. Additional nonpolymorphic molecules that are important to B lymphocyte functions are CD21 and CD40. The CD21 molecule is the complement receptor-2 molecule whose ligands are C3b and C3d. B lymphocyte responses to protein antigens are dependent on cytokines produced by activated T lymphocytes (CD4+). The CD40 molecule interacts with CD40 ligand on the surface of TH lymphocytes and functions to allow

B lymphocyte development into antibody-secreting plasma cells. A failure to express CD40 ligand has been associated with an inability to isotype switch, resulting in a hyper-IgM syndrome. B lymphocytes activated by antigen develop into antibody secreting plasma cells and memory lymphocytes of the same antigenic specificity.

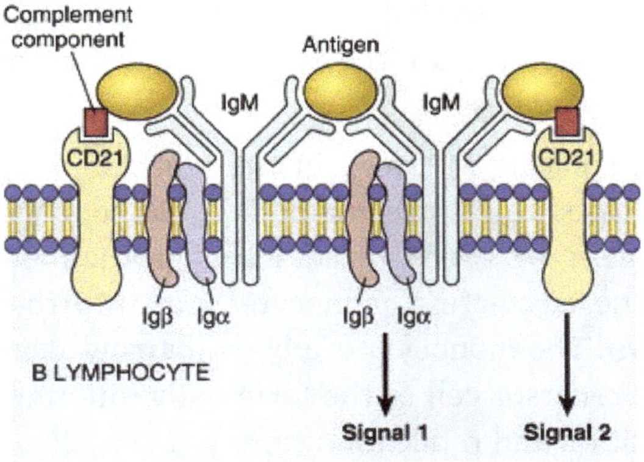

Fig. 7 The B lymphocyte antigen receptor complex.Membrane *IgM* (or IgD, not shown) and the signaling molecules *Iga* and *Igb. CD21,* also known as *complement receptor-2,* binds complement components and activates B lymphocytes. *Ig,* Immunoglobulin

Mononuclear Phagocytic System (Monocyte-Macrophage System)

The preferred term today for the functionally and phenotypically diverse population of mononuclear phagocytic cells is the *mononuclear phagocytic system* (MPS). It is also referred to as the monocyte-macrophage system. These cells have a broad range of functions contributing to immunity, inflammation, and tissue remodeling and repair. A brief history on the recognition of the defensive mechanism of phagocytosis not only facilitates our current understanding of how these cells play a crucial role in innate and adaptive immunity but also explains some of the terminology that often leads to confusion for students.

Elie Metchnikoff (1845-1916), a comparative developmental zoologist, is credited with recognizing and establishing the process of phagocytosis, an important defensive mechanism for organisms. He recognized the association between the systemic clearance of microorganisms and the presence of the microorganisms in the spleen and liver. Subsequent studies evaluating the systemic clearance of dyes suggested that Kupffer cells and endothelial cells lining the sinusoids of the liver were responsible because both cell types internalized the dyes. Because the investigators considered macrophages (Kupffer cells) and endothelial cells to have a common biologic function, phagocytosis, they proposed that they be encompassed as a system, the reticuloendothelial system. We now understand that the mechanism of uptake by endothelial cells is not by phagocytosis and as a result the term *reticuloendothelial system* is no longer used.

The term mononuclear phagocytic system was developed to differentiate lymphoid cells (mononuclear T and B lymphocytes), granulocytes (polymorphonuclear leukocytes), and endothelial cells from the lineage-committed precursors in the bone marrow, blood monocytes and tissue macrophages, and dendritic cells that currently comprise the MPS. It is very likely that as we learn more about the precursors and differentiated cells that constitute the MPS, there will be proposals for new, more specific classification schemes.

In general, a circulating MPS cell in the blood is designated as a monocyte, whereas the tissue-based cell is designated as a macrophage. The blood monocyte-to-tissue macrophage is well recognized, although the mechanisms that allow for differentiation of the circulating monocyte pool into the tissue-based pool are still largely unknown. The monocyte is a bone marrow–derived cell of the myeloid lineage that is the precursor cell to the terminally differentiated macrophage that has limited recirculation and replication capacity.

The myeloid dendritic cell represents a specific type of mononuclear cell present in nonlymphoid tissues with unique migratory properties and is discussed separately. As opposed to granulocytic myeloid cells, macrophages are long-lived (days to months) and can exist as quiescent "resident" cells widely distributed throughout the body. It is becoming increasingly clear that there is heterogeneity in the circulating monocyte pool that corresponds with the ultimate tissue localization of resident macrophages. The phenotypic characterization of the cells the MPS contains is often used in an attempt to identify specific populations of MPS. Morphologically, monocytes are variably sized with an irregular shape, oval or kidney-shaped nucleus, prominent cytoplasmic vesicles, and a high cytoplasm to nucleus ratio. These features are not unique to monocytes, and as a result, they are difficult to distinguish from circulating dendritic cells, activated lymphocytes, and NK cells based on morphology or by light scatter (flow cytometry). This section covers basic concepts attributable to monocytes, tissue macrophages, and myeloid dendritic cells and refers to specific organ systems. See additional chapters in the section on pathology of organ systems for details on organ-specific cells of the MPS. Certain organ systems have specific names for their resident macrophages, whereas other organ systems only refer to them as macrophages (Table 2).

Table 2. Nomenclature and Location of Nonlymphoid Monocyte-Macrophage Cell Types

Organ/Tissue	Name	Location
Lung	Alveolar macrophages	Alveolar spaces
	Pulmonary intravascular macrophages	Capillaries of the lung
Connective tissues	Histiocytes	Interstitium

Organ/Tissue	Name	Location
Kidney	Mesangial cells	Glomerular tuft
Brain	Microglial cells	Neuroparenchyma and
		perivascular areas
Bone	Osteoclasts	Bone marrow
Blood	Monocytes	Circulation
Liver	Kupffer cells	Hepatic sinusoids

Growth and differentiation of monocytes is regulated by specific growth factors, such as IL-3, colony-stimulating-factor-1 (CSF-1), granulocyte-macrophage CSF (GM-CSF), IL-4, and IL-13, and inhibitors such as type I interferons and transforming growth factor-β (TGF-β). CSF-1 is the most important because it controls the proliferation, differentiation, and survival of the monocyte. Monocytes represent approximately 4% to 10% of blood leukocytes and are identified in mammals, birds, amphibians, and fish. They are largely viewed as accessory cells that importantly link inflammation and innate immune responses to adaptive immunity.

Hematopoietic stem cells (HSC) give rise to the common myeloid progenitor (CMP), the precursor cell to the granulocyte/macrophage progenitor (GMP) and macrophage/dendritic cell progenitor (MDP). The MDP is the common progenitor cell for monocytes, macrophages, and conventional dendritic cells. Monocytes express the CSF-1 receptor (CD115) and the chemokine receptor CX3CR1, are differentiated from polymorphonuclear cells (PMNs), NK cells, and lymphoid cells, and do not express CD3, CD19, or CD15. Monocyte heterogeneity based on surface marker expression and function has identified subsets that are an area of intense investigation and are best characterized in humans and rodents. Subpopulations of blood monocytes can be phenotyped based on the expression of surface markers CD14 and CD 16 (FcγR-III). Two additional subpopulations of blood monocytic cells are the myeloid blood dendritic cells, which are negative for CD14 and CD16. In the mouse, the main subset of $CD115^+$ monocytes are characterized as large cells expressing Ly6C, the chemokine receptor CCR2 and the adhesion molecule L-selectin (CD62L), and CX3CR1.

These are referred to as inflammatory monocytes or inflammatory-monocyte-derived macrophages that are preferentially recruited to inflamed tissues and lymph nodes where they produce high levels of TNF-α and IL-1. The emigration of Ly6C+ monocytes from the bone marrow to the periphery depends on the chemokine receptor CCR2 and its ligands CCL7 and CCL2. Ly6C negative monocytes have less of an influence on inflammatory reactions and appear to function more importantly as tissue resident cells and as cells involved in healing and regeneration associated with vascular injury.

In those species characterized to date, there appear to be two major functional subpopulations of monocytes, one that is recruited and differentiated into macrophages at the site of inflammation and expresses higher levels of MHC class II and adhesion molecules and one that is responsible for repopulating resident tissue macrophages. Both populations can give rise to dendritic cells (see Fig. 5-8). Classification schemes are forever evolving, and there are definite species differences that may explain species differences in rates of infection and types of clinical disease associated with specific microbial agents. Similar phenotypic and functional heterogeneity exists with tissue-based macrophages.

The MPS of hematopoietic and lymphoid organs is diverse with functionally and phenotypically distinct parallel subpopulations in humans, rodents, and pigs. In primary lymphoid organs, mature macrophages are involved in the production, differentiation, and destruction of all lineages of hematopoietic cells in the bone marrow, and in positive and negative selection processes in the thymus. In secondary lymphoid organs, macrophages are uniquely positioned to enhance their phagocytic properties to endogenous and exogenous material and to influence other cell types through their products. The resident macrophages in the spleen differ in microscopic localization, phenotype, and function.

The reason for this complexity is largely attributable the spleen's role as a hematopoietic organ and as a secondary lymphoid organ. Distinct subpopulations of macrophages are present in the red pulp, white pulp, and marginal zone with some recognized species differences. The red pulp macrophage functions in the phagocytosis of hematogenous pathogens and senescent erythrocytes. Erythrophagocytosis primarily occurs in the spleen and liver and allows for the removal of senescent erythrocytes and recycling of iron, often evident as cytoplasmic accumulations of pigments. The white pulp macrophages are also actively phagocytic, and a morphologically distinct cell, the "tingible body macrophage," can often be easily identified histologically and represents macrophages involved in the uptake and removal of apoptotic T and B lymphocytes.

The marginal zone of the spleen provides a complex environment for the interface for the red and white pulp, specifically an important transit area for cells leaving circulation and entering the white pulp, and for B lymphocyte differentiation. The development of granulomatous inflammatory reactions in the spleen as a response to hematogenous microorganisms often begins in the marginal zone. The two subpopulations of macrophages present in the marginal zone are the metallophilic macrophage and the marginal zone macrophage.

Marginal zone macrophages express high levels of PRRs and scavenger receptors that facilitate the clearance of pathogens from the circulation. The function of metallophilic macrophages is unknown. Tissue macrophages are derived from a combination of precursors in the blood (monocytes) and from local proliferation of precursors that varies for individual organ systems.

Much has been written about the relationship between monocytes, macrophages, and dendritic cells. The inclusion of dendritic cells as a component of the MPS is in part attributable to the fact that they are derived from a common myeloid precursor, influenced by similar growth factors (e.g., CSF-1), express common surface markers, and have no unique properties as antigen-presenting cells that allow them to be differentiated from macrophages.

Like macrophages, dendritic cells in specific organ systems may have a specific name or designated only as dendritic cells preceded by the organ or in some instances a specific anatomic location within an organ. Dendritic cell subsets are also an intense area of investigation with regards to phenotypic and functional heterogeneity. The so-called conventional dendritic cells are present as immature cells in the interstitial tissues of all organs except the brain.

Macrophages

Mononuclear phagocytic cells include circulating monocytes and tissue-based macrophages. In the spleen, macrophages are located in the marginal zone, white pulp, and red pulp, where they function primarily as phagocytic cells. In the lymph node, macrophages are located in the subcapsular sinus, which is analogous to the marginal zone of the spleen, and the medulla. These physical locations, the subcapsular sinus of lymph nodes and marginal zone of the spleen, facilitate their exposure to potential antigens. Nonlymphoid tissue-based macrophages have different functions and are named according to the tissue in which they reside (see Table 2). Macrophages express Fc receptors (FcR) for antibody and can phagocytose antigens opsonized by antibody or complement components. Another primary function is their involvement in the immune response as antigen-presenting cells. In this instance, they phagocytose antigen and process it into peptide fragments, which are then presented to T lymphocytes, and the induction of cell-mediated immune responses. Although all nucleated cells express MHC class I molecules and could be considered antigen-presenting cells, only three cell types normally express MHC class II molecules and are regarded as the major antigen-presenting cells. They are the macrophage, dendritic cell, and B lymphocyte. Whereas B lymphocytes and dendritic cells constitutively express MHC class II molecules, macrophages express MHC class molecules on activation.

Macrophages also have an important role in the generation of a cell-mediated immune response and are essential to type IV hypersensitivity reactions. Activated T_H1 lymphocytes synthesize IFN-γ, a potent activator of macrophages. Under the influence of IFN-γ, macrophages have increased phagocytic activity and are more efficient at killing.

Dendritic Cells

Dendritic cells comprise a distinct population of cells that are characterized by elongate cell processes. Most dendritic cells are antigen-presenting cells, which process antigens and present fragments to T lymphocytes. They are more efficient than macrophages and B lymphocytes at antigen presentation. Antigen-presenting dendritic cells are nonphagocytic, bone marrow–derived cells. They are the most important antigen-presenting cell for initiating primary immune responses to protein antigens.

Antigen-presenting dendritic cells express a number of molecules, such as TLRs and mannose receptors, that make them efficient at capturing and responding to antigens. They also express high concentrations of MHC class II molecules and B7 co-stimulatory molecules. By expressing chemokine receptors similar to T lymphocytes, they have the ability to localize in T lymphocyte regions of lymphoid tissue. By colocalizing to these areas, they are uniquely positioned to present antigens to recirculating T lymphocytes.

Antigen-presenting dendritic cells function to capture antigen and then migrate to T lymphocyte areas of secondary lymphoid organs, where they present fragments of the antigen on their surface and increase their expression of co-stimulatory molecules that activate T lymphocytes. Specifically, migrating dendritic cells, derived from Langerhans' cells that have captured antigen, enter the lymph node through efferent lymphatics and localize in lymphoid organs, where they present antigenic peptides to T lymphocytes that facilitate B lymphocyte activation and the production of antibody-secreting plasma cells. In addition to their function as antigen-presenting cells, they are also important in the process of negative selection in the thymus and in the maintenance of peripheral tolerance.

The four types of antigen-presenting dendritic cells and their locations are listed in Table 3. Circulating dendritic cells, also known as *veiled cells,* make up less than %1 of peripheral blood mononuclear cells. The second type of dendritic cell, the follicular dendritic cell, is primarily located in lymphoid follicles. These cells are not derived from the bone marrow, do not express MHC class II molecules, and do not function as an antigen-presenting cell. Follicular dendritic cells have FcR and receptors for C3b. They store antigen-antibody and antigen-C3b complexes and are thought to be involved in the development and maintenance of memory B lymphocytes.

Table 3. Antigen-Presenting Dendritic Cells and Their Primary Location

Dendritic Cells	Location
Langerhans' cells	Skin, mucous membranes, iris, ciliary body
Interstitial dendritic cells	Most major organs
Interdigitating dendritic cells	T lymphocyte area of secondary lymphoid tissue and thymic medulla
Circulating dendritic cells	Peripheral blood

Natural Killer Cells

NK cells are nonspecific cytotoxic cells that are important in early responses to tumor cells and viral infections. NK cells are bone marrow–derived, large granular lymphocytes that make up 5% to 15% of the peripheral blood mononuclear cells. Their size, slightly larger than that of a small lymphocyte, and the presence of abundant granular cytoplasm distinguish them from T lymphocytes.

They are commonly referred to as large granular lymphocytes. The cytoplasm of NK cells and CTL (T_c) is characterized by cytotoxic granules that contain perforin and granzymes, two potent pathways mediating lysis of the target cell. NK cells and T lymphocytes express numerous similar surface molecules and kill virus infected cells and tumor cells by similar mechanisms. Two membrane molecules, CD16 and CD56, are commonly used to identify NK cells. NK cells express FcγR (CD16) and the β-subunit of the IL-2 receptor (CD2).

They do not express antigen-specific TCR or CD3 molecules. In contrast to cytotoxic lymphocytes, NK cells are not MHC restricted, are constitutively cytolytic, and do not develop memory cells. Because NK cells are activated early in an immune response and do not require a previous sensitization phase to develop memory cells after activation, they are the cytotoxic cell of innate immunity, the counterpart to the adaptive immune response's CTL (T_c).

Although NK cells do not express any antigen-specific molecules, they are very efficient at recognizing and killing altered or virally infected cells. NK cell activity is regulated through activating and inhibitory receptor molecules expressed on their cell surface. These NK cell receptor molecules fall into two distinct categories: the immunoglobulin-like NK receptors and the C-type lectin-like NK receptors. Ligands for these receptors are cell surface molecules whose expression has been altered as a result of infection or damage. Ligands for activating receptors that stimulate NK cell activity commonly include viral and stress-induced proteins. Ligands for inhibitory receptors that block NK cell activity most commonly involve class I MHC molecules. A decreased expression of class I MHC molecules makes cells susceptible to NK cell–mediated lysis.

A decrease in MHC class I expression often occurs in virus-infected cells and in neoplastic cells, making them susceptible to attack by NK cells. Normal cells are protected from NK cell killing because all nucleated cells express class I MHC molecules. This is an oversimplification of the "opposing-signals" model of NK cell regulation of how cytotoxic activity is limited to altered self-cells. Recent studies on the molecular mechanisms of NK cell regulation indicate that the absence of an inhibitory stimulus by itself is insufficient for triggering NK cell killing. NK cells also require triggering of activating receptors.

Several activating receptors have been identified. One is the NKG2D receptor, a C-type lectin-like molecule that recognizes a number of stress-induced proteins. These stress-induced proteins are normally only constitutively expressed in the intestinal epithelium or as a result of cellular distress caused by infection or neoplastic transformation. There are a number of additional activating receptors, some of which recognized viral proteins, that are structurally similar to class I MHC molecules.

Because NK cells express FcγR (CD16), they can also function in antibody-dependent cellular cytotoxicity (ADCC). In the case of NK cells, ADCC allows for antibody-bound targets to be identified and targeted for NK cell–induced lysis.

NK cells also facilitate the early response to viral infections not only by responding to cytokines produced early in a viral infection, but also by producing cytokines that help direct the immune response. NK cells are activated by IFN-α and IFN-β, released by virus-infected cells, and by IL-12, released by macrophages. After activation, NK cells have the ability to produce IFN-γ, a major cytokine directing the development of T_H1-type immune response early in the infection. IL-2 and IL-15 stimulate NK cell proliferation, and IL-12 enhances NK cell killing.

CYTOKINES: MESSENGER MOLECULES OF THE IMMUNE SYSTEM

General Properties of Cytokines

Cytokines make up a vast group of low molecular weight soluble glycoprotein proteins that are produced by immune and nonimmune cells, are largely produced locally, and act locally to direct the immune response. The expression of cytokine receptors and their respective ligands is highly regulated and contributes to the complexity of the systemic organization of the immune response. Cytokines are involved in every aspect of leukocyte biology and the immune response and are essential to leukocyte development, recirculation, differentiation, and activation and in maintaining self-tolerance. Cytokines can influence the cytokine-producing cell itself (autocrine), other cells present locally (paracrine), or distant cells (endocrine). Cytokines use common signal transducing pathways, converting an extracellular signal through a cell surface receptor to activate or inhibit the target cell.

The nomenclature of cytokines has evolved from a system that originally named them according to their cellular source (e.g., lymphokine from lymphocytes and monokines from monocytes) to one that named them according to not only the cellular source but also the target cell (e.g., interleukin, a cytokine produced by a leukocyte that influences another leukocyte) or to the primary function (e.g., chemokine, a cytokine that affects chemotaxis). As cytokines were characterized, it became apparent that they have pleiotropic, redundant, synergistic, and antagonistic features that do not allow for such a simplistic classification scheme. More recently, cytokines and their receptors have been classified based on their molecular structure and common signaling pathways.

Many cytokines share a similar, α-helix structure that is also shared by their respective receptors and are classified as type I cytokines and receptors. As is discussed later, the classification of cytokines and cytokine receptors according to their structural similarities allowed for the identification of the cause of the profound cytokine defects associated with X-linked severe combined immunodeficiency disease in humans and dogs. Unfortunately, type I cytokines also have now been found to include other regulatory proteins such as growth hormone, prolactin, erythropoietin, thrombopoietin, and leptin. Type II cytokines include type I interferons (IFN-α and IFN-β), type II interferon (IFN-γ), and the IL-10 family of cytokines.

The breadth and depth of knowledge regarding the function, regulation, and control of cytokines is overwhelming; however, an overview of the major cytokines and their primary functions is important for understanding the pathogenic mechanism of many disease processes.

Cytokines that broadly influence innate and adaptive immune responses include IL-1, interferons (type 1), IL-6, and TNF-α. These cytokines are produced and influence a wide array of cell types. Cytokines that are involved in hematopoiesis and lymphocyte development include IL-2, IL-3, IL-4, IL-5, IL-12, IL-15, TGF-β, and GM-CSF to mention a few.

Chemokines are a large group of cytokines that influence leukocyte development, trafficking, and function. They are organized into subfamilies, with distinct functions, based on the position of cysteine residues. The C-X-C subfamily of chemokines is primarily produced by activated macrophages and tissue cells (e.g., endothelium), and the C-C subfamily is largely produced by activated T lymphocytes. Chemokines are responsible for the anatomic localization ("homing") of lymphocytes within lymphoid and nonlymphoid tissue. Chemokines and the other proinflammatory cytokines. The most important functional group of cytokines related to the pathogenesis of a number of diseases of immunity are those involved in the regulation of T_H lymphocytes. As discussed previously, T_H lymphocytes are classified based on their functional capacity and ability to elicit primarily an antibody response or a cell-mediated immune response rather than on their expression of specific cell markers.

T_H1 lymphocytes are activated by IL-12 and IL-18 and produce primarily IL-2, IFN-γ, and TNF-β to direct a cell-mediated immune response. T_H2 lymphocytes are activated by IL-4 and produce primarily IL-3, IL-4, IL-5, IL-6, IL-10, and IL-13 to direct a humoral immune response. As discussed later in the chapter, the type of response (T_H1 versus T_H2 type) may determine if a diseased state will occur. IL-15 regulates the growth and activity of NK cells.

Some cytokines, such as IL-10 and TGF-β, downregulate immune responses. In summary, cytokines produced by the T_H1 or T_H2 subset of lymphocytes not only promote the activation and functional capacities of the subset that produces them (autocrine effect) but also inhibit the development and activity of the other subset. This is known as cross-regulation and has important implications with regard to protective immune responses and adverse immune responses, as is discussed later.

Finally, a number of cytokine inhibitors were identified, and one of the more studied ones includes a factor called IL-1 receptor antagonist, which is produced by macrophages, hepatocytes, and keratinocytes. This factor inhibits the local and systemic effects of IL-1 by blocking the IL-1 receptor. Another group of inhibitors are the soluble cytokine receptors, which are the enzymatic product of cleavage of the extracellular domain of cytokine receptors that bind their respective cytokines, preventing interaction with the membrane-bound receptor form.

The best characterized soluble cytokine receptor is the soluble IL-2 receptor. A number of pathogenic organisms have adapted this as an evasion strategy by producing cytokine-binding proteins or mimics to influence the development of the immune response. Although soluble receptors have been identified in a number of human diseases, their exact role remains to be determined.

STRUCTURE AND FUNCTION OF HISTOCOMPATIBILITY ANTIGENS

The MHC represents a complex of genes that encode specialized molecules involved in intercellular recognition and the distinguishing of self from nonself. These cell surface molecules have immunologic and nonimmunologic functions. The histocompatibility designation originated from the identification of these molecules in determining the compatibility of transplanted tissues. The MHC is an essential component in humoral and cell-mediated immunity.

Most T lymphocytes only recognize fragments of antigen when they are bound to MHC molecules, and this requirement is the basis for MHC restriction. The repertoire of MHC molecules is genetically controlled and determines an individual's ability or inability to respond to specific antigens. MHC molecules are present throughout vertebrates and are maintained in gene clusters, each of which encodes different MHC products, which are linked. The primary function of cell surface MHC molecules is to bind peptide fragments of foreign proteins for presentation to antigen-specific T lymphocytes. There are three major classes of genes, and these encode for MHC molecules that are grouped according to their structure, tissue distribution, and function. Class I and class II genes encode cell surface molecules. Class III genes encode components of the complement system, enzymes 21-hydroxylase A and B, cytochrome p450, TNF-α and TNF-β, and heat shock protein 70.

MHC class I molecules are present on all nucleated cells (and platelets in some species). Their major function is the presentation of peptide fragments of antigens to CTL (T_c) ($CD8^+$). This requirement results in $CD8^+$ lymphocytes being MHC class I restricted. MHC class I molecules are further subdivided into highly polymorphic loci, referred to as Ia, and relatively nonpolymorphic loci, referred to as Ib, Ic, and Id. Each class I molecule is composed of a heterodimer consisting of a polymorphic α-chain that is linked to a nonpolymorphic β_2-microglobulin. The extracellular region of the α-chain consists of three domains (α_1, α_2, and α_3). The α_1 and α_2 domains form a groove where the peptide fragments bind the MHC molecule (Fig. 8). Although MHC class I molecules differ in their ability to bind peptide fragments, they are not as restrictive as antibodies and TCRs. The intracellular processing of antigen into peptide fragments, the association of those fragments with MHC class I molecules, and their transport to the cell surface is a complex process.

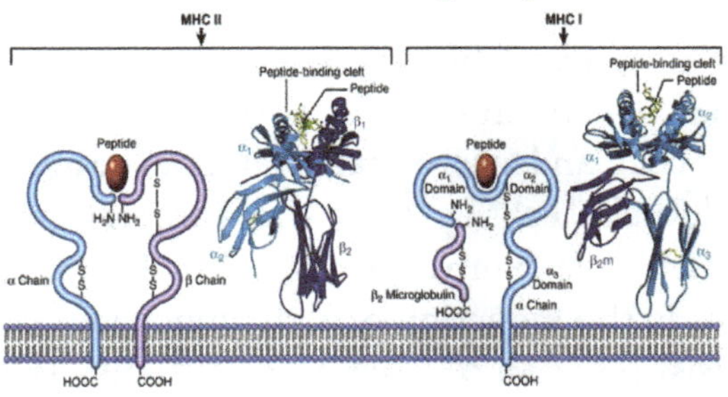

Fig. 8 Schematic diagram and crystal structures of class I and II major histocompatibility complex (MHC) molecules

Antigen uptake by antigen-presenting cells is by phagocytosis or endocytosis. Antigen processing is the degradation of an antigen into peptide fragments, which are complexed with MHC molecules. Antigen presentation is the transport of the peptide-MHC complex to the membrane, where they are displayed. Antigens can arise intracellularly (endogenous) and extracellularly (exogenous), and the immune system most effectively eliminates these antigens through the elaboration of CTL (T_c) or secretion of antibody. The immune system uses two different processing pathways for antigen processing and antigen presentation. Intracellular antigens are processed in a cytosolic pathway and presented in association with MHC class I molecules. Extracellular antigens are processed in an endocytic pathway and presented in association with MHC class II molecules. Endogenous antigens are degraded into small peptide fragments within the cytoplasm by the proteasome complex. Peptide fragments are transported to the endoplasmic reticulum (ER) by an adenosine triphosphate–binding peptide transporter (TAP). Within the ER, the newly synthesized MHC class I α-chain and associated β_2-microglobulin bind the antigenic peptide and form a complex that is transported from the ER to the Golgi and then to the plasma membrane for presentation to $CD8^+$ CTL (T_c).

The antigen recognition molecule of the cytotoxic T lymphocyte (T_c) recognizes the MHC-peptide complex by means of its CD8 molecule, which functions as a co-receptor, binding to the nonpolymorphic α_3 domain of the MHC class I heavy chain. Because CTL (T_c) only recognize peptides when they are presented as a complex with MHC class I molecules, they are referred to as being MHC class I restricted. MHC restriction is the result of positive selection of lymphocytes during T lymphocyte development in the thymus.

Portions of some antigens, those portions not processed for presentation, and in some cases, entire antigens are completely degraded by exopeptidases of the antigen-presenting cell into amino acids and do not initiate an immune response. Endogenous antigens are most frequently encountered during viral infections and thus CTL (T_c) are an important defense mechanism for eliminating virally infected cells.

Class II molecules have a variable tissue distribution depending on the species of domestic animal, but in general they are present on antigen-presenting cells (B lymphocytes, dendritic cells, and macrophages) and can be induced on T lymphocytes, keratinocytes, and endothelial cells by IFN-γ. There are significant species differences with regard to the constitutive expression of MHC molecules. The major function of MHC class II molecules is the induction of T_H lymphocytes. Class II MHC molecules are heterodimers consisting of an α-chain and a β-chain. The antigen-binding site of the class II molecule, unlike that of the class I molecule, is formed by portions of both the α_1 and β_1 domain.

Additionally, as with the class I MHC molecules, polymorphism of the class II MHC molecules is associated with determining an individual's response to antigens of infectious organisms (see next section). Peptides that bind to class II MHC molecules are in general derived from exogenous antigens, which have been internalized and processed within endosomes and lysosomes of antigen-presenting cells.

Antigen-presenting cells can internalize antigen by phagocytosis or endocytosis (receptor mediated or pinocytosis). Macrophages are the only cell type capable of both because other antigen-presenting cells are poorly phagocytic. Extracellular antigens are processed into peptide fragments in an endocytic pathway and presented in association with MHC class II molecules on the cell membrane. During the synthesis of a class II molecule within the ER, it associates with another protein called the *invariant chain,* which prevents the molecule from binding endogenously derived peptides.

The complex is then transported from the ER to the Golgi complex and into an endocytic compartment (vesicles) that contains the antigenic peptide fragments derived from exogenous antigens. Proteolytic cleavage of the invariant chain allows for the association of the peptide fragment with the class II MHC molecule. The peptide-class II MHC complex is then transported to the cell surface for presentation to $CD4^+$ T_H lymphocytes. The CD4 molecule acts as a coreceptor for induction of T_H lymphocyte activation. Because T_H lymphocytes only recognize peptides when they are presented as a complex with class II MHC molecules, they are referred to as *class II MHC restricted.* It is worth mentioning that of the two scientists, Peter Doherty and Rolf Zinkernagel, who received the Nobel Prize in Medicine in 1996 for discovering MHC restriction, Dr. Doherty is an Australian veterinarian.

MHC molecules are important in regulating T lymphocyte development in the thymus and in the peripheral lymphoid tissues determining specific responses to different forms of antigens. During the development and maturation process in the thymus, only T lymphocytes capable of recognizing self-MHC molecules are selected (positive selection) for export to the peripheral lymphoid tissues. These developmental processes influence an individual's T lymphocyte repertoire, which is the functional population that influences immunity.

An individual's ability to mount an effective immune response is determined in part by his or her ability to recognize endogenous and exogenous antigens and their MHC haplotype. Thus, in one case, the association of an antigenic peptide fragment with a specific MHC molecule may result in a protective antibody response with elimination of an infectious agent, whereas in another case, the association of an antigenic peptide fragment with a specific MHC molecule may result in an inappropriate immune response to an innocuous antigen, producing an allergic reaction.

The organization (chromosomal location) and characterization (e.g., number of loci) of the MHC of each species of domestic animals appears to be fairly conserved and present in higher vertebrates and mammals. Most mammalian species studied have class I, II, and III genes, with differences between species being the arrangement and number of genetic loci comprising the MHC. In general, class I genes are more closely related within a species than between species, and the avian MHC is smaller and less complex, with many genes found in the mammalian MHC being absent. Although it is beyond the scope of this chapter to discuss the details regarding the differences between domestic species, the preceding overview is relevant to most domestic species.

Major Histocompatibility Complex and Disease Association

The MHC influences transplant acceptance or rejection, immune responsiveness, and the pathogenesis of a number of diseases. The MHC represents a complex of genes that encode specialized molecules involved in antigen presentation and thus regulate immune responses. The ability of the immune system to respond to an antigen is determined in part by the binding of peptide fragments to MHC molecules, which are then presented on the surface of antigen-presenting cells.

There is a growing body of information associating certain MHC alleles with increased or decreased susceptibility to certain diseases (Table 2). Because the MHC genes of most domestic species are not well characterized, it is difficult to distinguish if the observed effects are due to the MHC itself or to other tightly linked genes. These conclusions are generally the result of an observation that some MHC alleles occur at a higher frequency among individuals affected with the disease, as compared with the general population. The association of an increased risk with certain MHC alleles is never the sole basis for determining if an individual will develop the disease, as often other hereditary and environmental factors also play an important role.

The diseases most often associated with certain MHC alleles have a pathogenesis that incorporates a significant immunologic component. The types of diseases identified are diverse; however, they frequently include autoimmune, infectious, and allergic diseases. Additionally, MHC diversity may increase or decrease the susceptibility to infectious diseases. There is evidence that MHC polymorphisms may significantly impact disease resistance and is best illustrated in species in which there is a loss of MHC diversity attributed to a limited breeding pool of animals. In the case of the cheetah and Florida panther, the current breeding stocks of both species are derived from a limited genetic pool, thus resulting in reduced MHC diversity. In both species, there is an increased susceptibility to infectious agents that is not seen in other species of big cats.

Although there are a number of hypotheses to account for the role of MHC molecules in disease susceptibility, the actual mechanisms remain elusive. The most often hypothesized mechanism is attributed to the role of MHC alleles in determining responsiveness or nonresponsiveness to a particular pathogen. On the one hand, through antigen presentation and activation of cytotoxic or T lymphocytes, it determines whether a protective immune response is generated to a particular pathogen. On the other hand, certain MHC alleles may encode molecules that are used by infectious agents, as in the case of receptors for viruses or bacterial toxins, and facilitate their infectivity or pathogenicity.

DISORDERS OF THE IMMUNE SYSTEM

As has been discussed, immunity is a complex defensive system of recognition and effector mechanisms for protecting the host from infectious pathogens and cancer. During the normal immune response, there are mechanisms for eliminating the inciting foreign antigen, and associated with this is some degree of tissue damage that elicits an inflammatory response of appropriate duration and severity for the antigen. However, there are a number of instances in which the immune response elicits an inflammatory response that is not appropriate to the inciting antigen and these fall into three general categories. The largest category is the hypersensitivity reactions, which are associated with a large number of diseases covered throughout this text.

The second category is the autoimmune diseases, in which the immune response is inappropriately directed at a self-antigen, resulting in damage to normal organs or tissue. The third category is the immunodeficiency diseases, in which a genetic or acquired defect results in an inability to mount an immune response and thus control infections, resulting in severe systemic inflammation. The chapter now focuses on general features of immunologic tissue injury, with discussion of some specific immunologic diseases that are attributable to disorders of the immune system. Finally, we conclude with a discussion of amyloidosis, a condition that is the result of a number of mechanisms, some of which have an immunologic basis.

MECHANISMS OF IMMUNOLOGIC TISSUE INJURY: HYPERSENSITIVITY REACTIONS

A hypersensitivity reaction is defined as the altered reactivity to a specific antigen that results in pathologic reactions upon the exposure of a sensitized host to that specific antigen. The designation of these immune responses as "hyper" is somewhat of a misnomer because the reactions elicited are better characterized as inappropriate or misdirected responses. An immune response can be either beneficial or harmful. By characterizing hypersensitivity responses as inappropriate or misdirected, we are not implying that these responses are any different from those that occur as a normal "beneficial" defense mechanism. To state it more clearly: If the immune response is beneficial it is immunity and if it is harmful, it is hypersensitivity.

All hypersensitivity reactions are characterized by sensitization and effector phases. The sensitization phase requires that the host must have had either a previous exposure or a prolonged exposure to the antigen so that he or she can develop an immune response to the inciting antigen. The pathology associated with hypersensitivity reactions occurs in the effector phase and is most commonly manifested as an inflammatory reaction or as cell lysis.

Hypersensitivity reactions have historically been classified on the basis of the immunologic mechanism that mediates the disease as type I, type II, type III, or type IV. Types I, II, and III are mediated by antibody, and type IV is mediated by macrophages and T lymphocytes. Type I is also known as *immediate type hypersensitivity* and most often is the result of an IgE response that is directed against an environmental or exogenous antigen (also known as an *allergen*). The result is the release of vasoactive mediators from IgE-sensitized mast cells, and these mediators produce an acute inflammatory response.

Type II is also known as cytotoxic hypersensitivity and most often occurs when IgG or IgM is directed against either an altered self-protein or a foreign antigen bound to a tissue or cell. The result can lead to either destruction of the tissue or cell by ADCC, complement-mediated lysis, or altered cellular function without evidence of tissue or cell damage. Type III is also known as *immune complex hypersensitivity* and is due to the formation of insoluble antibody-antigen complexes (also known as *immune complexes*).

The result is activation of the complement system and the development of an inflammatory reaction at the sites of immune complex deposition. Type IV is also known as *delayed-type hypersensitivity* (DTH) and is the result of activation of sensitized T lymphocytes to a specific antigen. The resulting immune response is either mediated by direct cytotoxicity or by the release of cytokines that act primarily through macrophages. This original classification, as proposed by Gell and Coombs, was based largely on the primary initiating event involved in the individual reactions and not on the actual pathogenesis as it relates to what is seen clinically or pathologically.

Although the original classification of hypersensitivity reactions is still valid, "newer" versions that are based on the pathogenesis better illustrate the complexity of these reactions and the specific pathology (lesions) associated with them. In humans, genetic mapping studies of most diseases characterized by a hypersensitivity reaction suggest that there are disease-associated susceptibility genes, further supporting the complex pathogenesis of these diseases. Finally, the pathogenesis of many diseases rarely involves a single hypersensitivity reaction, and in fact, some diseases may begin as an immediate hypersensitivity but progress to be predominantly DTH. For clarity, the hypersensitivity diseases are discussed in the context of their predominant mechanism except when it is appropriate to elaborate on the progression of a disease.

CHAPTER 3

ANTIGENS AND ANTIBODIES

An antigen is a foreign substance that enters your body. This can include bacteria, viruses, fungi, allergens, venom and other various toxins. An antibody is a protein produced by your immune system to attack and fight off these antigens.

Antigens are molecules capable of stimulating an immune response. Each antigen has distinct surface features, or epitopes, resulting in specific responses.

Antibodies (immunoglobins) are Y-shaped proteins produced by B cells of the immune system in response to exposure to antigens. Each antibody contains a paratope which recognizes a specific epitope on an antigen, acting like a lock and key binding mechanism. This binding helps to eliminate antigens from the body, either by direct neutralization or by 'tagging' for other arms of the immune system.

Antibodies are also called immunoglobulins or Ig. They are Y-shaped proteins made by your immune system's B lymphocytes or B cells.

B cells attack and eliminate viruses and other toxins outside the cell. They do this by making specific antibodies for a single type of antigen.

These tailored antibodies lock on to their specific antigens and tag them for attack. Antibodies also block these antigens, keeping them away from your healthy cells. Ultimately, antibodies kill these antigens, stopping infection.

The main types of antibodies (immunoglobulins) include:

- **IgG.** These are the most abundant types of antibodies in your plasma. They detoxify harmful substances and provide long-term protection.
- **IgM.** These are the first antibodies made by B cells in response to antigens.
- **IgA.** These antibodies collect antigens and remove them from your body in your mucus or other body fluids.
- **IgE.** These antibodies trigger allergies and protect against parasites. Small amounts are in your skin, lungs, and mucosal membranes.
- **IgD.** These antibodies bind to B cells and signal them to release IgM antibodies.

Each antibody guards against its target antigen, and many types of antibodies are found throughout your body. They play a vital role in your body's defense against illness and disease.

HOW DO ANTIBODIES FIGHT OFF ANTIGENS?

The molecules on the surfaces of antigens differ from those found naturally in your body. So, when an antigen enters your body, your immune system recognizes it right away. In order to attack this antigen invader, your immune system calls out for antibody protection.

Where are antibodies produced?

Antibodies are produced by B cells (specialized white blood cells). When an antigen comes into contact with a B cell, it causes the B cell to divide and clone. These cloned B cells — or plasma cells — release millions of antibodies into your bloodstream and lymph system.

Antibodies are located in various areas of your body, including your skin, lungs, tears, saliva and even breast milk. In fact, high amounts of antibodies are present in colostrum (a thick fluid secreted by the breasts for a few days after giving birth). That's why breastfeeding (chestfeeding) can boost your baby's immune system.

T-CELL ANTIGEN RECEPTORS

Structure of the T-cell receptor

T-cell antigen receptors are found only on the cell membrane. For this reason, T-cell receptors were difficult to isolate in the laboratory and were not identified until 1983. T-cell receptors consist of two polypeptide chains. The most common type of receptor is called alpha-beta because it is composed of two different chains, one called alpha and the other beta. A less common type is the gamma-delta receptor, which contains a different set of chains, one gamma and one delta. A typical T cell may have as many as 20,000 receptor molecules on its membrane surface, all of either the alpha-beta or gamma-delta type.

The T-cell receptor molecule is embedded in the membrane of the cell, and a portion of the molecule extends away from the cell surface into the area surrounding the cell. The chains each contain two folded domains, one constant and one variable, an arrangement similar to that of the chains of antibody molecules. And, as is true of antibody structure, the variable domains of the chains form an antigen-binding site. However, the T-cell receptor has only one antigen-binding site, unlike the basic antibody molecule, which has two.

Many similarities exist between the structures of antibodies and those of T-cell receptors. Therefore, it is not surprising that the organization of genes that encode the T-cell receptor chains is similar to that of immunoglobulin genes. Similarities also exist between the mechanisms B cells use to generate antibody diversity and those used by T cells to create T-cell diversity. These commonalities suggest that both systems evolved from a more primitive and simpler recognition system.

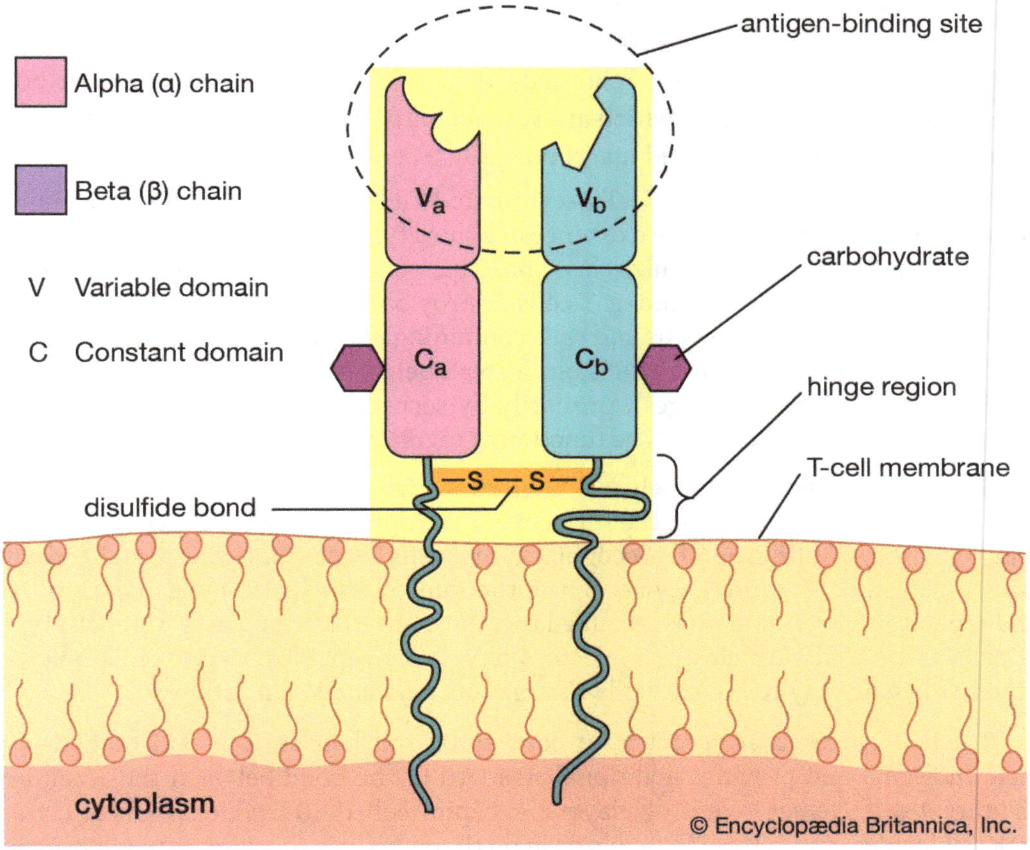

Fig. 1. T-cell antigen receptor

FUNCTION OF THE T-CELL RECEPTOR

Despite the structural similarities, the receptors on T cells function differently from those on B cells. The functional difference underlies the different roles played by B and T cells in the immune system. B cells secrete antibodies to antigens in blood and other body fluids, but T cells cannot bind to free-floating antigens. Instead they bind to fragments of foreign proteins that are displayed on the surface of body cells. Thus, once a virus succeeds in infecting a cell, it is removed from the reach of circulating antibodies only to become susceptible to the defense system of the T cell.

But how do fragments of a foreign substance come to be displayed on the surface of a body cell? First, the substance must enter the cell, which can happen through either phagocytosis or infection. Next, the invader is partially digested by the body cell, and one of its fragments is moved to the surface of the cell, where it becomes bound to a cell-surface protein. This cell-surface protein is the product of one of a group of molecules encoded by the genes of the major histocompatibility complex (MHC). In humans MHC proteins were first discovered on leukocytes (white blood cells) and therefore are often referred to as HLA (human leukocyte antigens). There are two major types of MHC molecules: class I molecules, which are present on the surfaces of virtually all cells of the body that contain nuclei—that is, most body cells—and class II molecules, which are restricted to the surfaces of most B cells and some T cells, macrophages, and macrophage-like cells.

Two main types of mature T cells—cytotoxic T cells and helper T cells—are known. Some scientists hypothesize the existence of a third type of mature T cell called regulatory T cells. Some T cells recognize class I MHC molecules on the surface of cells; others bind to class II molecules. Cytotoxic T cells destroy body cells that pose a threat to the individual—namely, cancer cells and cells containing harmful microorganisms. Helper T cells do not directly kill other cells but instead help activate other white blood cells (lymphocytes and macrophages), primarily by secreting a variety of cytokines that mediate changes in other cells. The function of regulatory T cells is poorly understood.

To carry out their roles, helper T cells recognize foreign antigens in association with class II MHC molecules on the surfaces of macrophages or B cells. Cytotoxic T cells and regulatory T cells generally recognize target cells bearing antigens associated with class I molecules. Because they recognize the same class of MHC molecule, cytotoxic and regulatory T cells are often grouped together; however, populations of both types of cells associated with class II molecules have been reported. Cytotoxic T cells can bind to virtually any cell in the body that has been invaded by a pathogen.

T cells have another receptor, or coreceptor, on their surface that binds to the MHC molecule and provides additional strength to the bond between the T cell and the target cell. Helper T cells display a coreceptor called CD4, which binds to class II MHC molecules, and cytotoxic T cells have on their surfaces the coreceptor CD8, which recognizes class I MHC molecules. These accessory receptors add strength to the bond between the T cell and the target cell.

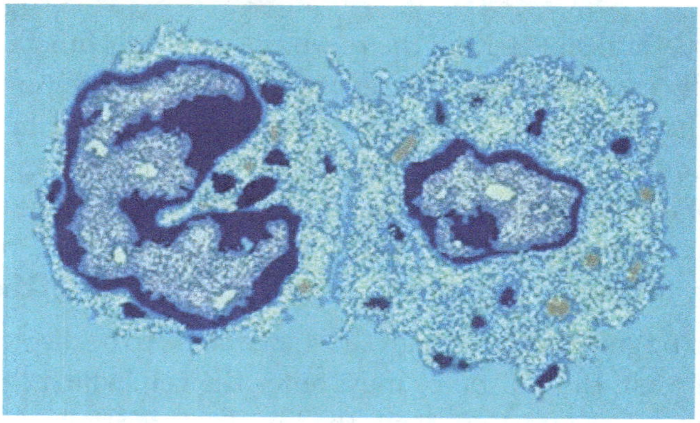

Fig. 2. Cytotoxic T cell

The T-cell receptor is associated with a group of molecules called the CD3 complex, or simply CD3, which is also necessary for T-cell activation. These molecules are agents that help transduce, or convert, the extracellular binding of the antigen and receptor into internal cellular signals; thus, they are called signal transducers. Similar signal transducing molecules are associated with B-cell receptors.

LIFE CYCLE OF T AND B LYMPHOCYTES

T cells

When T-cell precursors leave the bone marrow on their way to mature in the thymus, they do not yet express receptors for antigens and thus are indifferent to stimulation by them. Within the thymus the T cells multiply many times as they pass through a meshwork of thymus cells. In the course of multiplication they acquire antigen receptors and differentiate into helper or cytotoxic T cells. As mentioned in the previous section, these cell types, similar in appearance, can be distinguished by their function and by the presence of the special surface proteins, CD4 and CD8.

Most T cells that multiply in the thymus also die there. This seems wasteful until it is remembered that the random generation of different antigen receptors yields a large proportion of receptors that recognize self antigens—i.e., molecules present on the body's own constituents—and that mature lymphocytes with such receptors would attack the body's own tissues.

Most such self-reactive T cells die before they leave the thymus, so that those T cells that do emerge are the ones capable of recognizing foreign antigens. These travel via the blood to the lymphoid tissues, where, if suitably stimulated, they can again multiply and take part in immune reactions.

The generation of T cells in the thymus is an ongoing process in young animals. In humans large numbers of T cells are produced before birth, but production gradually slows down during adulthood and is much diminished in old age, by which time the thymus has become small and partly atrophied. Cell-mediated immunity persists throughout life, however, because some of the T cells that have emerged from the thymus continue to divide and function for a very long time.

B cells

B-cell precursors are continuously generated in the bone marrow throughout life, but, as with T-cell generation, the rate diminishes with age. Unless they are stimulated to mature, the majority of B cells also die, although those that have matured can survive for a long time in the lymphoid tissues. Consequently, there is a continuous supply of new B cells throughout life. Those with antigen receptors capable of recognizing self antigens tend to be eliminated, though less effectively than are self-reactive T cells. As a result, some self-reactive cells are always present in the B-cell population, along with the majority that recognize foreign antigens.

MICROBIAL ANTIGENS

Bacterial Antigens

Bacteria are single-celled prokaryotic organisms consisting of a cytoplasm containing the essential elements of cell structure surrounded by a lipid-rich cytoplasmic membrane. Outside the cytoplasmic membrane is a thick, carbohydrate-rich cell wall. The major components of the bacterial surface thus include the cell wall and its associated protein structures, the capsule, the pili, and the flagella. The cell wall of Gram-positive organisms is largely composed of peptidoglycan (chains of alternating *N*-acetyl glucosamine and *N*-acetyl muramic acid cross-linked by short peptide side chains) (see Fig. 3).

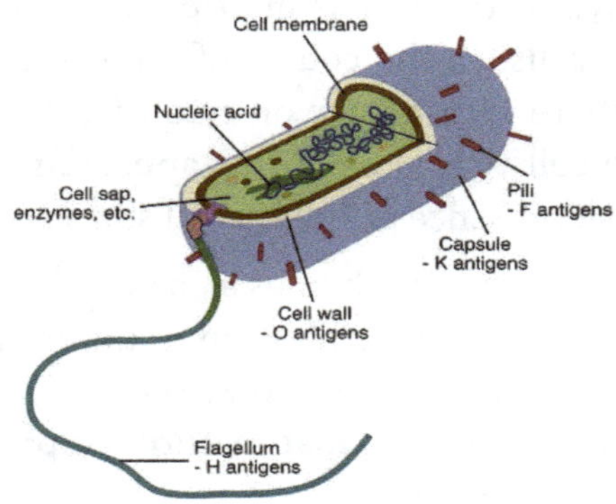

Fig. 3. The structure of a typical bacterium and the location of its most important antigens

Gram-positive cell walls also contain lipoteichoic acids that are involved in the transport of ions across the cell wall. The cell wall in Gram-negative organisms, in contrast, consists of a thin layer of peptidoglycan covered by an outer membrane consisting of a lipopolysaccharide. Most of the antigenicity of Gram-negative bacteria is associated with the lipopolysaccharide. This consists of an oligosaccharide attached to a lipid (lipid A) and to a series of repeating trisaccharides. The structure of these trisaccharides determines the antigenicity of the organism. Many bacteria are classified according to this antigenic structure. For example, the genus *Salmonella* contains a major species, *Salmonella enterica*, that is classified into more than 2300 serovars based on antigenicity. These polysaccharide antigens are called O antigens.

The outer cell wall lipopolysaccharides of Gram-negative bacteria bind to toll-like receptors (TLRs) and other pattern-recognition receptors and induce the production of inflammatory cytokines when an animal is infected. These cytokines cause a fever and sickness, so bacterial lipopolysaccharides are also called endotoxins.

Bacterial capsules consist mainly of polysaccharides that are usually good antigens. The capsules protect bacteria against phagocytosis and intracellular destruction, whereas anticapsular antibodies can overcome the effects of the capsule and protect an infected animal. Capsular antigens are collectively called K antigens.

Pili and fimbriae are short projections that cover the surfaces of some Gram-negative bacteria; they are classified as F or K antigens. Pili bind bacteria together and play a role in bacterial conjugation and movement. Fimbriae bind bacteria to cell surfaces. Antibodies to fimbrial proteins may be protective since they can prevent bacteria from sticking to body surfaces. Bacterial flagella are long filaments used for bacterial movement. They consist of a single protein called flagellin. Flagellar antigens are collectively called H antigens.

Other significant bacterial antigens include the porins, the heat-shock proteins, and the exotoxins. The porins are proteins that form pores on the surface of Gram-negative organisms. Heat-shock proteins are generated in large amounts in stressed bacteria. The exotoxins are toxic proteins secreted by bacteria or released into the surrounding environment when they die. Exotoxins are highly immunogenic proteins and stimulate the production of antibodies called antitoxins. Many exotoxins, when treated with a mild protein-denaturing agent such as formaldehyde, lose their toxicity but retain their antigenicity. Toxins modified in this way are called toxoids. Toxoids may be used as vaccines to prevent disease caused by toxigenic bacteria such as *Clostridium tetani*. Bacterial nucleic acids rich in unmethylated CpG sequences serve both as effective antigens for the adaptive immune system and as potent stimulators of innate immunity acting through TLRs.

Viral Antigens

Viruses are very small organisms that can grow only inside living cells. They are thus "obligate," intracellular parasites. Viruses usually have a relatively simple structure consisting of a nucleic acid core surrounded by a protein layer. This protein layer is termed the capsid, and it consists of multiple subunits called capsomeres. Capsid proteins are good antigens, highly capable of stimulating antibody formation. Some viruses may also be surrounded by an envelope containing lipoproteins and glycoproteins. A complete viral particle is called a virion. When a virus infects an animal, the virion proteins are processed and trigger adaptive immune responses

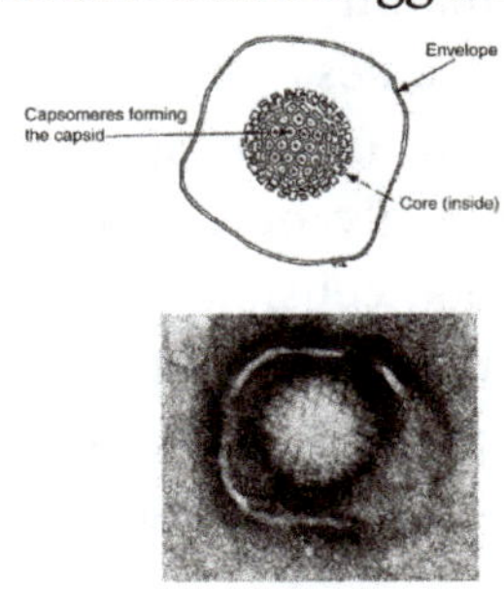

Fig. 4. The structure of a virus. This is an electron micrograph of equine herpesvirus type 4 magnified 184,000 times. The virus is negatively stained; that is, the electron-dense "dye" has filled the low areas on the virion, leaving the higher areas unstained.

Viruses, however, are not always found free in the circulation but live within cells, where they are protected from the unwelcome attentions of antibodies. Indeed, viral nucleic acid can be integrated into a cell's genome. In this situation, the viral genes code for new proteins, some of which are expressed on the surface of infected cells. These proteins, although they are synthesized inside an animal's own cells, can still bind to antigen receptors and provoke adaptive immunity. These newly synthesized foreign proteins are called endogenous antigens to distinguish them from the foreign antigens that enter from the outside and are called exogenous antigens.

OTHER MICROBIAL ANTIGENS

In addition to bacteria and viruses, animals may be invaded by fungi, protozoan parasites, arthropods, and even parasitic worms (helminths). Each of these organisms consists of many different structures composed of proteins, carbohydrates, lipids, and nucleic acids. Many of these can serve as antigens and trigger adaptive immunity. However, their antigenicity does vary, and the adaptive responses triggered by these organisms are not always successful in protecting an animal or eliminating the invader.

Nonmicrobial Antigens

Invading microorganisms are not the only source of foreign material entering the body. Food contains many foreign molecules that under some circumstances may trigger immune responses and cause an allergic reaction. Likewise, inhaled dusts can contain antigenic particles such as pollen grains, and these may enter the body through the respiratory system. Foreign molecules may be injected directly into the body through a snake or mosquito bite, or by a veterinarian. Furthermore, foreign proteins may be injected into animals for experimental purposes. Organ grafts are an effective way of administering a large amount of foreign material to an animal.

Cell Surface Antigens

The outer membrane of every mammalian cell consists of a fluid lipid bilayer with a complex mixture of protein molecules embedded in it. Most of these proteins can act as antigens if they are injected into another species or even into a different individual of the same species. For example, glycoproteins known as blood-group antigens are found on the surface of red blood cells. Early attempts to transfuse blood between unrelated individuals usually met with disaster because the transfused cells were rapidly destroyed. Investigation revealed that the problem was due to the presence of naturally occurring antibodies against these foreign red cell glycoprotein antigens.

Nucleated cells, such as leukocytes, possess hundreds of different protein molecules on their surface. These proteins are good antigens and readily provoke an immune response when injected experimentally into a different species. These surface molecules are classified by the CD system. Other cell surface proteins may provoke an immune response (such as graft rejection) if transferred into a genetically different individual of the same species. The cell surface proteins that trigger graft rejection are called histocompatibility antigens.

HOW ANTIGEN-BINDING RECEPTORS ARE MADE

One of the central problems encountered in understanding adaptive immunity is to explain how lymphocytes recognize the enormous diversity of microbes that may invade the body. Given that microorganisms change rapidly, the immune system must be able to respond not only to existing organisms but also, within reason, to newly evolved organisms.

The ability of the adaptive immune responses to respond specifically to an enormous number of foreign antigens implies the existence of an enormous number of different lymphocytes, each with its own specific antigen receptors. This then raises the question, How do lymphocytes generate such an enormous diversity of antigen-specific receptors?

The ability of a receptor to bind an antigen is determined by the shape of its binding site. This shape depends on the folding of its peptide chains, which is governed, in turn, by their amino acid sequences.

Each amino acid in a peptide chain exerts an influence on its neighboring amino acids, which determines their relative configuration. The shape of a peptide chain therefore represents the contributions of all amino acids in the chain as the peptide assumes its most energetically favorable conformation. The folding of a protein is determined by its amino acid sequence, and that sequence is determined by the sequence of bases in the DNA coding for that protein. The diversity of antigen receptors implies either a corresponding diversity in the genes coding for these receptors or a mechanism that generates diversity from a limited pool of receptor genes. This second mechanism is now known to be the method employed by the adaptive immune system.

Receptor-Antigen Binding

When an antigen and its receptor bind, they interact through the chemical groups on the surface of the antigen and on the complementarity determining regions (CDRs) of the receptor. In classic chemical reactions, molecules are assembled through the establishment of firm, covalent bonds. These bonds can be broken only by the input of a large amount of energy, energy that is not readily available in the body. In contrast, the formation of noncovalent bonds provides a rapid and reversible way of forming complexes and permits reuse of molecules in a way that covalent bonding would not allow. However, noncovalent bonds act over short intermolecular distances and, as a result, form only when two molecules approach each other very closely. The binding of an antigen to a BCR or TCR is exclusively noncovalent, so the strongest binding occurs when the shape of the antigen and the shape of the receptor conform to each other. This requirement for a close conformational fit has been likened to the specificity of a key for its lock.

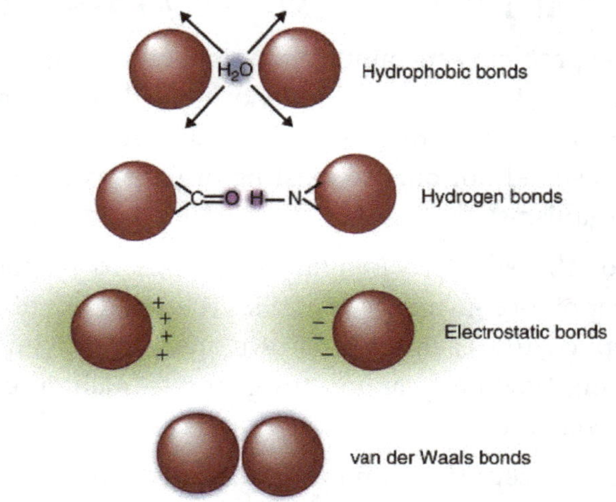

Fig. 5. Noncovalent bonds that link an antigen with its receptor arranged in order of relative importance. All these bonds are effective only over a very short distance. It is therefore essential that the shape of the antigen and its receptor site match very well if strong binding is to be achieved.

The major bonds formed between an antigen and its receptor are hydrophobic (Fig. 5). When antigen and antibody molecules come together, they exclude water molecules from the area of contact. This frees some water molecules from constraints imposed by the proteins and is therefore energetically stable. (The bond can be likened to two wet glass microscope slides stuck together. Anyone who has tried to separate two wet glass slides can confirm the effectiveness of this type of bonding.)

A second type of binding between an antigen and its receptor is through hydrogen bonds. When a hydrogen atom covalently bound to one electronegative atom (e.g., an–OH group) approaches another electronegative atom (e.g., an O=C—group), the hydrogen is shared between the two electronegative atoms. This situation is energetically favorable and is called a hydrogen bond. The major hydrogen bonds formed in antigen-receptor interaction are O–H–O, N–H–N, and O–H–N. Hydrogen bonds are already present between proteins and water molecules in aqueous solution, so the binding of an antigen to its receptor by hydrogen bonds requires relatively little net energy change.

Electrostatic bonds formed between oppositely charged amino acids may contribute to antigen-receptor binding, but the charge on many protein groups is commonly neutralized by electrolytes in solution. As a result, the importance of electrostatic bonding is unclear.

When two atoms approach very closely, a nonspecific attractive force, called a van der Waals force, becomes operative. It occurs as a result of a minor asymmetry in the charge of an atom because of the position of its electrons. This force, although very weak, may become collectively important when two large molecules come into contact. It can therefore contribute to antigen-receptor binding.

The binding of a receptor to its antigen is therefore mediated by multiple noncovalent bonds. Each bond is relatively weak in itself, but collectively the bonds may have a significant binding strength. All these bonds act only across short distances and weaken rapidly as that distance increases. Electrostatic bond and hydrogen bond strengths are inversely proportional to the square of the distance between the interacting molecules; the van der Waals forces and hydrophobic bonds are inversely proportional to the seventh power of that distance. Thus the strongest binding between an antigen and its receptors occurs when their shapes match perfectly and multiple noncovalent bonds form. Antigens can bind to receptors when they fit less than perfectly, although the strength of this binding will be much reduced.

ANTIGEN RECEPTOR GENES

The information needed to make all proteins, including antigen receptors, is stored in an animal's genome. All that is required for the production of these molecules is that the necessary genes be turned on.

Once the appropriate genes are activated, they can be transcribed into RNA and translated into the appropriate receptor protein on B or T cells. It has been estimated that mammals can produce up to 10^{15} different antigen receptors to be expressed on B and T cells.

Multiple genes code for each receptor peptide chain. Several genes code for each variable region, whereas only one codes for a constant region. As a result, the single constant-region gene can be combined with any one of several different variable-region genes to make a complete receptor chain (Fig. 6). Instead of having genes for all possible receptor chains, it is only necessary to have genes for all the variable regions and to join these to an appropriate constant-region gene as required. In addition, antigen receptor chains may be paired in different combinations to yield even greater diversity, a process called combinatorial association.

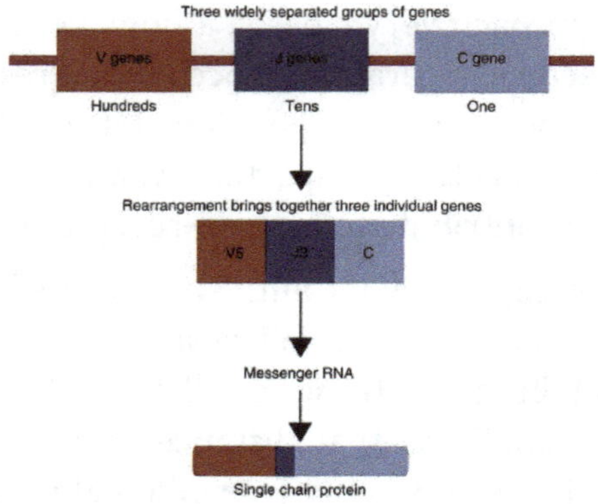

Fig. 6. Antigen receptor chains are coded for by three genes originating in three widely separated groups. The genes for a complete receptor chain are assembled by joining one gene selected from each group.

IMMUNOGLOBULIN/B CELL RECEPTOR DIVERSITY

To make as many different antibodies as possible, it is necessary to diversify the amino acid sequences of the variable domains in both light and heavy chains. Since these amino acid sequences are determined by the nucleotide sequences in the genes coding for these variable regions, mechanisms must exist for generating this nucleotide sequence diversity. In practice, gene diversity is generated through three distinct mechanisms: gene recombination, somatic mutation, and gene conversion.

All three mechanisms alter and diversify antibody gene sequences in such a way that an incredibly diverse array of antigen receptors is generated. The relative importance of each of these mechanisms differs among species, and the diversity-generating mechanisms that operate in humans and mice are not the same as those that operate in domestic mammals. The assembly of these diverse antigen receptors is carefully controlled during lymphocyte development by such factors as DNA methylation, chromatin structure, and location within the nucleus.

GENE RECOMBINATION

Gene recombination results from the random selection of one gene from each of several groups of genes followed by recombining these selected genes to generate sequence diversity. It is well seen in the genes that code for immunoglobulins.

Three gene loci code for immunoglobulin peptide chains, and each is found on a different chromosome (Fig. 7). One locus, called *IGK*, codes for ê light chains; one, called *IGL*, codes for ë light chains; and one, called *IGH*, codes for heavy chains.

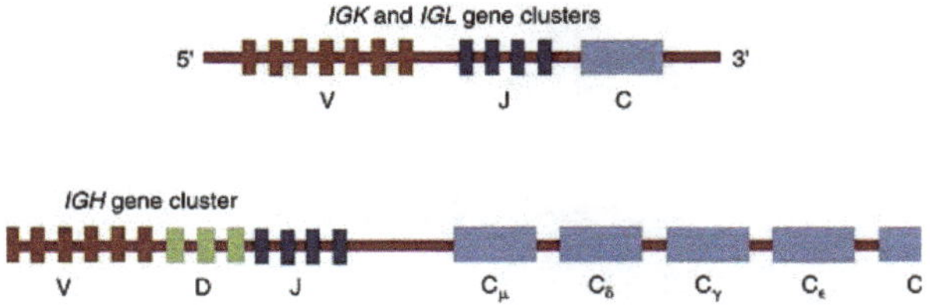

Fig. 7. Genes coding for immunoglobulin light chains and heavy chains. Note that there are two distinct light chain loci, one coding for kappa chains and one coding for lambda chains. These are located on different chromosomes. The precise number of V, D, and J genes varies among species.

GENERATION OF JUNCTIONAL DIVERSITY

Gene Rearrangement

The most obvious way to generate V-region diversity is to randomly select one V gene from the available pool and join it to one randomly selected J gene—a process called recombination. Since many different V and J genes are available, the number of possible combinations can be very large. For example, if there are 100 V genes and 10 J genes, then 100 × 10 = 1000 different V regions can be constructed.

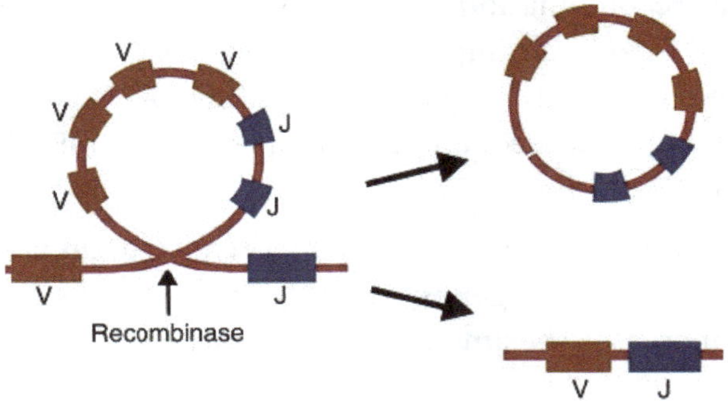

Fig. 8. One of the most important mechanisms of deleting unwanted genes is by looping out. In this case, unwanted V genes form a loop that is then cut off by a recombinase enzyme and the cut ends joined together. As a result, the desired V gene is linked directly to a J gene. The excised loop is destroyed.

Light chain assembly requires the combination of one V, one J, and one C gene. During B cell development, the intervening genes are looped out, excised, and discarded. The V and J genes have sites at each end that guide the cutting enzymes (Fig. 8). The looped-out genes are chopped off, and the free ends of the DNA are rejoined so that the V and J genes form a continuous sequence. Two sets of enzymes are used in this process. Recombinases cut the DNA at two points, thus excising unwanted genes. Following this, DNA repair enzymes join the two free ends to reform a continuous sequence. If these enzymes are defective, antibodies (and TCRs) cannot be made. In foals with severe combined immunodeficiency, for example, there is a defect in the DNA repair enzyme that joins the cut ends. As a result, these foals cannot make either TCRs or BCRs and thus have no functional B or T cells.

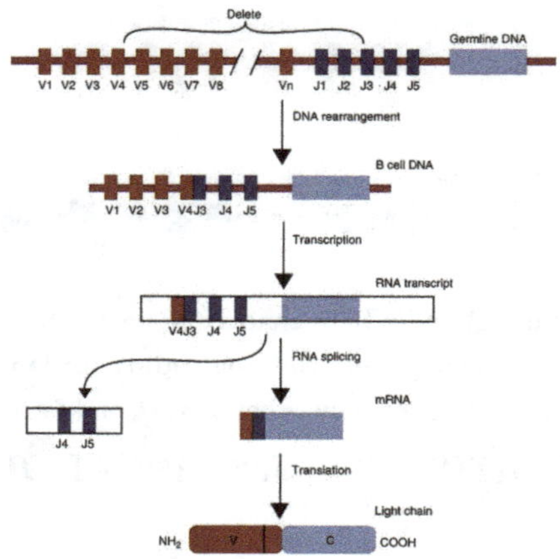

Fig. 9. Construction of an immunoglobulin light chain. Selected V and J genes are first joined as the intervening genes are deleted. The VJ and C genes remain separated until RNA splicing occurs. At that time the intervening RNA segments are deleted leaving the V, J, and C genes together in the mRNA. DNA rearrangement occurs during early B cell development so that each individual B cell is committed to making a single form of light chain for its antigen receptor.

Light chain gene recombination occurs in two stages. Randomly selected V and J genes are first joined to form a complete V-region gene. The joined V-J genes remain separated from the C gene until messenger RNA (mRNA) is generated. At that time the unwanted J genes are excised, and the complete V-J-C mRNA is then translated to form a light chain (Fig. 9).

When a heavy chain V region is assembled, its construction requires the splicing together of *IGHV*, *IGHD*, and *IGHJ* genes (Fig. 10). This use of three randomly selected genes enormously increases the amount of variability.

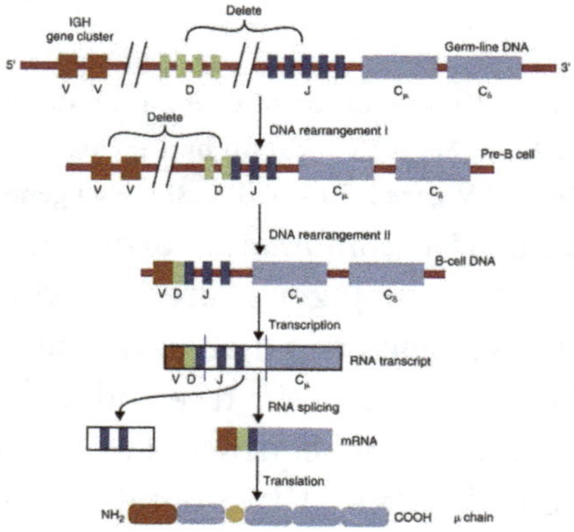

Fig. 10. Production of a complete immunoglobulin heavy chain gene. Two DNA rearrangement events are required to link V, D, and J genes together. The first event joins selected D and J genes; the second event adds a selected V gene.

For example, if a pool of 100 V, 10 J, and 10 D genes are recombined, then 100 × 10 × 10 = 10,000 different V regions can be constructed. The recombination of these genes also occurs in a specific order. Thus *IGHD* is first joined to *IGHJ*, then V genes are attached to make a complete V-region gene. After transcription, any unwanted J genes are deleted, the C gene mRNA is attached, and the completely assembled V-D-J-C mRNA is translated to form a heavy chain.

Base Deletion

Although random recombination of genes generates much V-region diversity, additional mechanisms increase this diversity still further. For example, endonucleases can remove nucleotides randomly from the cut ends of the genes. As a result, the precise nucleotide at which V and J genes join can vary, leading to changes in the nucleotide sequence at the splice site and variations in the amino acid sequence in the V region.

Base Insertion

In immunoglobulin heavy chain gene processing, additional nucleotides may be inserted at the V-D and D-J splice sites. Some of these nucleotides (N-nucleotides) are added randomly by an enzyme called terminal deoxynucleo-tidyltransferase (TdT). Up to 10 N-nucleotides may be inserted between V and D and between D and J.

Although the random selection of genes from two or three different pools generates a large number of different combinations, not all of these combinations will produce usable antibodies. Some combinations may result in a nucleotide sequence that cannot be translated into protein. These are called nonproductive rearrangements. For example, nucleotides are read as triplets called codons, each of which codes for a specific amino acid. If the codons are to be read correctly, then the sequence must be in the correct reading frame. If nucleotides are inserted or deleted so that the codon reading frame is changed, the resulting gene may code for a totally different amino acid sequence. If this frameshift results in inappropriate splicing, translation is prematurely terminated. It is probable that nonproductive rearrangements are produced in two of three attempts during B cell development. When this happens, the B cell has several additional opportunities to produce a functional antibody. For example, immature B cells initially rearrange one of the *IGK* genes (Fig. 11).

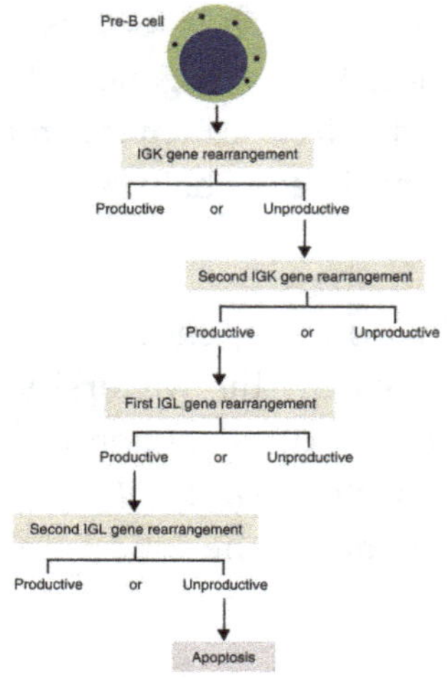

Fig. 11. During its development, each B cell has four attempts to make a productive gene rearrangement coding for a functional immunoglobulin. If it fails in all four attempts, the cell undergoes apoptosis.

If this fails to produce a functional light chain, they switch to the other *IGK* allele for a second attempt. If this does not work, the B cell will use one of the *IGL* alleles, and if this fails, the second *IGL* allele represents the last resort. If all these efforts fail to produce a functional light chain, the B cell cannot make a functional immunoglobulin. It will undergo apoptosis without participating in an immune response.

The sequence of events described previously has been worked out in mice and humans and may not apply to domestic mammals. One obvious difference lies in the use of κ and λ light chains. In mice, rabbits, pigs, and humans, ê chains are preferentially used (95% in mice, 90% in rabbits, 60% in pigs, 60% in humans). In the other domestic species, ë light chains predominate (98% in ruminants, 60% to 90% in horses). The reasons for these differences are unknown.

It should also be pointed out that immunoglobulin gene rearrangement is not entirely random. For example, in rabbits, mice, and humans the most 32 *IGHV* genes tend to be used most often. This preferential use of certain genes results from a combination of factors, including the recombination signal sequences, the accessibility of the genes to the recombinase enzyme, sequences at the splicing sites, and way in which DNA can fold.

THE IMPORTANCE OF ANTIGENS AND ANTIBODIES

The red cells of an individual contain antigens on their surfaces that correspond to their blood group and antibodies in the serum that identify and combine with the antigen sites on the surfaces of red cells of another type. The reaction between red cells and corresponding antibodies usually results in clumping—agglutination—of the red cells; therefore, antigens on the surfaces of these red cells are often referred to as agglutinogens.

Antibodies are part of the circulating plasma proteins known as immunoglobulins, which are classified by molecular size and weight and by several other biochemical properties. Most blood group antibodies are found either on immunoglobulin G (IgG) or immunoglobulin M (IgM) molecules, but occasionally the immunoglobulin A (IgA) class may exhibit blood group specificity. Naturally occurring antibodies are the result of immunization by substances in nature that have structures similar to human blood groups. These antibodies are present in an individual despite the fact that there has been no previous exposure to the corresponding red cell antigens—for example, anti-A in the plasma of people of blood group B and anti-B in the plasma of people of blood group A. Immune antibodies are evoked by exposure to the corresponding red cell antigen. Immunization (i.e., the production of antibodies in response to antigen) against blood group antigens in humans can occur as a result of pregnancy, blood transfusion, or deliberate immunization. The combination of pregnancy and transfusion is a particularly potent stimulus. Individual blood group antigens vary in their antigenic potential; for example, some of the antigens belonging to the Rh and ABO systems are strongly immunogenic (i.e., capable of inducing antibody formation), whereas the antigens of the Kidd and Duffy blood group systems are much weaker immunogens.

The blood group antigens are not restricted solely to red cells or even to hematopoietic tissues. The antigens of the ABO system are widely distributed throughout the tissues and have been unequivocally identified on platelets and white cells (both lymphocytes and polymorphonuclear leukocytes) and in skin, the epithelial (lining) cells of the gastrointestinal tract, the kidney, the urinary tract, and the lining of the blood vessels. Evidence for the presence of the antigens of other blood group systems on cells other than red cells is less well substantiated. Among the red cell antigens, only those of the ABO system are regarded as tissue antigens and therefore need to be considered in organ transplantation.

CHEMISTRY OF THE BLOOD GROUP SUBSTANCES

The exact chemical structure of some blood groups has been identified, as have the gene products (i.e., those molecules synthesized as a result of an inherited genetic code on a gene of a chromosome) that assist in synthesizing the antigens on the red cell surface that determine the blood type. Blood group antigens are present on glycolipid and glycoprotein molecules of the red cell membrane. The carbohydrate chains of the membrane glycolipids are oriented toward the external surface of the red cell membrane and carry antigens of the ABO, Hh, Ii, and P systems. Glycoproteins, which traverse the red cell membrane, have a polypeptide

The genes responsible for inheritance of ABH and Lewis antigens are glycosyltransferases (a group of enzymes that catalyze the addition of specific sugar residues to the core precursor substance). For example, the *H* gene codes for the production of a specific glycosyltransferase that adds L-fucose to a core precursor substance, resulting in the H antigen; the *Le* gene codes for the production of a specific glycosyltransferase that adds L-fucose to the same core precursor substance, but in a different place, forming the Lewis antigen; the *A* gene adds *N*-acetyl-D-galactosamine (H must be present), forming the A antigen; and the *B* gene adds D-galactose (H must be present), forming the B antigen.

The P system is analogous to the ABH and Lewis blood groups in the sense that the P antigens are built by the addition of sugars to precursor globoside and paragloboside glycolipids, and the genes responsible for these antigens must produce glycosyltransferase enzymes.

The genes that code for MNSs glycoproteins change two amino acids in the sequence of the glycoprotein to account for different antigen specificities. Additional analysis of red cell membrane glycoproteins has shown that in some cases the absence of blood group antigens is associated with an absence of minor membrane glycoproteins that are present normally in antigen-positive persons.

METHODS OF BLOOD GROUPING

Identification of blood groups

The basic technique in identification of the antigens and antibodies of blood groups is the agglutination test. Agglutination of red cells results from antibody cross-linkages established when different specific combining sites of one antibody react with antigen on two different red cells. By mixing red cells (antigen) and serum (antibody), either the type of antigen or the type of antibody can be determined depending on whether a cell of known antigen composition or a serum with known antibody specificity is used.

backbone to which carbohydrates are attached. An abundant glycoprotein, band 3, contains ABO, Hh, and Ii antigens. Another integral membrane glycoprotein, glycophorin A, contains large numbers of sialic acid molecules and MN blood group structures; another, glycophorin B, contains Ss and U antigens.

In its simplest form, a volume of serum containing antibody is added to a thin suspension (2–5 percent) of red cells suspended in physiological saline solution in a small tube with a narrow diameter. After incubation at the appropriate temperature, the red cells will have settled to the bottom of the tube. These sedimented red cells are examined macroscopically (with the naked eye) for agglutination, or they may be spread on a slide and viewed through a low-power microscope.

An antibody that agglutinates red cells when they are suspended in saline solution is called a complete antibody. With powerful complete antibodies, such as anti-A and anti-B, agglutination reactions visible to the naked eye take place when a drop of antibody is placed on a slide together with a drop containing red cells in suspension. After stirring, the slide is rocked, and agglutination is visible in a few minutes. It is always necessary in blood grouping to include a positive and a negative control for each test.

An antibody that does not clump red cells when they are suspended in saline solution is called incomplete. Such antibodies block the antigenic sites of the red cells so that subsequent addition of complete antibody of the same antigenic specificity does not result in agglutination. Incomplete antibodies will agglutinate red cells carrying the appropriate antigen, however, when the cells are suspended in media containing protein. Serum albumin from the blood of cattle is a substance that is frequently used for this purpose. Red cells may also be rendered specifically agglutinable by incomplete antibodies after treatment with such protease enzymes as trypsin, papain, ficin, or bromelain.

After such infections as pneumonia, red cells may become agglutinable by almost all normal sera because of exposure of a hidden antigenic site (T) as a result of the action of bacterial enzymes. When the patient recovers, the blood also returns to normal with respect to agglutination. It is unusual for the red cells to reflect antigenicity other than that determined by the individual's genetic makeup. The presence of an acquired B antigen on the red cells has been described occasionally in diseases of the colon, thus allowing the red cell to express an antigenicity other than that genetically determined. Other diseases may alter immunoglobulins; for example, some may induce the production of antibodies directed against the person's own blood groups (autoimmune hemolytic anemia) and thus may interfere with blood grouping. In other diseases a defect in antibody synthesis may cause the absence of anti-A and anti-B antibody.

DIFFERENCE BETWEEN ANTIBODY AND ANTIGEN

Antigen and antibodies are two very different entities. In a nutshell, an antibody is a glycoprotein which is produced in response to and counteract a particular antigen. On the other hand, an antigen is a foreign substance (usually harmful) that induces an immune response, thereby stimulating the production of antibodies.

Difference Between Antigen and Antibody

Antigen	Antibodies
Also called	
Also called Immunogens	Also called Immunoglobulins
Molecular Type	

Antigen	Antibodies
Antigens are usually lipids. However, they	All antibodies are proteins
can also be proteins, carbohydrates and nucleic acids	
Effect	
Antigens cause allergic reactions or even illnesses	Protects against the effects of the antigen either by lysis or immobilization of the particle
Specific Binding Site	
Epitopes are regions of the antigen where interacts with the antibodies	Paratopes are variable regions of an antibody that binds to an epitope.
Origins	
Antigens have origins outside the body	Antibodies always originate within the body

IMMUNOGLOBULIN INTERSECTION

Immunoglobulins, also known as antibodies, are glycoprotein molecules produced by plasma cells (white blood cells). They act as a critical part of the immune response by specifically recognizing and binding to particular antigens, such as bacteria or viruses, and aiding in their destruction. The antibody immune response is highly complex and exceedingly specific. The various immunoglobulin classes and subclasses (isotypes) differ in their biological features, structure, target specificity, and distribution. Hence, the assessment of the immunoglobulin isotype can provide useful insight into the complex humoral immune response. Assessment and knowledge of immunoglobulin structure and classes is also important for selection and preparation of antibodies as tools for immunoassays and other detection applications.

Soluble vs. membrane-bound immunoglobulins

Immunoglobulins occur in two main forms: soluble antibodies and membrane-bound antibodies (the latter contain a hydrophobic transmembrane region). Alternative splicing regulates the production of secreted antibodies and surface-bound B cell receptors in B cells.

Membrane-bound immunoglobulins are associated non-covalently with two accessory peptides, forming the B-cell antigen receptor complex. The first antigen receptors expressed by B cells are IgM and IgD. The receptor is a prototype of the antibody that the B cell is prepared to produce. The B cell receptor (BCR) can only bind antigens. It is the heterodimer of Ig alpha and Ig beta that enables the cell to transduce the signal and respond to the presence of antigens on the cell surface. The signal generated causes the growth and proliferation of the B cell and antibody production inside the plasma cell.

IMMUNOGLOBULIN CLASSES (ISOTYPES)

The various antibodies produced by plasma cells are classified by isotype, each of which differs in function and antigen responses primarily due to structure variability. Five major antibody classes have been identified in placental mammals: IgA, IgD, IgE, IgG, and IgM. This classification is based on differences in amino acid sequence in the constant region (Fc) of the antibody heavy chains. IgG and IgA are further grouped into subclasses (e.g., in human IgG1, IgG2, IgG3, IgG4, IgA1, and IgA2) based on additional small differences in the amino acid heavy chain sequences.

Based on differences in the amino acid sequence in the constant region of the light chain, immunoglobulins can be further sub-classified by determination of the type of light chain (kappa light chain or lambda light chain). A light chain has two successive domains: one constant domain and one variable domain. The ratio of these two light chains differs greatly among species, but the light chains are always either both kappa or both lambda, never one of each. Determination of individual subclasses is relevant in assessing primary immunodeficiencies or immune responses, especially if the total IgG or IgA concentration is not altered or elevated.

ISOTYPE CLASS SWITCHING

One of the primary functions of B cells in adaptive immunity is that of effecting a humoral response through the secretion of specific antibodies to address invading bodies and their toxic products. Some of these cells can undergo a "class switch" that causes expression of a new antibody isotype. For example, the antibody isotype could switch from an IgM to an antibody of all possible classes (e.g., IgG1, . . . IgG4, IgE). During this switch, the constant region of the heavy chain is changed, but not the variable region of the heavy chain. This switch does not affect the antibody's specificity for its antigen, but it does alter the effector functions that each class of antibody can execute. The antibody class switch is critically dependent on the type of cytokine that is present. Various cytokines, such as IL-4, IL-5, IFN-gamma, and TGF-beta, are known to be responsible for class switching. At a certain stage, the cell will lose its ability to undergo a switch to a class that has been generated before.

Why knowing the isotype matters

Immune responses can vary with each antigen presented to the immune system, so quantifying specific antibody levels helps to interpret the immune response after immunization or vaccination. Assessing human monoclonal antibody levels is also used widely as a diagnostic indicator to determine immunoglobulin-deficiency disorders, such as autoimmune diseases and gastrointestinal conditions that can be characterized by specific isotype deficiencies or varying concentrations of one or more isotypes. Disease states can range from the absence of one isotype class or subclass to a total deficiency of immunoglobulin classes.

The various isotypes also differ in their ability to bind to certain resins. Knowing the isotype is essential to assess the optimal purification techniques in order to gain maximum yield and purity of a desired antibody.

IMMUNOGLOBULIN MEASUREMENT

Measurement of individual immunoglobulins is performed for 2 reasons:

Detection of immunodeficiency

The most commonly used test is measurement of IgG in foals, llamas and calves for failure of transfer of passive immunity. There are many different immunodeficient states that have been reported in animals. Some are inherited,, e.g. severe combined immunodeficiency in Basset Hounds and Arabian or Arabian cross horses, whereas others are acquired, e.g. selective IgM deficiency in horses with lymphoma.

Determination of the nature of a paraprotein in monoclonal gammopathies

Monoclonal gammopathies are a group of disorders that are characterized by the clonal proliferation of B-lymphocytes. These cells secrete large amounts of a single immunoglobulin, which can result in clinical signs of excessive bleeding, renal failure and hyperviscosity. In dogs, monoclonal gammopathies occur typically with lymphoid neoplasia, especially multiple myeloma, chronic lymphocytic leukemia and lymphoma. In addition, monoclonal gammopathies can be idiopathic or occur secondary to canine Ehrlichiosis, Leishmania infection, or chronic pyoderma.

In most of these reactive plasma cell proliferations, the monoclonal immunoglobulin is IgG, whereas IgG, IgM or IgA can comprise the monoclonal protein in the neoplastic conditions. Therefore, quantification of the immunoglobulin class in a documented monoclonal gammopathy (by serum protein electrophoresis) may be helpful for the differential diagnosis of these conditions. In neoplastic conditions such as lymphoma and multiple myeloma, excessive amounts of a single immunoglobulin are produced. The type of immunoglobulin involved can be determined by quantifying the different immunoglobulins using radial immunodiffusion (Fig. 12). Therefore, RID should only be performed after a monoclonal gammopathy has been confirmed on serum protein electrophoresis.

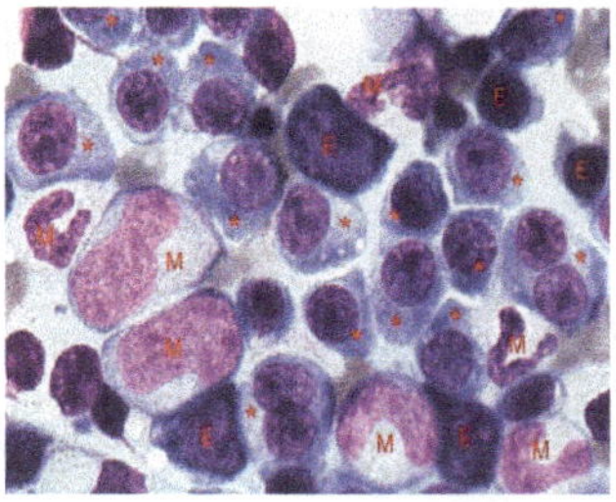

Fig. 12. Bone marrow cytology in a dog with multiple myeloma. There are large numbers of plasma cells (*) in the aspirate, some of which are binucleate. Hematopoietic cells (both myeloid [M] and erythroid [E]) are found in normal numbers and maturation sequence.

In the past, immunoelectrophoresis was used to detect the immunoglobulin class, however this test is qualitative, insensitive, and cumbersome. It has been replaced by immunoglobulin quantification by single radial immunodiffusion (RID), which we use here at Cornell University. In this technique, agarose gel is impregnated with antibody against the species-specific immunoglobulin. The patient's serum is placed in a well and diffuses through the gel. When a zone of antibody-antigen equivalence is reached, a precipitin ring forms. This takes up to 48 hours to occur. The width of the ring is compared to a standard curve run on the same gel and is converted into a immunoglobulin value in mg/dL. It must be noted that in monoclonal gammopathies, that the provided result for the monoclonal immunoglobulin is semi-quantitative. Because these proteins are abnormal, an exact quantification cannot be provided. In these situations, we use a combination of the RID result with the electrophoresis to give an indication of the amount of paraprotein.

It is important to know that there are different sources of these RID kits. The immunoglobulin results cannot be compared between kits, due to the use of different standards. Therefore, it is essential to use the same laboratory for immunoglobulin measurement and to interpret the results in relation to the laboratory's reference ranges. Comparing the immunoglobulin results of the same animal from different laboratories using different kits is invalid.

We currently offer immunoglobulin quantification in dogs, cats, horses, cattle and llamas (for the latter, IgG only). We have established our own reference intervals for dogs and cats, using RID kits from VMRD or Triple J Farms. These are valid for adult animals only (growing animals usually have lower immunoglobulins and if a young animal is being tested, several age-matched control animals should be submitted concurrently). Our reference intervals for other species are provided by the manufacturer and are age-dependent, therefore it is imperative to provide an age when submitting these samples.

CHAPTER

4 THE COMPLEMENT SYSTEM

INTRODUCTION

The complement system helps or "complements" the ability of antibodies and phagocytic cells to clear pathogens from an organism. It is part of the immune system called the " innate immune system " that is not adaptable and does not change over the course of an individual's lifetime. However, it can be recruited and brought into action by the adaptive immune system.

The complement system consists of a number of small proteins found in the blood, generally synthesized by the liver, and normally circulating as inactive precursors (pro-proteins). When stimulated by one of several triggers, proteases in the system cleave specific proteins to release cytokines and initiate an amplifying cascade of further cleavages.

The end result of this activation cascade is massive amplification of the response and activation of the cell-killing membrane attack complex. Over 25 proteins and protein fragments make up the complement system, including serum proteins, serosal proteins, and cell membrane receptors. They account for about 5% of the globulin fraction of blood serum.

Three biochemical pathways activate the complement system: the classical complement pathway, the alternative complement pathway, and the lectin pathway. The following are the basic functions of the complement: opsonization (enhancing phagocytosis of antigens); chemotaxis (attracting macrophages and neutrophils); cell lysis (rupturing membranes of foreign cells); and clumping (antigen-bearing agents).

The proteins and glycoproteins that constitute the complement system are synthesized by the liver hepatocytes. But significant amounts are also produced by tissue macrophages, blood monocytes, and epithelial cells of the genitourinal tract and gastrointestinal tract. The three pathways of activation all generate homologous variants of the protease C3-convertase. The classical complement pathway typically requires antigen, antibody complexes for activation (specific immune response), whereas the alternative and mannose-binding lectin pathways can be activated by C3 hydrolysis or antigens without the presence of antibodies (non-specific immune response). In all three pathways, C3-convertase cleaves and activates component C3, creating C_{3a} and C_{3b}, and causing a cascade of further cleavage and activation events. C_{3b} binds to the surface of pathogens, leading to greater internalization by phagocytic cells by opsonization. C5a is an important chemotactic protein, helping recruit inflammatory cells.

C_{3a} is the precursor of an important cytokine (adipokine) named ASP and is usually rapidly cleaved by carboxypeptidase B. Both C_{3a} and C5a have anaphylatoxin activity, directly triggering degranulation of mast cells, as well as increasing vascular permeability and smooth muscle contraction. C5b initiates the membrane attack pathway, which results in the membrane attack complex (MAC), consisting of C5b, C6, C7, C8, and polymeric C9.

MAC is the cytolytic endproduct of the complement cascade; it forms a transmembrane channel, which causes osmotic lysis of the target cell. Kupffer cells and other macrophage cell types help clear complement-coated pathogens. As part of the innate immune system, elements of the complement cascade can be found in species earlier than vertebrates, most recently in the protostome horseshoe crab species, putting the origins of the system back further than was previously thought.

In the classical pathway, C1 binds with its C_{1q} subunits to Fc fragments (made of CH2 region) of IgG or IgM, which forms a complex with antigens. C_{4b} and C_{3b} are also able to bind to antigen-associated IgG or IgM, to its Fc portion.

Such immunoglobulin-mediated binding of the complement may be interpreted, as that the complement uses the ability of the immunoglobulin to detect and bind to non-self antigens as its guiding stick. The complement itself is able to bind non-self pathogens after detecting their pathogen-associated molecular patterns (PAMPs); however, utilizing specificity of antibody, complements are able to detect non-self enemies much more specifically. There must be mechanisms that complements bind to Ig but would not focus its function to Ig but to the antigen.

The complement system bridges innate and acquired immunity by

- Augmenting antibody (Ab) responses and immunologic memory
- Lysing foreign cells
- Clearing immune complexes and apoptotic cells

Complement components have many biologic functions (e.g., stimulation of chemotaxis, triggering of mast cell degranulation independent of immunoglobulin E [IgE]).

COMPLEMENT ACTIVATION

There are three pathways of complement activation:

- Classical
- Lectin
- Alternative

Classical pathway components are labeled with a C and a number (eg, C1, C3), based on the order in which they were identified. Alternative pathway components are often lettered (e.g., factor B, factor D) or named (e.g., properdin).

Classical pathway activation is either

- Antibody-dependent, occurring when C1 interacts with antigen-IgM or aggregated antigen-IgG complexes
- Antibody-independent, occurring when polyanions (e.g., heparin, protamine, DNA and RNA from apoptotic cells), gram-negative bacteria, or bound C-reactive protein reacts directly with C1

This pathway is regulated by C1 inhibitor (C1-INH). Hereditary angioedema is due to a genetic deficiency of C1-INH.

Lectin pathway activation is antibody-independent; it occurs when mannose-binding lectin (MBL), a serum protein, binds to mannose, fucose, or *N*-acetylglucosamine groups on bacterial cell walls, yeast walls, or viruses. This pathway otherwise resembles the classical pathway structurally and functionally.

Alternate pathway activation occurs when components of microbial cell surfaces (eg, yeast walls, bacterial cell wall lipopolysaccharide [endotoxin]) or immunoglobulin (eg, nephritic factor, aggregated IgA) cleave small amounts of C3. This pathway is regulated by properdin, factor H, and decay-accelerating factor (CD55). The three activation pathways converge into a final common pathway when C3 convertase cleaves C3 into C_{3a} and C_{3b} (see figure Complement activation pathways). C3 cleavage may result in formation of the membrane attack complex (MAC), the cytotoxic component of the complement system. MAC causes lysis of foreign cells.

Factor I, with cofactors including membrane cofactor protein (CD46), inactivates C_{3b} and C_{4b}.

COMPLEMENT DEFICIENCIES AND DEFECTS

Deficiencies or defects in specific complement components have been linked to specific disorders; the following are examples:

- Deficiency in C1, C2, C3, MBL, MBL-associated serine protease 2 (MASP-2), factor H, factor I, or complement receptor 2 (CR2): Susceptibility to recurrent bacterial infections

- Deficiency of C5, C9, factor B, factor D, or properdin: Susceptibility to neisserial infections
- Defects in C1, C4, and C5: Systemic lupus erythematosus
- Defects in CR2: Common variable immunodeficiency
- Defects of CR3: Leukocyte adhesion deficiency type 1
- Mutations in the genes for factor B, factor H, factor I, membrane cofactor protein (CD46), or C3: Development of the atypical variant of hemolytic uremic syndrome

BIOLOGIC ACTIVITIES OF COMPLEMENT

Complement components have other immune functions that are mediated by complement receptors (CRs) on various cells. Several CRs use molecules that have been assigned a CD number.

- CR1 (CD35) promotes phagocytosis and helps clear immune complexes.
- CR2 (CD21) regulates antibody production by B cells and is the Epstein-Barr virus receptor.
- CR3 (CD11b/CD18), CR4 (CD11c/CD18), and C_{1q} receptors play a role in phagocytosis.
- C_{3a}, C5a, and C_{4a} (weakly) have anaphylatoxin activity: They cause mast cell degranulation, leading to increased vascular permeability and smooth muscle contraction.
- C_{3b} acts as an opsonin by coating microorganisms and thereby enhancing their phagocytosis.
- C3d enhances antibody production by B cells.
- C5a is a neutrophil chemoattractant; it regulates neutrophil and monocyte activities and may cause augmented adherence of cells, degranulation and release of intracellular enzymes from granulocytes, production of toxic oxygen metabolites, and initiation of other cellular metabolic events.

The mammalian immune system is a remarkable complex of biochemical processes enabling efficient detection and prosecution of pathogens that threaten host viability. The incredible complexity of mammalian immune systems is required to provide adequate defense in spite of the impressive number of pathogens and host processes that cause disease. Immune processes have traditionally been divided into two broad, but interconnected, subsystems on the basis of their functions in host defense. The adaptive immune system is organized around two classes of specialized lymphocytes, T and B cells, which display an extremely diverse repertoire of antigen-specific recognition receptors that enable specific identification and elimination of pathogens, as well as adaptive immune measures that ensure tailored immune responses, as well as long-lived immunological memory against reinfection.

In contrast, the innate arm of immunity is composed of those immunological effectors that provide robust, immediate, and nonspecific immune responses. These include evolutionarily primitive humoral, cellular, and mechanical processes that nevertheless play a vital role in the protection of the host from pathogenic challenge.

The complement system comprises a far-reaching and vital component of innate immunity and represents one of the major effector mechanisms of the innate immune system. Discovered in 1896 by Bordet as a heat-labile component of serum, it was so named for its ability to 'complement' the antibacterial properties of antibody in the heat-stabile fraction of serum.

It is now appreciated that complement is a complex network of plasma and membrane-associated serum proteins which can elicit highly efficient and tightly regulated inflammatory and cytolytic immune responses to infectious organisms (bacteria, viruses, parasites), tissue damaged by physical, chemical, or neoplastic insults, and other surfaces identified as 'nonself'.

For many years after its discovery, the role of complement in immunity was thought to be confined to innate immune responses with no impact on adaptive immune responses, in much the same way as innate immunity, in general, was relegated to those functions of immunity that involved prevention and confinement of infection while adaptive immunity provided effectors required to clear the infection.

The ability to separate the functions of the two arms of immunity was called into question as early as the 1970s, and since then the body of knowledge illustrating the interplay between the adaptive and innate wings of immunity has grown dramatically.

Similarly, the ability of complement to not only affect robust innate immune responses but also to interface with and influence T- and B-cell biology and adaptive responses has become increasingly appreciated. This review attempts to summarize the roles that complement biology plays in the immune response, both in the innate detection and elimination of pathogenic infections and in the modulation of adaptive immune responses.

COMPLEMENT ACTIVATION DURING NORMAL HOMEOSTASIS AND PATHOGEN INFECTION

The central component of the complement system is C3. The activation of each of the three pathways (CP, LP, and AP) results in cleavage of inactive C3 protein into the functional fragments C_{3a} and C_{3b}. C_{3a} is an inflammation mediator and C_{3b} is an opsonin, which can bind covalently and tag any surface in the immediate proximity to the site of its generation.

COMPLEMENT TICK-OVER IN THE ALTERNATIVE PATHWAY

In the plasma, during normal physiological conditions, the dominant active complement pathway is the AP. The AP monitors for pathogen invasion by maintaining a low level of constitutive activation by a process known as tick-over. Tick-over is the spontaneous hydrolysis of a labile thioester bond, which converts C_3 to a bioactive form $C_3(H_2O)$ in the fluid phase. The rate of hydrolysis of C_3 to $C_3(H_2O)$ can be accelerated by interactions between C_3 and a number of biological and artificial interfaces, including gas bubbles, biomaterial surfaces, and lipid surfaces and complexes.

Upon hydrolysis, the thioester domain (TED) of C_3 undergoes a dramatic structural change that exposes a binding site for another member of the AP called Factor B (FB). The $C_3(H_2O)$-bound FB is then cleaved by a serine protease (SP) Factor D (FD) allowing formation of a fluid phase C_3 convertase complex $C_3(H_2O)$Bb. $C_3(H_2O)$ Bb is able to interact and cleave native C_3 molecules to C_{3a} and C_{3b}. During normal physiological conditions, this C_3 convertase constantly generates small amounts of C_{3b}, which is able to bind covalently via its TED domain to any adjacent surface containing hydroxyl groups.

Nevertheless, not all hydroxyl groups attract equally C_{3b} (12). The -OH in the 6th position appears to be more reactive than the average -OH group in sugars. Therefore, the particular sugars composition of the pathogen surface will determine the efficacy of complement activation. C_{3b} will bind covalently to a surface that is located within about 60 nm from the convertase, due to the fact that the half-life of the thioester in C_{3b} is ~60 μs with a poor attachment efficiency of 10% (1_3). On host cells, bound C_{3b} molecules are rapidly inactivated by an army of membrane-expressed or fluid phase-recruited complement regulators. A tick-over mechanism for spontaneous activation of the CP has also been suggested, but the molecular interactions of this process are not well understood.

CLEARANCE OF APOPTOTIC CELLS

Apoptosis, programed cellular death, is a process of normal cellular homeostasis and in healthy individuals everyday billions of cells die by this mechanism. Complement activation occurs on apoptotic cells with low levels of C_{3b} deposition to facilitate their elimination without releasing danger signals, which could lead to further immune responses. This complement activation occurs by membrane alterations and by decreased expression of complement regulators on the membrane of apoptotic compared to resting cells. The silent clearance of the apoptotic cells is assured by the binding of the initiators of the CP (C_{1q}) and LP [Mannose-Binding Lectin (MBL) and ficolins]. These initiator proteins interact with receptors on phagocytic cells (immature dendritic cells or macrophages), which elicit immune tolerance and prevent immune responses toward self-antigens.

PATHOGEN ELIMINATION

On pathogens that lack specific regulators of complement, C_{3b} interacts with FB and FD to form a surface-bound C_3 convertase as part of the AP, which cleaves C_3 into C_{3a} and C_{3b}. Maximum complement activation is achieved during pathogen recognition leading to a pro-inflammatory milieu, contributing to generation of an adaptive immune response and rapid elimination of the pathogen. Complement-derived anaphylatoxins have potent inflammatory mechanisms including recruitment of phagocytes to the site of infection and activation of leukocytes, endothelial cells, or platelets. Upon activation, terminal complement components also have direct lytic capacity to kill pathogens.

The CP and LP have a critical role in pathogen recognition and initiation of the complement cascade. However, the AP assures more than 80% of the terminal complement activity during pathogen recognition (21). Additional AP C3 convertases are formed on the C_{3b} molecules generated either by CP activation or the AP C3 convertases. This chain reaction amplifies opsonization of the target and increases generation of anaphylatoxins. This amplification loop augments the effect of all pathways and is the heart of the complement cascade (22).

STRUCTURAL BASIS OF COMPLEMENT ACTIVATION AND REGULATION

Target Recognition and Initiation of Complement Pathways

The CP and LP have clearly identified recognition molecules, C_{1q}, MBL, and ficolins, which trigger each pathway only when and where it is necessary. The recognition event induces a structural change in the recognition molecule, which in turn induces the activation of enzymes able to cleave the subsequent molecules in the cascade and generate the central enzymatic complexes of complement, CP and AP C_3 convertases. The AP lacks a traditional target recognition molecule as an initiator. However, several molecules, such as properdin and P-selectin, can recruit $C_3(H_2O)$ and C_{3b} to the cell surface and serve as local initiators of the AP.

RECOGNITION MOLECULES OF THE CLASSICAL AND LECTIN COMPLEMENT PATHWAYS

Complement pathway and LP are triggered after interaction of a pattern-recognition molecule with the target structure. The recognition molecule of the CP, C_{1q}, has an extra-hepatic origin and is produced mainly by immature dendritic cells, monocytes, and macrophages. It has a complex, described as a "bouquet of flowers" topology, composed of 18 chains of three types (A, B, and C), forming six globular target recognition domains (gC_{1q}) attached to a collagen-like region (CLR). Each gC_{1q} domain carries a Ca^{2+} ion, which maintains domain stability and regulates the electrostatic field. C_{1q} recognizes mostly charged patterns and can bind to more than 100 different target molecules, including IgG and IgM containing immune complexes and surface-bound pentraxins [C-reactive protein (CRP), pentraxin 3 (PTX-3)]. Therefore, CP can be activated in either an immune complex-dependent and -independent manner. Mapping of the target molecule-binding sites on gC_{1q} by a site-directed mutagenesis, revealed that charged residues on the apex of the gC_{1q} heterotrimer (with participation of all three chains), as well as, the side of the B-chain are crucial for binding to IgG, IgM, CRP, and PTX-3. These binding sites are not identical, but partially overlapping. C_{1q} recognizes pathogen-associated molecular patterns including lipopolysaccharide (LPS) and bacterial porins.

The gC_{1q} domain also recognizes molecules, exposed on the surface of dying cells, including phosphatidylserine, double stranded DNA, glyceraldehyde-3-phosphate dehydrogenase (GAPDH) (38), annexins A2 and A5, and calreticulin. The most well-characterized target recognition molecule of the LP is the MBL, which recognizes carbohydrates. MBL has a similar overall structure to C_{1q}, but exists in multiple oligomeric forms (trimers, tetramers, and higher ordered oligomers). C_{1q} and MBL associate in a Ca-dependent manner with SP complexes, consisting of C_{1r} and C_{1s} for the CPand MBL-associated serine proteases (MASP) for the LP. In absence of Ca^{2+} ions (such as in plasma samples collected in EDTA), C_{1q} and MBL cannot interact with $C_{1r2}C_{1s2}$ and MASPs, respectively and CP and LP activation is prevented. In the presence of Ca^{2+} ions, after activation, SPs cleave subsequent complement components C_4 and C_2. The resulting complex C_{4b2a} is the C_3 convertase for CP and LP. This C_3 convertase has enzymatic activity and is able to cleave the central complement component C_3 to bioactive fragments C_{3a} and C_{3b}.

THE CLASSICAL PATHWAY

- Free immunoglobulin molecules can not bind or activate complement components.
- When immunoglobulin binds to the antigen, the complement-binding site is exposed (because of conformational changes).
- In classical pathway, first complement component C_1 binds to CH_3 domain of IgM or CH_2 domain of IgG molecule. The C1 molecule is composed of three separate proteins C_{1q}, C_{1r} and C_{1s} bound together by calcium (Ca^{++}) dependent bonds.
- The C_{1q} subunit is made up of an umbrella like radial array of six chains that are connected to central stalk by a collagen like arm and each has globular

head, which recognizes and binds to Fc region of immunoglobulin heavy chain.

- Each F_c region of an immunoglobulin has one C_{1q} binding site and for activation of C_{1q} at least two heavy chain (F_c region) must bind.
- Since IgG has one Fc region, at least two molecule of IgG must be brought close together before C_{1q} can bind and this is possible when they bind to a multivalent antigen.
- IgM being a pentamer, one single molecule can activate C1.Thus IgM is more efficient complement fixing antibody than IgG.
- C_{1r} and C_{1s} are serine esterases and they form a tetramer complex containing two molecule of each and located between C_{1q} strands. Binding of C_{1q} to two or more Fc regions leads to enzymatic activation of C_{1r} that cleaves and activates C_{1s}.
- The activation is normally prevented by a protein C_1 inhibitor (C_1 - INH), it also removes C_{1r} and C_{1s} from the complex but this inhibition is overcome when immunoglobulin is bound to antigen.
- Activated C_{1s} cleaves the next protein in the cascade, C_4 to generate C_{4b} (the small fragment C_{4a} leaves the major fragment C_{4b} and the removal of C_{4a} activates and expose a thioester bond on the C_{4b} molecule that generates a reactive carbonyl (=C=0) group and binds C_{4b} to target cell surface (i.e. antigen).
- The C_2 glycoprotein binds C_{4b} to form C_{4b2} in presence of Mg^{++} ions. Activated C_{1s} splits bound C_2 into C_{2a} (larger fragment) and C2b (smaller, soluble fragment). The C_2 must be bound to C4 before it is cleaved and this is called substrate modulation. The C_{4b2a} complex is the classical pathway C_3 convertase. The C_{4b2a} protease breaks down C3 into C_{3a} and C_{3b}. The small fragment C_{3a} is removed and C_{3b} form covalent bonds with target cell surface or with the antibody where complement activation was initiated. Once C_{3b} is deposited, it can bind to factor B and generate more C_3 convertase by the alternative pathway. Thus a single molecule of C_{4b2a} complex can lead to the deposition of hundred or thousands of molecules of C_{3b} on the cell surface where complement is activated. C_{4b2a3b} complex function as the classical pathway C_5 convertase and cleaves C_5 and initiate the terminal steps of complement of activation.
- The classical pathway was first identified and characterized.

THE ALTERNATIVE (INDIRECT) COMPLEMENT PATHWAY

- In alternative pathway C_3 is activated and form a stable attachment of C_{3b} to microbial cell surface without the involvement of antibody.

- Normally C_3 in plasma breaks down spontaneously into C_{3a} and C_{3b}. The newly formed C_{3b} binds covalently through thioester bonds to the surface of cells including microbes.
- Under normal condition cell bound C_{3b} binds to H factor.
- H factor binds with sialic acid or other neutral and anionic polysaccharides present in cell surfaces.
- Binding of H factor activate I factor (protease) and C_{3b} is destroyed thus complement activation stops.
- Since mammalian cell surface glycoproteins are heavily sialylated, it does not trigger the alternative complement pathway.
- Bacterial cell walls, bacterial lipopolysaccharides, viruses, aggregated immunoglobulin (IgA), cobra venom etc. permit activation of C_{3b}. Thus activation can occur by both immunologically and non immunologically.
- The bound C_{3b} binds to a plasma protein called B factor and once bound, factor B is cleaved by a plasma serine protease (called factor D) to generate a bound fragment called B_b (also a soluble fragment B_a).
- Factor D acts only on B factor after it is bound to C_{3b} (another example of substrate modulation).
- The complex C_{3b}Bb is the alternative pathway C3 convertase and cleaves C3 to C_{3b} and C_{3a}. C_{3a} is released and C_{3b} remain attached to cells. Half-life of C_{3b} is only 5 minutes.
- Another protein called properdin (factor P) binds to the complex to form C_{3b} BbP and increase the half-life to 30 minutes. Microbial cells favour the attachment of Properdin.
- C_{3b} may also be generated by other protease from activated phagocytic cells and there is generation of C_{3b} at the site of inflammation.
- Some C_{3b} molecules generated by alternative pathway bind to C_3 convertase itself and form $C_{3b}Bb_{3b}$, which function as the alternative pathway C5 convertase and cleave C_5 to initiate the terminal steps of complement activation.
- The Lectin Pathway/Mannose - Binding Pathway
- When macrophages ingest bacteria or other foreign materials, they are stimulated to secrete IL-1, IL-6 and TNF-a.
- These three cytokines act on hepatocytes and stimulate them to secrete acute phase proteins, one such protein is Lectin (mannose binding protein).
- Mannose is a major component of bacterial cell wall glycoproteins.

- The mannose binding protein (MBP or MBL) binds to bacteria in blood stream and acts as opsonin.
- MBP is structurally similar to C_{1q}, and activate classical pathway of complement by activating C_{1r}-C_{1s} complex or MBP associated serine esterase.
- In cattle, buffalo and other bovidae, there are at least three other mannose-binding proteins and one such is conglutinin.
- Conglutinin can bind to cell bound C_{3b} (C_{3b} has mannose rich oligosaccharide side chains) and clump or conglutinate C_{3b} coated particles.

TERMINAL PATHWAY OF COMPLEMENT ACTIVATION

- Once C5 binds to C_{3b}, C5convertase generated by classical pathway (C_{4b2a}), alternative pathway (C_{3b}Bb) or mannose binding pathway cleaves C5 to small peptide C5a (released) and C5b, which attach to C_{3b}.
- This cleavage exposed a site on C5b and binds C6 and C7 to form C5b67.
- The C5b67 can detach itself from C_{3b} and insert into the lipid bilayer of nearby cell or microbial membrane.
- Once it is inserted into lipid bilayer, it binds to one C8 molecule and multiple C9 molecules (about 12 to 18) to form a complex [C5b678 (9) n] of tubular tranmembrane pore called the membrane attack complex (MAC).
- The MAC form a large doughnut shaped structure that inserts itself into a cell membrane and forms a tranmembrane channel and cause osmotic lysis of the target cell.

TERMINAL PATHWAY

The formation of C5 convertase is the first step of the terminal pathway. This convertase is either formed by components of the classical/lectin pathway (C_{4b2a3b}) or the alternative pathway (C_{3b}2BbP) that cleaves C_5 to C_{5a} and C_{5b}.

When the C_{5a} is released it acts as a potent anaphylatoxin. C_{5b} is the first component of the self-assembly of Membrane Attack Complex (MAC) or its soluble counterpart soluble Terminal Complement Complex (sTCC).

Although self-assembly, the process is highly regulated and performed in a highly regular order.

MAC is a supramolecular construction composed of C_{5b}, C_6, C_7, C_8 and several molecules of C_9. In the first step C_{5b} in complex with C6 bind C7 which change the structure of C_7 allowing for the whole complex to be inserted in the target membrane and serve as a receptor for C_8.

The whole complex can then bind several molecules of C_9 (n=1-18) resulting in the trans-membrane MAC lesion.

Post-traumatic inflammation and secondary tissue damage after SCI is characterized by, among other things, complement activation, expression of inflammatory cytokines and chemokines, the up-regulation of adhesion molecules, and the infiltration of neutrophils and macrophages. Complement activation products play known roles in promoting the expression of these inflammatory molecules and the recruitment and activation of leukocytes. A key role for complement in SCI has been shown by the demonstration that deficiency of C_3 or inhibition of C_3 activation, the point of convergence for all three complement activation pathways, protects against inflammation and injury. The classical, alternative, and terminal complement pathways are activated in rodent SCI, as demonstrated by the deposition of C_{1q} and C_4 (classical), f_B (alternative) and C_9 (terminal) on neurons, oligodendrocytes, and injured axons.

However, C_{1q} deficiency improves histological and functional locomotor outcome after SCI, indicating that the classical pathway play a key role in tissue damage. There is strong evidence that activation of the classical pathway is mediated by antibodies that are produced after SCI. After contusion injury, there is an accumulation of intraspinal antibody-secreting B cells, and antibody and C_{1q} colocalize at the site of injury and demyelination, while B cell deficiency confers neuroprotection and there is only minimal C_{1q} deposition in the spinal cords of B cell-deficient mice.

Further linking antibody-mediated complement activation to SCI pathology, it has been shown that the injection of isolated SCI antibodies into intact spinal cords causes complete transient paralysis in wt mice, while C_3 deficient mice exhibit significantly reduced hind limb deficits and pathology.

In the present study, we show that fB-deficient mice have an improved outcome after SCI. The level of protection afforded to fB-deficient mice was similar to that seen in our previous study using C_3-deficient mice. These data indicate a dependence on the alternative pathway for complement-mediated SCI. Together with the previous findings described above using B cell and C_{1q}-deficient mice, it is likely that the alternative pathway plays a critical role in amplifying antibody-mediated classical pathway initiated complement activation. In this context, reduced pathology and improved locomotor recovery in f_B-deficient mice was associated with significantly reduced C3 and MAC deposition compared to wt control mice, even though the classical (and lectin) pathway is intact in fB-deficient mice. A similar dependence on both antibody-mediated lectin pathway activation and alternative pathway activation has been described in models of intestine ischemia and reperfusion injury.

In a more clinically relevant paradigm, we demonstrated that specific inhibition of the alternative pathway with anti-f_B mAb was also protective against SCI, and to a similar level as fB deficiency. Selective inhibition of the alternative pathway while leaving the classical and lectin pathways intact has potential benefits over inhibiting all pathways at the C_3 activation step. Complement is an important component of host defense, and the classical and lectin pathways provide important contributions to defense against some pathogens. Thus, compared with C3 inhibition, alternative pathway inhibition would be less generally immuno-suppressive and may have less potential for increasing the incidence of sepsis or infection. Complement is also implicated in neuroprotective and regenerative mechanisms. Activated microglia and macrophages have been shown to be important for neuron protection and axon growth in animal models, and complement activation products, in particular C5a, can recruit and activate these cells. A recent study demonstrated that the treatment of rats 14 days post-SCI with a C5a receptor antagonist reduced locomotor recovery and myelination. Complement also participates in phagocytic clearance of apoptotic cells and cellular debris via their opsonization with C_{1q} and C_3 activation products, and interfering with this clearance pathway can impair axon growth. Thus, compared with total complement blockade, allowing activation of the classical (or lectin) pathway while inhibiting alternative pathway amplification could feasibly improve the balance between the neurodegenerative and neuroprotective effects of complement inhibition.

The exacerbated injury and impaired recovery of locomotor function in CD59a-deficient mice, together with increased deposits of the MAC (C_9) in these mice compared to wt control treated mice, indicate an important contribution of the terminal pathway and the MAC to secondary neuronal injury after trauma. Furthermore, significant functional deficit persisted in CD59-deficient mice at 21 days after injury compared with controls. It is possible that neoepitope expression and cell lysis resulting from enhanced MAC formation in CD59-deficient mice could result in enhanced complement activation. However, while there were significantly increased deposits of C9 in CD59-deficient mice at both 24 and 72 hours post-SCI compared with wt treated control mice, CD59 deficiency had little effect on C3 or fB deposition. Previous studies using CD59a-deficient mice have similarly implicated the MAC in spinal cord demyelination and axonal injury in murine acute experimental allergic encephalomyelitis, as well as in axonal damage during Wallerian degeneration (peripheral nerve injury).

The alternative and terminal complement pathways have also been implicated in causing neuropathology in a different model of traumatic neuroinflammation, traumatic brain injury. In these previous studies, CD59a deficiency impaired neurological outcome and increased neuronal cell death and brain tissue destruction compared to wt mice, whereas fB deficiency was protective.

The anti-f_B mAb used in the current study has also previously been shown to be protective in a model of traumatic brain injury. Administration of anti-fB mAb at 1 and 24 hours after traumatic brain injury resulted in significantly reduced neuronal cell death and tissue injury compared to controls for up to 7 days after injury (most distal time point analyzed). Of note, it was shown in this previous study that anti-fB mAb significantly reduced serum alternative pathway activity 24 hours after injury, but that alternative pathway activity returned to normal by 7 days, even with repeated mAb injection.

In agreement with this previous data, we also found that anti-fB mAb significantly reduced serum alternative pathway activity 24 hours after administration. Together with our data showing that anti-fB mAb administered 12 or more hours after SCI is not protective, these data together indicate that short term inhibition of the alternative pathway early after SCI is key to reducing injury and improving functional recovery and that continued complement inhibition is unlikely to have any further beneficial effect.

Neutrophils and macrophages are recruited to the spinal cord after SCI, and their infiltration and activation is strongly linked with neuronal and glial cell death. We previously demonstrated that C_3 deficiency reduced neutrophil numbers in the spinal cord at 24 and 72 hours postinjury. C_{1q} deficiency, however, did not effect neutrophil infiltration after SCI (at either 24 or 72 hours). In the current study, we show that compared with control-treated mice, there are significantly reduced neutrophil numbers in fB-deficient and fB-inhibited mice at both time points post-SCI.

We similarly showed reduced macrophage/microglia numbers in fB-deficient or fB-inhibited mice compared with controls at 72 hours postinjury, whereas it was previously shown that C_{1q} deficiency was (interestingly) associated with increased macrophage infiltration. Together, these data indicate a key role for the alternative pathway in neutrophil and macrophage infiltration after SCI. It is interesting that unlike fB deficiency, CD59 deficiency did not significantly effect the number of macrophages at 72 hours postinjury.

Neutrophils, on the other hand, were present in significantly higher numbers in CD59-deficient mice compared to wt treated controls at 72 hours after injury. The MAC can influence cellular infiltration when deposited in sublethal quantities in cell membranes by inducing the expression of adhesion molecules, cytokines, and chemokines, including IL-8. Why there is an apparent difference in CD59-deficient mice on neutrophil and macrophage infiltration at 72 hours postinjury (compared to controls) is not clear, but a consequence could be the protraction of neutrophil mediated inflammatory events and a reduction in macrophage-mediated protective events.

In addition to showing that the complement inhibitor CD59 plays an important role in providing protection against SCI, the data have potential clinical implications. As discussed above, for reasons relating to the protective roles of complement that are relevant for SCI patients, there are potential benefits of selectively inhibiting the alternative pathway of complement to reduce secondary damage and improve functional recovery after SCI. However, the MAC plays a very limited known role in host defense and immune homeostatic/repair mechanisms, and because our data indicate that the MAC is a significant contributor to pathology in SCI, selective inhibition of the terminal pathway could potentially have even greater benefit over blocking complement at an early step in any pathway.

BIOLOGICAL EFFECTS OF COMPLEMENT ACTIVATION

Cell lysis

The most important purpose of complement activation is to lyse the microbes that have entered into the host.

Complement activation leads to the lysis of bacterial, viral, fungal, protozoal, and many other cells through the membrane attack complexes.

However, cells such as cancer cells are more resistant to complement mediated lysis. Furthermore, many nucleated cells can endocytose the MACs into the cell so that the MACs don't form the pores. Some nucleated cells can also repair the damage caused by the MACs.

This explains the inability of monoclonal antibodies to lyse some cancer cells:

Inflammation

During complement activation, some of the complement components are split into complement fragments. In general, the larger fragments continue the complement cascade, while the smaller fragments play important roles in inflammation.

Complement fragments act as anaphylatoxins:

C_{3a}, C_{4a}, and C5a fragments formed during complement activation are generally called anaphylatoxins. (Anaphylatoxins are complement fragments, which cause mast cell degranulation and smooth muscle contraction.) These fragments bind to their respective receptors (C_{3a}, C_{4a}, or C_{5a} receptors) on mast cells in the inflammatory site and basophils in blood.

↓

Consequently, mast cells and basophils release histamine and other inflammatory mediators.

↓

The inflammmatory mediators induce smooth muscle contraction and increase the vascular permeability. Increase in vascular permeability results in an influx of fluid and leukocytes from blood vessels into the site of inflammation.

↓

C5a is the most important anaphylatoxin. C5a binds to C5a receptors on mast cells and induce the mast cells to release histamine and other inflammatory mediators. C5a also binds to C5a receptors on neutrophils and monocytes and attract them to the inflammatory site. Thus C5a also acts as a chemotactic factor for neutrophils and monocytes. C5a also induces neutrophil adhesion, which results in neutrophil aggregation. C5a can also stimulate neutrophil oxidative mechanism leading to the production of toxic oxygen species, which act against microbes.

Complement fragments act as opsonins:

In Greek, the word 'opsonin' means 'to make tastier'.) Opsonization is a process by which phagocytosis is facilitated by antibody and C_{3b} bound to the surface of the microbes. C_{3b}, C_{4b}, and iC_{3b} complement fragments have opsonizing actions. C_{3b} is an important opsonin.

These fragments formed during complement activation coat the target cell surfaces (such as microbial surfaces) or the antigen- antibody complexes (immime complexes). Phagocytic cells such as neutrophils and macrophages have receptors for C_{3b}, C_{4b}, and iC_{3b}. Binding of phagocytic cells through these receptors result in the bridging of microbes to the phagocytic cells. Consequently, the phagocytic cells engulf the microbes and destroy them.

REMOVAL OF CIRCULATING IMMUNE COMPLEXES BY COMPLEMENT

The binding of antibodies to antigens results in the formation of antigen-antibody complexes or immune complexes. In certain autoimmune diseases and certain microbial infections large amounts of immune complexes are formed. The immune complexes that circulate in blood are called circulating immune complexes. The presence of large amounts of immune complexes in circulation is harmful to the host because the immune complexes may deposit in tissues and initiate inflammatory reactions at the deposited site, leading to immune complex mediated host tissue damage.

Activation of complement system helps in the removal of circulating immune complexes by the following mechanisms:

Binding of antibody to antigen (and the consequent formation of antigen-antibody complexes) led to the activation of classic pathway of complement system. C_{3b} formed during complement activation coats the immune complexes.

↓

Erythrocytes and platelets have C_{3b} receptors on their surface. The C_{3b} coated immune complexes bind to the erythrocytes and platelets through the C_{3b} receptors.

↓

The erythrocytes and platelets carry the immune complexes to the spleen and liver. The macrophages in liver and spleen strip the immune complexes on the surface of erythrocytes and platelets and phagocytose the immune complexes, resulting in the removal of immune complexes from the circulation.

COMPLEMENT IN INDUCTION OF SECONDARY B CELL IMMUNE RESPONSES

Germinal centers of lymphoid tissues (such as lymph nodes) are packed with B cells, T cells and follicular dendritic cells. Follicular dendritic cells have receptors for complement fragments (and Fc region of antibody). Follicular dendritic cells bind to complement fragments coating the immune complexes through their complement receptors. (The dendritic cells capture the antigen-antibody complexes through their F_c receptors also.)

The captured antigen- antibody complexes are displayed on the surface of dendritic cells for extended periods (even many months). Specific surface immunoglobulin (sig) receptors (on memory B cells) for the antigen in the antigen-antibody complex bind to the antigen in the antigen-antibody complex. The memory B cell is activated and divides to produce plasma cells. The plasma cells produce large amounts of antibodies specific to the antigen in the immune complex. Thus the complement fragments play an important role in the development of secondary B cell immune responses against antigens.

Biological Effects of Complement

The main role of complement is to amplify the humoral immune response. The complement through its various prod-ucts participates in the inflammatory response, opsonization of antigen, viral neutralization, and clearance of immune complexes as follows:

Chemotaxis

- C5a is a chemotactic molecule specifically recognized by polymorphonuclear leukocytes or phagocytic cells. This substance causes leukocytes to migrate to a tissue in which an antigen-antibody reaction is taking place. At that site, a phagocytic cell recognizes opsonized particles and ingests them.
- C5a not only has a chemotactic effect on neutrophils, but also activates these cells causing their reversible aggregation and release of stored enzymes, including proteases.
- C5a also enhances the adhesiveness of neutrophils to the endothelium.

Opsonization

Complement plays an important role in opsonization of pathogenic bacteria and viruses. Bacteria and viruses are easily phagocytosed by phagocytic cells in the presence of complement component C_{3b}. This is because the receptors for the C_{3b} component are present on the surface of many phagocytes.

HYPERSENSITIVITY REACTIONS

Complement participates in type II (cytotoxic) and type III (immune-complex) hypersensitivity reactions. The C_{3a}, C_{4a}, and C5a components stimulate degranulation of mast cells with release of mediators, such as histamine. The C_{3a} frag-ments bind to receptors on basophils and mast cells and induce the release of stored vasoactive amines (e.g., histamine) and heparin. The release of histamine into the tissues results in increased capillary permeability and smooth muscle contrac-tion. Fluid is released into the tissue, thereby causing edema and swelling.

There is some evidence that C_{3a} and C5a may also act directly on endothelial cells, causing increased vascular perme-ability. The end result is very similar to the classical anaphy-lactic reaction that takes place when IgE antibodies bound to the membranes of mast cells and basophils react with the cor-responding antigens. For this reason, C_{3a} and C5a are called as anaphylatoxins.

Cytolysis

Complement mediates cytolysis. Insertion of C5b-9 com-plex (MAC) into the cell membrane leads to killing or lysis of erythrocytes, bacteria, and tumor cells. The insertion of the MAC complex results in disruption of the mem-brane, thereby leading to entry of water and electrolytes into the cell.

ENHANCEMENT OF ANTIBODY PRODUCTION

The binding of C_{3b} to the surface receptors on the activated B cells markedly enhances the production of antibodies in comparison to that of B cells activated by antigen alone. Hence, deficiency of C_{3b} leads to reduced production of antibodies. Therefore, low concentration of both C_{3b} and antibodies affects host defense, resulting in severe pyogenic infections.

Deficiency of Complement

Complement plays an important role in the well-being of humans. Deficiency of various components may result in many diseases as follows:

- Inherited deficiency of C1 esterase inhibitors causes angio-edema. The low level of C1 esterase inhibitors leads to over-production of esterase. This leads to an increase in release of anaphylatoxins, which cause capillary permeability and edema.
- Acquired deficiency of DAF results in an increase in com-plement-mediated hemolysis. The condition manifests clinically as paroxysmal nocturnal hemoglobinuria.

- Inherited or acquired deficiency of C5-8 components greatly enhances susceptibility to Neisseria bactere-mia and other infections. Deficiency of C3 leads to severe recurrent pyogenic sinusitis and respiratory infections.
- The synthesis of sufficient quantities of complement is reduced in the patients with severe liver disease, such as chronic hepatitis or alcoholic cirrhosis. These patients, therefore, are highly susceptible to infections caused by pyogenic bacteria.

TEST OF COMPLEMENT FUNCTION

A complement test is a blood test that measures the activity of a group of proteins in the bloodstream. These proteins make up the complement system, which is one part of the immune system.

The complement system helps antibodies fight off infections and destroy substances that are foreign to the body. These foreign substances may include viruses, bacteria, and other germs. The complement system is also involved in how autoimmune disease and other inflammatory conditions work. When a person has an autoimmune disease, the body views its own tissues as foreign and makes antibodies against them. There are nine major complement proteins, labeled C1 through C9. However, this system is very complex. Currently, over 60 known substances in the immune system combine with complement proteins when activated.

A total complement measurement checks the activity of the main complement components by gauging the total amount of complement protein in your blood. One of the more common tests is known as a total hemolytic complement, or a CH50 measurement.

Complement levels that are too low or too high can cause problems.

PURPOSE OF A COMPLEMENT TES

A common use for a complement test is to diagnose autoimmune diseases or other immune function conditions. Certain diseases can have abnormal levels of a particular complement.

A doctor can use a complement test to monitor the progress of a person undergoing treatment for an autoimmune disease such as systemic lupus (SLE) or rheumatoid arthritis (RA). It can also be used to gauge the effectiveness of ongoing treatments for autoimmune disorders and certain kidney conditions. The test may also be used to identify individuals at high risk of complications in certain diseases.

Types of complement tests

A total complement measurement checks how well the complement system is functioning.

A doctor often orders total complement tests for people with a family history of complement deficiency and those who have symptoms of:

- RA
- hemolytic uremic syndrome (HUS)
- kidney disease
- SLE
- myasthenia gravis, a neuromuscular disorder
- an infectious disease, such as bacterial meningitis
- cryoglobulinemia, which is the presence of abnormal proteins in the blood

Specific complement tests, such as C2, C3, and C4 tests, may help evaluate the course of certain diseases. Depending on your symptoms and history, your doctor will order either a total complement measurement, one of the more targeted tests, or all three. A blood draw is all that's necessary.

HOW DO YOU PREPARE FOR A COMPLEMENT TEST?

A complement test requires a routine blood draw. No preparation or fasting is necessary.

How is a complement test performed?

A healthcare provider will follow these steps to perform the blood draw:

- They disinfect an area of skin on your arm or hand.
- They wrap an elastic band around your upper arm to allow more blood to fill the vein.
- They insert a small needle into your vein and draw the blood into a small vial.
- When the vial is full, they remove the elastic band and needle and place a small bandage over the puncture site.
- There may be some soreness of the arm where the needle entered the skin. You may also experience some mild bruising or throbbing after the blood draw.
- Risks of a complement test
- The blood draw carries few risks. Rare risks from a blood draw include:
    - excessive bleeding
    - lightheadedness
    - fainting
    - infection, which can happen any time the skin is broken.

CHAPTER

SEROLOGICAL TESTING 5

Serological test, also called serology test or antibody test, any of several laboratory procedures carried out on a sample of blood serum (the clear liquid that separates from the blood when it is allowed to clot) for the purpose of detecting antibodies or antibody-like substances that appear specifically in association with certain diseases. There are different types of serological tests—for example, flocculation tests, neutralization tests, hemagglutinin-inhibition tests, enzyme-linked immunosorbent assays (ELISAs), and chemiluminescence immunoassays.

Among flocculation tests, complement-fixation tests are the most common. These are based on the precipitation, or flocculation, that takes place when an antibody and specially prepared antigens (substances that provoke antibody production in the body) are mixed together. Neutralization tests depend on the capacity of an antibody to neutralize the infectious properties of the infectious organisms. Hemagglutinin-inhibition tests are based on the ability of viruses to cause the red blood cells of certain animal species to agglutinate (congeal, or clump together); this agglutination will be prevented by the antibody. ELISAs make use of fluorescent, light (chemiluminescent), or colorimetric signal detection; the signals are produced by enzymatic reactions that occur during the detection and quantification of a specific antigen or antibody in a solution. Chemiluminescence immunoassays are based on the detection of light signals emitted through chemical reactions between enzymes or chemical probes that bind to antibodies.

The interpretation of an antibody test result can be complex because antibody testing is used for many reasons. Depending on the antibodies tested for, antibody testing can be used for (1) diagnosis of infection, (2) identification of previous exposure to pathogens (particularly in unvaccinated animals), and (3) assessment of immunity prior to or following vaccination (Table 1). Clinicians should understand when and why to perform antibody testing and use this knowledge to make evidence-based decisions prior to vaccination.

Hemagglutination inhibition (for FPV) and serum neutralization (for FHV-1, FCV, and rabies) are the reference standards to determine the presence of effective antibody-mediated immunity. These test methodologies can only be performed in a laboratory setting using live cell cultures (i.e., they cannot be performed in a practice using rapid patient-side test kits). These diagnostic tests are predominantly research tools used in vaccine efficacy and prevalence studies.

It is important when attempting to demonstrate protective immunity in a patient using an in-clinic antibody test kit that the performance of the kit be compared against the appropriate reference standard in order to demonstrate correlationwith protective immunity.

The presence of anti-FPV antibodies correlates strongly with protection (Table 1). Currently, experts recommend antibody testing for FPV to assess immunity and inform decisions about whether to vaccinate. Rapid in-clinic test kits to detect antibodies to FPV, FHV-1, and FCVare available to veterinarians in North America and have been validated in two different studies using the appropriate reference tests. Of concern, however, was the occurrence of some anti-FPV antibody false-positive results in one study, which in practice would lead to some unprotected cats not being vaccinated.

Table 1. Possible Uses of In-Clinic Serology Testing

Pathogen	Usefulness of Antibody Testing
FPV	Useful for assessment of immunity because presence of antibodies correlates strongly with protection. Result can be used to decide whether to vaccinate (i.e., only vaccinate antibody-negative cats)
FHV-1	Not reliable for assessment of immunity. Effective immunity against FHV-1 requires both an antibody and cell-mediated immune response. Result should not be used to decide whether to vaccinate
FCV	Not reliable for assessment of immunity. Effective immunity against FCV requires both an antibody and cell-mediated immune response. Result should not be used to decide whether to vaccinate
FeLV	Useful for assessment of exposure and/or diagnosis of infection (in combination with other testing methodologies). Recently a rapid in-clinic test kit to detect antibodies to FeLV transmembrane protein (p15E) was released in Europe.
	A positive p15E antibody result cannot differentiate between exposure and infection. FeLV-vaccinated cats usually have low levels of antibodies to p15E. Results from FeLV antigen testing (and not antibody testing) should be used to decide whether to vaccinate. Rapid in-clinic FeLV test kits detect soluble p27 antigen in whole blood, serum, or plasma and are not affected by FeLV vaccination.
	The AAFP recommends testing all cats for FeLV p27 antigen prior to initial vaccination. There is no proven benefit to vaccinating infected cats.

Pathogen	Usefulness of Antibody Testing
FIV	Useful for diagnosis of infection. Between 2002 and 2015, an inactivated whole-virus vaccine was available in North America that interferes with antibody results using some test kits. FIV-vaccinated cats may test antibody positive for more than 7 years after the last vaccination.
Pathogen	Usefulness of Antibody Testing
	Additionally, cats may travel from locations where the vaccine is still in use to the USA, Canada, and other countries where the vaccine is not available. Rapid in-clinic test kits able to differentiate between FIV-infected and FIV-vaccinated cats are available.
Rabies	Vaccination against rabies is essential in regions where it is required by statute/law or where the virus is endemic and should follow label recommendations. Serum neutralization results cannot be used to decide whether to vaccinate against rabies.

FELINE LEUKEMIA VIRUS (FELV)

Serologic testing for FeLV is important to identify infected cats and prevent transmission of the virus. Testing is also recommended before vaccination against FeLV, because vaccination of infected cats will not limit development or transmission of disease. The time between infection and the presence of detectable antigen varies but is likely to be within 28–30 days. Vaccination against FeLV will not yield a positive test result when antigen tests are used, nor will the presence of maternally derived antibodies in kittens. Testing serum, plasma, or whole blood is considered more reliable than testing saliva or tears. Most test kits have positive and negative controls incorporated into the kit, so technical problems with running the test may be detected.

A negative result on a screening test is very reliable; however, false-positive results may occur with the tests of soluble antigen, especially in a population of cats with a low incidence of disease. A true positive result may reflect either transient or persistent viremia, so clinical decisions should not be based on a single test result.

Confirmation of positive results, especially in asymptomatic cats, should be pursued by additional testing such as soluble antigen testing using a kit from a different manufacturer or immunofluorescent antigen testing on blood or bone marrow. Cats with discordant results should be retested using both test methods in 60 days and should probably be considered potentially infective until their status is clarified.

Some cats previously thought to have cleared infection have been identified using real-time PCR, which is a very sensitive method to detect cell-associated FeLV proviral DNA or viral RNA. These cats are proviral DNA positive but FeLV antigen negative and are unlikely to shed virus or develop clinical disease. However, proviral FeLV could be transmitted in blood transfusions, so potential feline blood donors should be PCR negative for FeLV.

FELINE IMMUNODEFICIENCY VIRUS (FIV)

Because the concentration of FIV antigen in the blood of infected cats is often very low, in-house diagnostic tests are designed to detect anti-FIV antibodies rather than antigen. Test kits yield a positive or negative result for antibody rather than a titer. Antibodies usually develop within 60 days of infection, but this period is quite variable, and a few infected cats do not develop detectable antibody levels. Once present, antibodies appear to be present for >2 yr, except for those transiently detectable in kittens that have maternally derived antibodies. A kitten <6 mo of age that tests positive should be retested after 6 mo of age for this reason. If the test is still positive, the kitten is most likely infected.

With the currently available ELISA in-house test kits, sensitivity is high. However, these tests cannot distinguish between antibodies produced in response to vaccination with FIV vaccine and those produced by natural infection. An ELISA test that appears to successfully discriminate between antibodies produced in response to vaccination and those produced in natural infections has been developed but is not available for commercial use. A reasonable approach is to use the in-house test as a screening test. A negative result is a fairly reliable indicator that the cat is not infected. Positive results, especially in asymptomatic cats, should be confirmed by another test such as Western blot if available. Kittens born to vaccinated queens are antibody-positive for a variable length of time.

CANINE PARVOVIRUS (CPV)

Both ELISA and immunomigration test kits are available for detection of CPV antigen in feces. These tests are fairly specific for the virus, but dogs that have been recently vaccinated may transiently shed antigens detected by the test kits. The sensitivity is somewhat lower for several reasons.

Fecal shedding occurs for only ~7–10 days, beginning on day 3–5 after exposure, so virus is not always detectable in dogs with clinical signs. Blood in the feces as well as the formation of antigen-antibody complexes, with antibodies from the blood or exudate present in the gut, may be associated with false-negative results. It appears that in-house test kits may have decreased sensitivity to the new CPV2c strain.

Although in-house test kits for diagnosis of CPV are not licensed for use in cats, several studies have shown they can be used to detect feline panleukopenia virus in cat feces. The specificity and sensitivity are not known. Some cats test positive after vaccination, even when inactivated virus vaccines are used.

In-house tests for assay of anti-CPV antibodies have become available to evaluate the need for revaccination and the presence of possibly interfering maternal antibodies. These tests are not intended to diagnose parvovirus infection and do not distinguish between natural exposure and vaccine-induced antibodies.

Currently available test kits include ELISA and immunochromatographic tests. They are semiquantitative and use color changes in positive control wells compared with color changes in samples to determine relative antibody levels. The level of anti-CPV antibody protective against infection is not known, but results are interpreted based on protective titers measured by other methods. PCR is widely available for detection of virus in feces.

CANINE DISTEMPER VIRUS (CDV)

In-house test kits for determination of antibodies to CDV are available, usually in combination with canine parvovirus antibody testing. These tests are semiquantitative ELISA for anti-canine distemper IgG in serum or plasma. They may be used to evaluate the need for revaccination and to determine the level of maternal antibody present in puppies. They are less useful for diagnosis of infection with CDV. An immunochromatography-based assay for CDV antigen has been developed and has good sensitivity and specificity, especially when conjunctival swabs are the sample used; sensitivity and specificity are somewhat less for blood and nasal swabs. This assay is not currently available as an in-house test kit.

Borrelia burgdorferi

Lyme disease is caused by the tickborne spirochete *B burgdorferi*. In general, diagnostic tests for this infection have had several potential problems, including relatively high levels of positive results in clinically healthy animals, persistence of antibodies after apparent resolution of clinical disease, interpretation of antibody titers in vaccinated dogs, and the fact that detectable antibody may not be present until 4–6 wk after exposure. An in-clinic ELISA test kit for detection of anti-*B burgdorferi* antibodies in serum or plasma minimizes some of these problems by using a synthetic peptide (C_6) based on a conserved *B burgdorferi*-specific protein. This protein is important in inducing a humoral immune response by 3–5 wk after natural infection in dogs. Vaccination does not induce a cross-reactive immune response to this antigen, so assays using the C_6 protein are able to distinguish vaccine-induced antibodies from those produced in response to natural infections. C_6-based assays are also more specific than previous tests, because there is no cross-reactivity with other tickborne agents or with autoimmune antibodies.

A currently available in-house test assay for anti–*B burgdorferi* antibodies is a screening test that gives only a positive or negative result and is thus not quantitative. Although licensed for dogs, this test kit also has been validated in cats and horses. Quantitative assays, performed in reference laboratories, can be used to monitor treatment efficacy (i.e., detection of decreasing antibody titers), but these results are not always conclusive.

Ehrlichia canis

Canine ehrlichiosis is a tickborne disease caused by one of several species of *Ehrlichia*. It can be associated with thrombocytopenia, anemia, and neutropenia as well as other nonspecific clinical signs. Although identification of *Ehrlichia* morulae in leukocytes can be diagnostic for this infection, serologic assay for detection of antibodies is more common and has better sensitivity. In-house tests for ehrlichiosis are either qualitative (giving only a positive or negative result) or semiquantitative tests for antibodies to *E canis*. Those currently available are ELISA to be performed on serum, plasma, or whole blood. The test kits use either recombinant analogues of major outer membrane proteins of *E canis* or whole *E canis* proteins as the antigen. The different *Ehrlichia* species stimulate antibodies that appear to cross-react in these assays, for the most part. Because anti"*E canis* antibodies may be very long-lived and may be present in subclinical infections, detection of these antibodies does not distinguish between exposure and *Ehrlichia*-induced illness and cannot reliably indicate success of response to therapy.

Brucella canis

B canis is not a problem in some countries, and tests are not always readily available. However, infection may be subclinical, or it may cause a variety of clinical signs, including abortion, infertility, and discospondylitis. Infection most often occurs during mating; thus, testing of breeding animals is important in disease prevention. A rapid slide agglutination test that includes a 2-mercaptoethanol (2-ME) step to reduce false-positive results by eliminating nonspecific IgM reactions is available as an in-house diagnostic kit. This assay detects serum antibody to surface antigens of the bacteria. Reports of sensitivity and specificity of this test vary depending on the confirmatory test used. ELISA and immunochromatographic assays have been developed for qualitative and semiquantitative tests for anti–*B canis* antibodies. Positive results obtained using any of these test kits should be confirmed with PCR or blood culture.

Heartworm Antigen—Dogs

Serologic testing for heartworm antigen in dogs is more sensitive than screening for microfilaremia and, in addition, can detect occult infections. Heartworm antigen is first detectable at ~5 mo after infection and will usually precede microfilaremia by a few weeks; however, this time frame may be shifted later in animals on macrocyclic lactone preventives and those with low numbers of worms. Antigen test formats available include ELISA and immuno-chromatographic assays. Serum or plasma may be used in all kits, and some may be performed using whole blood.

Some test kits can be stored at room temperature, whereas others must be stored refrigerated and brought to room temperature before use. Batch testing and single sample testing are both available. All of the test kits have very high specificity.

False-positive results are most often due to technical problems such as inadequate washing or failure to read the results at the optimal time. Manufacturer's instructions should be closely followed with any of the test formats.

Sensitivity varies from one test to another and is affected by worm load, worm gender (a female antigen is detected, thus male-only infections will not be detected), and maturity of female worms. None of these tests has 100% sensitivity. When unexpected false results are obtained on an antigen test, additional testing, using a different format, is recommended.

After adulticide treatment, antigenemia should become undetectable by 6 mo. However, it can take more than a month for some adult heartworms to die, so a positive antigen test at 5–6 mo after treatment does not necessarily indicate treatment failure. The test should be repeated 2–3 mo later.

Heartworm Antibody and Antigen—Cats

Heartworm disease in cats is substantially different from the disease in dogs, and recommendations for serologic testing are consequently different. Cats tend to have a much lower worm burden—often only one or two worms. Cats also have single-sex infections more frequently than do dogs.

Circulating microfilaremia is rare in cats, and microfilariae have a shorter life span. These differences are often attributed to a more effective feline immune response to heartworm infection. However, heartworms can cause serious disease in cats.

Heartworm antigen tests are less sensitive for detection of infection in cats than they are in dogs, with a reported sensitivity of 50%–80%. Therefore, a negative antigen test does not exclude heartworm infection. Antibody testing is also available and can be useful as a screening test, but the presence of antibody does not confirm feline heartworm disease.

Transient exposure to larvae will stimulate production of antibody; many early infections are cleared spontaneously, and adult heartworms never develop. A combination of testing for both heartworm antigen and anti-heartworm antibody results in much higher sensitivity and specificity than using either test method alone. Combination testing is warranted in cats with clinical signs of heartworm disease when results of a single test are not conclusive.

Test kits for detection of heartworm antigen and anti-heartworm antibody in cats are marketed in several formats. These can use either plasma or serum and are qualitative or semiquantitative.

Canine and Feline Pregnancy Diagnosis—Relaxin

The only known pregnancy-specific hormone in the bitch and queen is relaxin, which is produced by the placenta when a fertilized egg is implanted. Relaxin is first detectable in the plasma around day 20–25 after fertilization. It is not present in pseudopregnant or nonpregnant bitches or queens.

Relaxin levels peak by approximately day 40–50 of gestation and drop at parturition, but they may remain detectable for up to 50 days during lactation. In-clinic test kits to measure relaxin include microwell ELISA and immunomigration qualitative tests requiring serum, plasma, or whole blood. The assays appear to have very good specificity, ie, a detectable level of relaxin is not found in nonpregnant animals. False-negative results have been reported in some bitches carrying very small litters or in those with one or more nonviable puppies.

Canine and Feline Luteinizing Hormone—Ovulation Timing and Ovariectomy Status

In the bitch, serum luteinizing hormone (LH) is normally present in very low levels except for a dramatic rise just before ovulation. Ovulation occurs 2 days after this LH surge, and the LH level returns to baseline within 24-40 hr of peaking. Serum progesterone levels begin to rise at the time of the LH surge. A bitch will be fertile between 4–7 days after the LH surge, with the most fertile period on days 5 and 6. In addition, the LH surge determines the gestation period, with parturition occurring between day 64 and 66 after the surge. The LH surge may occur anywhere from 3 days before to 5 days after the onset of estrous behavior, so it cannot be reliably predicted by behavior.

Ovulation timing by measurement of LH requires daily testing, which usually begins when >50% of vaginal epithelial cells are cornified, based on vaginal cytology. There is occasionally a false LH peak not followed by ovulation, but it will also not be followed by an increase in progesterone. For that reason, assays of both LH and progesterone are recommended for most accurate ovulation detection. An increased LH concentration not followed by increased progesterone levels is considered a proestrus fluctuation, and testing for ovulation should continue.

A currently available in-clinic kit to measure LH concentrations in serum is essentially qualitative, with a serum level of <1 ng/mL being read as negative and a level of >1 ng/mL considered positive. The test is an immunochromatographic assay.

Ovariectomized bitches and queens have serum concentrations of LH >1 ng/mL. Because this LH concentration is also seen in intact bitches about to ovulate, a single high LH concentration does not confirm reproductive status, but a low LH concentration indicates a nonovariectomized animal.

Canine Ovulation Timing—Progesterone

Serum progesterone begins to increase after the LH surge with a modest increase on the day before ovulation and a further increase to 4–10 ng/mL on the day of ovulation. Progesterone continues to increase and stays increased throughout pregnancy or diestrus. As the rise in progesterone is more constant compared with LH, daily testing is not necessary. It is recommended that testing begin in late proestrus and continue every 2-3 days until a high range is reached, indicating ovulation.

The test kits for in-clinic progesterone testing are semiquantitative ELISA with preovulatory concentrations designated according to the kit used. Some kits are designed to give two additional progesterone ranges (intermediate and high), whereas others indicate only preovulatory and "ovulatory day or later" levels. In comparison with other test methods, the in-house test kits are less accurate, particularly in the range of roughly 1.5–10 ng/mL, which is the range of interest for earliest detection of ovulation. Accuracy is greater at higher progesterone levels. As mentioned above, measurement of both LH and progesterone is recommended for most accurate breeding management.

Thyroxine

Assay of total serum thyroxine (T_4) may be used as a screening test for canine hypothyroidism or as a diagnostic test for feline hyperthyroidism. (Also see The Thyroid Gland.) In addition, T_4 concentrations are measured when monitoring therapy for hypo- or hyperthyroidism. An in-house ELISA test kit, which uses an additional instrument to read results, provides semiquantitative information about T_4 concentration in canine and feline sera. The assay is run at one of two "dynamic ranges," depending on the predicted range of results. Published studies comparing this assay with other test methods for T_4 vary in their conclusions. It is recommended that T_4 concentrations be periodically measured in stored pooled serum of cats and dogs to monitor whether assay performance is consistent. It is probably still better to use a commercial laboratory for thyroxine measurement.

Almost all (99%) of total T_4 is bound to protein in the blood and therefore not biologically accurate. Free T_4 levels are a more accurate test of thyroid function in cats and dogs.

Foal Immunoglobulin (IgG)

Measurement of foal serum IgG concentration within the first 24 hr after birth can be useful in preventing disease related to failure of passive transfer of IgG in colostrum from mare to foal. Use of foal-side testing procedures can facilitate prompt diagnosis and treatment. A foal serum IgG level of >800 mg/dL is generally considered optimal, with <200 mg/dL indicating failure of passive transfer. Concentrations of 200–800 mg/dL are considered evidence of partial transfer.

Although radial immunodiffusion is considered the most accurate test for IgG concentration, it takes much longer (5–24 hr) than many of the other test methods and thus is not as useful as an indicator of the need for therapeutic intervention. More rapid screening tests include the zinc sulfate turbidity test, glutaraldehyde clot test, and ELISA test kits.

The zinc sulfate test estimates IgG in serum based on its precipitation when added to a zinc-containing solution. Turbidity generally becomes visible when IgG levels are 400–500 mg/dL. This test takes ~1 hr and may be performed with zinc sulfate solutions made in the clinic, or reagents for the test may be purchased as a test kit.

The glutaraldehyde clot test requires the addition of 1 volume of serum to 10 volumes of 10% glutaraldehyde and examination of the tubes at timed intervals up to 60 min. The presence of IgG in the serum causes a solid clot to form in the tube. Clot formation in <10 min generally correlates to an IgG concentration of >800 mg/dL, whereas a positive reaction within 60 min is interpreted as an IgG concentration of >400 mg/dL. Both of these test methods use serum, rather than plasma, so time for the blood to clot and separation of serum must be added to the time needed to perform the test.

ELISA test kits for in-house or foal-side testing can use either serum or whole blood as the sample and take ~10 min. Most are semiquantitative, with color changes corresponding to IgG concentrations of <400 mg/dL, 400–800 mg/dL, or >800 mg/dL. One quantitative handheld colorimetric immunoassay is currently available.

Reports of sensitivity and specificity among these methods vary. In general, sensitivity in identifying foals with IgG concentrations <400 mg/dL appears to be acceptable for all methods. Thus, there are few foals with total failure of passive transfer that would not be identified by any of these methods. Specificity is less acceptable for some of the methods, and treatment of some foals that did not need it might be instituted based on the results.

Calf Immunoglobulin

Measurement of IgG concentration in neonatal calf serum is important for the same reasons described for foals. However, IgG levels in calves are different from those in foals, with >1,000 mg/dL considered evidence of adequate passive transfer and <1,000 mg/dL indicating failure of passive transfer. Radial immunodiffusion is the gold standard for accurate measurement of serum IgG in calves (as in foals), but the length of time required to complete this assay makes it less useful than other methods. Other methods include zinc sulfate and sodium sulfite turbidity tests, glutaraldehyde coagulation test, measurement of total serum solids by refractometry, and a lateral flowthrough ELISA test kit.

The sodium sulfite and zinc sulfate turbidity tests are both based on the precipitation of high-molecular-weight proteins in these solutions. Serum is used as the sample, and tests are read after 15-30 min of incubation. Results of these tests vary in sensitivity and specificity depending on the endpoint chosen, and technical difficulties with reagents can decrease test performance. The glutaraldehyde clot test is performed as in foals, with no clot formation at 60 min indicating failure of passive transfer.

Measurement of serum total protein by refractometer is a fairly reliable indicator of adequate passive transfer in healthy, well-hydrated calves. A level of 5.2 g/dL is roughly equivalent to an IgG concentration of 1,000 mg/dL.

A commercially available ELISA test kit uses serum as the sample and takes ~20 min. The assay is qualitative in that it indicates an IgG concentration of >1,000 mg/dL or <1,000 mg/dL. Sensitivity and specificity are reasonably good, and this test is less influenced by factors such as calf dehydration or reagent instability than some other methods. Manufacturer recommendations for storing and using the kits must be followed.

CHAPTER 6

CELLS AND TISSUES OF THE IMMUNE SYSTEM

The key primary lymphoid organs of the immune system include the thymus and bone marrow, as well as secondary lymphatic tissues including spleen, tonsils, lymph vessels, lymph nodes, adenoids, skin, and liver.

The thymus "educates" T cells and provides an inductive environment for the development of T cells from hematopoietic progenitor cells. The thymus is largest and most active during the neonatal and pre-adolescent periods of development. By the early teens, the thymus begins to atrophy and thymic stroma is replaced by adipose tissue. Nevertheless, residual T-lymphopoiesis continues throughout adult life.

Bone marrow is the flexible tissue found in the interior of bones. In humans, red blood cells are produced in the heads of long bones. The red bone marrow is a key element of the lymphatic system, being one of the primary lymphoid organs that generate lymphocytes from immature hematopoietic progenitor cells. Bone marrow and thymus constitute the primary lymphoid tissues involved in the production and early selection of lymphocytes.

The lymphatic system is a part of the circulatory system, comprising a network of conduits called lymphatic vessels that carry a clear fluid, called lymph, unidirectionally towards the heart. The lymphatic system has multiple interrelated functions including the transportation of white blood cells to and from the lymph nodes into the bones, and the transportation of antigen -presenting cells (such as dendritic cells) to the lymph nodes where an immune response is stimulated. Lymphoid tissue is found in many organs, particularly the lymph nodes.

The spleen is similar in structure to a large lymph node and acts primarily as a blood filter. It synthesizes antibodies in its white pulp and removes antibody-coated bacteria along with antibody-coated blood cells by way of blood and lymph node circulation.

The palatine tonsils and the nasopharyngeal tonsil are lymphoepithelial tissues located near the oropharynx and nasopharynx. These immunocompetent tissues are the immune system's first line of defense against ingested or inhaled foreign pathogens. The fundamental immunological roles of tonsils aren't yet understood.

Lymph nodes are distributed widely throughout areas of the body, including the armpit and stomach, and linked by lymphatic vessels. Lymph nodes are garrisons of B, T and other immune cells. Lymph nodes act as filters or traps for foreign particles and are important in the proper functioning of the immune system. They are packed tightly with the white blood cells, called lymphocytes and macrophages.

The skin is one of the most important parts of the body because it interfaces with the environment, and is the first line of defense from external factors, acting as an anatomical barrier from pathogens and damage between the internal and external environment in bodily defense. Langerhans cells in the skin are part of the adaptive immune system.

The liver has a wide range of functions, including immunological effects—the reticuloendothelial system of the liver contains many immunologically active cells, acting as a "sieve" for antigens carried to it via the portal system.

IMMUNE SYSTEM CELLS

Leukocytes (white blood cells) are immune system cells involved in defending the body against infectious disease and foreign materials. Five different types of leukocytes exist, all produced and derived from a multipotent cell in the bone marrow known as a hematopoietic stem cell. The innate leukocytes include the phagocytes, mast cells, eosinophils, basophils, and natural killer cells. These cells identify and eliminate pathogens and are important mediators in the activation of the adaptive immune system.

Neutrophils and macrophages are phagocytes that travel throughout the body in pursuit of invading pathogens. Neutrophils are normally found in the bloodstream and are the most abundant type of phagocyte.

During the acute phase of inflammation neutrophils migrate toward the site of inflammation and are usually the first cells to arrive at the scene of infection. Macrophages reside within tissues and produce a wide array of chemicals.

They also act as scavengers, ridding the body of worn-out cells and other debris, and as antigen-presenting cells that activate the adaptive immune system. Dendritic cells are phagocytes in tissues that are in contact with the external environment, and are located mainly in the skin, nose, lungs, stomach, and intestines. These cells serve as a link between the bodily tissues and the innate and adaptive immune systems, as they present antigen to T-cells, one of the key cell types of the adaptive immune system.

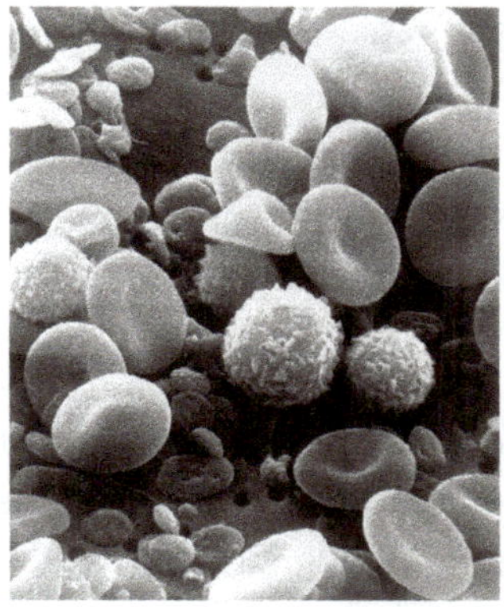

Fig. 1. Blood Cells: Red blood cells, several white blood cells including lymphocytes, a monocyte, a neutrophil, and many small disc-shaped platelets.

Mast cells reside in connective tissues and mucous membranes, and regulate the inflammatory response. They are most often associated with allergy and anaphylaxis.

Basophils and eosinophils are related to neutrophils. They secrete chemical mediators that are involved in defending against parasites, and play a role in allergic reactions, such as asthma. Natural killer cells are leukocytes that attack and destroy tumor cells, or cells that have been infected by viruses. The cells of the adaptive immune system are special types of leukocytes, called lymphocytes. B cells and T cells are the major types of lymphocytes and are derived from hematopoietic stem cells in the bone marrow.

T cells recognize a "non-self" target, such as a pathogen, only after antigens have been processed and presented in combination with a "self" receptor, called a major histocompatibility complex (MHC) molecule. There are two major subtypes of T cells: the killer T cell, which kills cells that are infected with viruses (and other pathogens) or are otherwise damaged or dysfunctional, and the helper T cell, which regulates both innate and adaptive immune responses and helps determine which immune responses the body makes to a particular pathogen. These cells have no cytotoxic activity and do not kill infected cells or clear pathogens directly. A third, minor subtype are the γ T cells that recognize intact antigens not bound to MHC receptors.

In contrast, the B cell antigen-specific receptor is an antibody molecule on the B cell surface, which recognizes whole pathogens without any need for antigen processing. Each lineage of B cell expresses a different antibody, so the complete set of B cell antigen receptors represent all the antibodies that the body can manufacture.

ANIMAL PRIMARY TISSUES

Multicellular, complex animals have four primary types of tissue: epithelial, connective, muscle, and nervous. Recall that tissues are groups of similar cells carrying out related functions. These tissues combine to form organs—like the skin or kidney—that have specific, specialized functions within the body. Organs are organized into organ systems to perform functions; examples include the circulatory system, which consists of the heart and blood vessels, and the digestive system, consisting of several organs, including the stomach, intestines, liver, and pancreas. Organ systems come together to create an entire organism.

Epithelial Tissues

Epithelial tissues cover the outside of organs and structures in the body and line the lumens of organs in a single layer or multiple layers of cells. The types of epithelia are classified by the shapes of cells present and the number of layers of cells. Epithelia composed of a single layer of cells are called *simple* epithelia; epithelial tissue composed of multiple layers is called stratified epithelia. Table 1 summarizes the different types of epithelial tissues.

Table 1 Different Types of Epithelial Tissues

Cell shape	Description	Location
squamous	flat, irregular round shape	simple: lung alveoli, capillaries stratified: skin, mouth, vagina
cuboidal	cube shaped, central nucleus	glands, renal tubules
columnar	tall, narrow, nucleus toward basetall, narrow, nucleus along cell	simple: digestive tract pseudostratified: respiratory tract
transitional	round, simple but appear stratified	urinary bladder

Squamous Epithelia

Squamous epithelial cells are generally round, flat, and have a small, centrally located nucleus. The cell outline is slightly irregular, and cells fit together to form a covering or lining. When the cells are arranged in a single layer (simple epithelia), they facilitate diffusion in tissues, such as the areas of gas exchange in the lungs and the exchange of nutrients and waste at blood capillaries.

Figure 2a illustrates a layer of squamous cells with their membranes joined together to form an epithelium. Image Fig. 2b illustrates squamous epithelial cells arranged in stratified layers, where protection is needed on the body from outside abrasion and damage. This is called a stratified squamous epithelium and occurs in the skin and in tissues lining the mouth and vagina.

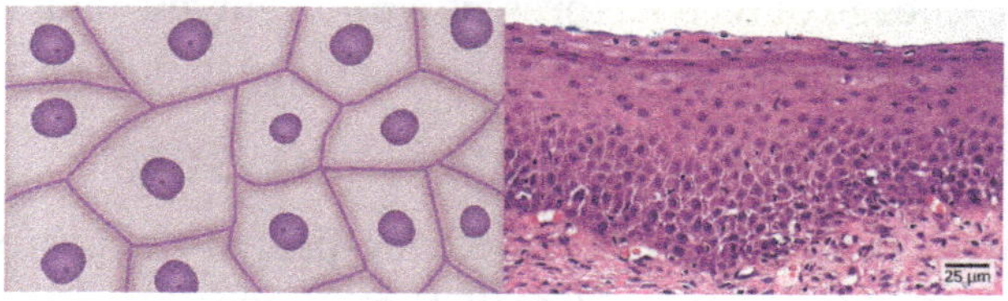

Fig. 2 Squamous epithelia cells (a) have a slightly irregular shape, and a small, centrally located nucleus. These cells can be stratified into layers, as in (b) this human cervix specimen.

Cuboidal Epithelia

Cuboidal epithelial cells, shown in Fig. 3, are cube-shaped with a single, central nucleus. They are most commonly found in a single layer representing a simple epithelia in glandular tissues throughout the body where they prepare and secrete glandular material. They are also found in the walls of tubules and in the ducts of the kidney and liver.

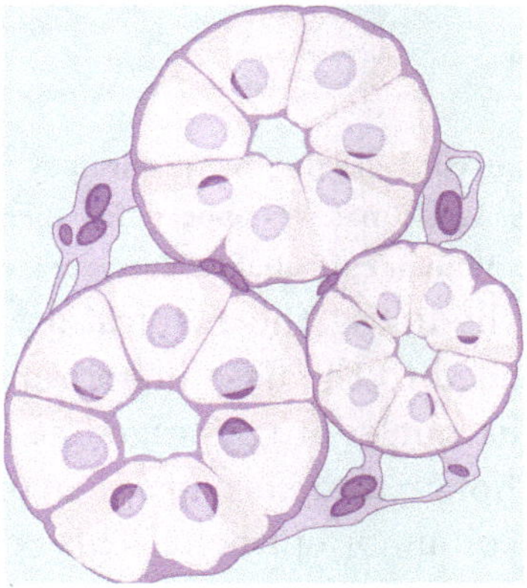

Fig. 3. Simple cuboidal epithelial cells line tubules in the mammalian kidney, where they are involved in filtering the blood.

Columnar Epithelia

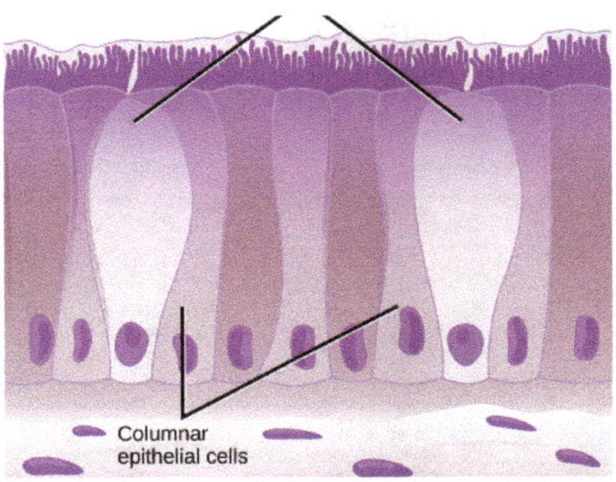

Fig. 4. Simple columnar epithelial cells absorb material from the digestive tract. Goblet cells secret mucous into the digestive tract lumen.

Columnar epithelial cells are taller than they are wide: they resemble a stack of columns in an epithelial layer, and are most commonly found in a single-layer arrangement. The nuclei of columnar epithelial cells in the digestive tract appear to be lined up at the base of the cells, as illustrated in Fig. 4. These cells absorb material from the lumen of the digestive tract and prepare it for entry into the body through the circulatory and lymphatic systems.

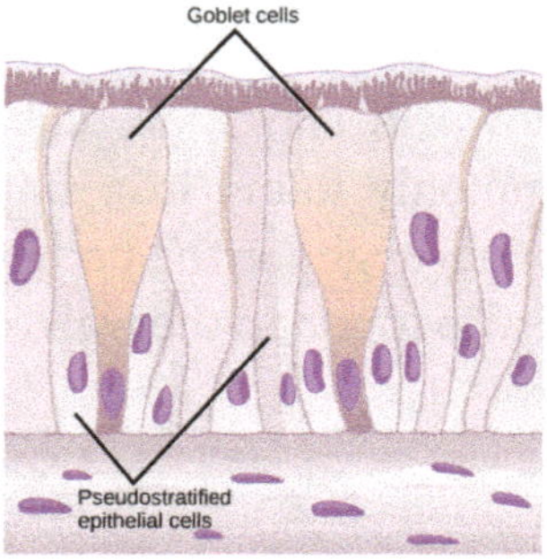

Fig. 5. Pseudostratified columnar epithelia line the respiratory tract. They exist in one layer, but the arrangement of nuclei at different levels makes it appear that there is more than one layer. Goblet cells interspersed between the columnar epithelial cells secrete mucous into the respiratory tract.

Columnar epithelial cells lining the respiratory tract appear to be stratified. However, each cell is attached to the base membrane of the tissue and, therefore, they are simple tissues. The nuclei are arranged at different levels in the layer of cells, making it appear as though there is more than one layer, as seen in Fig. 5. This is called pseudostratified, columnar epithelia. This cellular covering has cilia at the apical, or free, surface of the cells. The cilia enhance the movement of mucous and trapped particles out of the respiratory tract, helping to protect the system from invasive microorganisms and harmful material that has been breathed into the body. Goblet cells are interspersed in some tissues (such as the lining of the trachea). The goblet cells contain mucous that traps irritants, which in the case of the trachea keep these irritants from getting into the lungs.

Transitional Epithelia

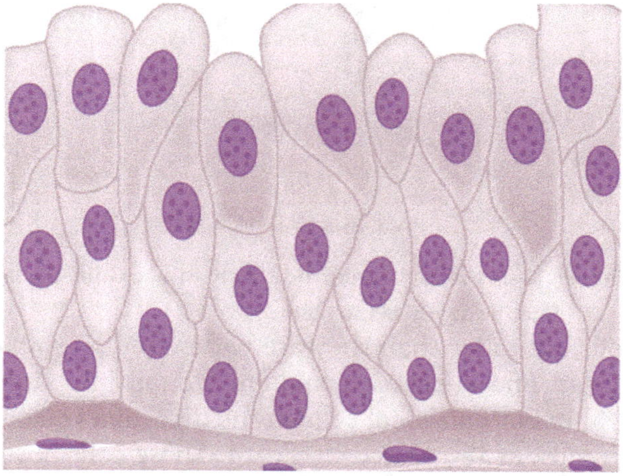

Fig. 6. Transitional epithelia of the urinary bladder undergo changes in thickness depending on how full the bladder is.

Transitional or uroepithelial cells appear only in the urinary system, primarily in the bladder and ureter. These cells are arranged in a stratified layer, but they have the capability of appearing to pile up on top of each other in a relaxed, empty bladder, as illustrated in Fig. 6. As the urinary bladder fills, the epithelial layer unfolds and expands to hold the volume of urine introduced into it. As the bladder fills, it expands and the lining becomes thinner. In other words, the tissue transitions from thick to thin.

Which of the following statements about types of epithelial cells is false?

- Simple columnar epithelial cells line the tissue of the lung.
- Simple cuboidal epithelial cells are involved in the filtering of blood in the kidney.
- Pseudostratisfied columnar epithilia occur in a single layer, but the arrangement of nuclei makes it appear that more than one layer is present.
- Transitional epithelia change in thickness depending on how full the bladder is.

Connective Tissues

Connective tissues are made up of a matrix consisting of living cells and a non-living substance, called the ground substance. The ground substance is made of an organic substance (usually a protein) and an inorganic substance (usually a mineral or water). The principal cell of connective tissues is the fibroblast. This cell makes the fibers found in nearly all of the connective tissues. Fibroblasts are motile, able to carry out mitosis, and can synthesize whichever connective tissue is needed. Macrophages, lymphocytes, and, occasionally, leukocytes can be found in some of the tissues. Some tissues have specialized cells that are not found in the others. The **matrix** in connective tissues gives the tissue its density. When a connective tissue has a high concentration of cells or fibers, it has proportionally a less dense matrix.

The organic portion or protein fibers found in connective tissues are either collagen, elastic, or reticular fibers. Collagen fibers provide strength to the tissue, preventing it from being torn or separated from the surrounding tissues. Elastic fibers are made of the protein elastin; this fiber can stretch to one and one half of its length and return to its original size and shape. Elastic fibers provide flexibility to the tissues. Reticular fibers are the third type of protein fiber found in connective tissues. This fiber consists of thin strands of collagen that form a network of fibers to support the tissue and other organs to which it is connected.

Loose/Areolar Connective Tissue

Loose connective tissue, also called areolar connective tissue, has a sampling of all of the components of a connective tissue. As illustrated in Fig. 7, loose connective tissue has some fibroblasts; macrophages are present as well.

Collagen fibers are relatively wide and stain a light pink, while elastic fibers are thin and stain dark blue to black. The space between the formed elements of the tissue is filled with the matrix. The material in the connective tissue gives it a loose consistency similar to a cotton ball that has been pulled apart. Loose connective tissue is found around every blood vessel and helps to keep the vessel in place. The tissue is also found around and between most body organs. In summary, areolar tissue is tough, yet flexible, and comprises membranes.

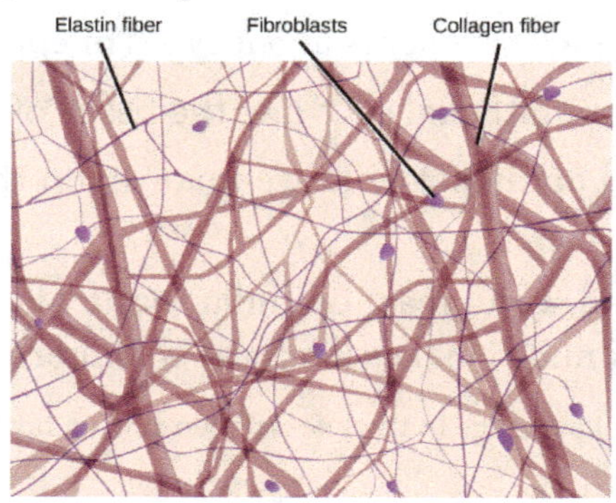

Fig. 7. Loose connective tissue: Loose connective tissue is composed of loosely-woven collagen and elastic fibers. The fibers and other components of the connective tissue matrix are secreted by fibroblasts.

Fibrous Connective Tissue

Fibrous connective tissues contain large amounts of collagen fibers and few cells or matrix material. The fibers can be arranged irregularly or regularly with the strands lined up in parallel. Irregularly arranged fibrous connective tissues are found in areas of the body where stress occurs from all directions, such as the dermis of the skin. Regular fibrous connective tissue, shown in Fig. 8, is found in tendons (which connect muscles to bones) and ligaments (which connect bones to bones).

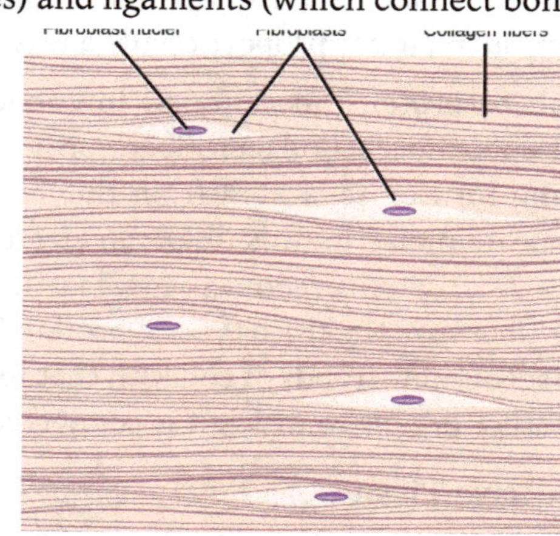

Fig. 8. Fibrous connective tissue: Fibrous connective tissue from the tendon has strands of collagen fibers lined up in parallel. This arrangement helps the tissue resist tension that occurs from all directions.

Cartilage

Cartilage is a connective tissue with a large amount of the matrix and variable amounts of fibers. The cells, called **chondrocytes**, make the matrix and fibers of the tissue. Chondrocytes are found in spaces within the tissue called **lacunae.**

A cartilage with few collagen and elastic fibers is hyaline cartilage, illustrated in Fig. 9. The lacunae are randomly scattered throughout the tissue and the matrix takes on a milky or scrubbed appearance with routine histological stains. Sharks have cartilaginous skeletons, as does nearly the entire human skeleton during a specific pre-birth developmental stage. A remnant of this cartilage persists in the outer portion of the human nose. Hyaline cartilage is also found at the ends of long bones, reducing friction and cushioning the articulations of these bones.

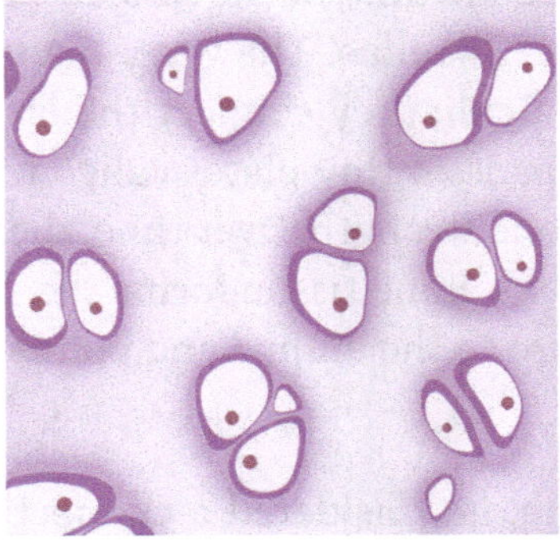

Fig. 9. Hyaline cartilage consists of a matrix with cells called chondrocytes embedded in it. The chondrocytes exist in cavities in the matrix called lacunae.

Elastic cartilage has a large amount of elastic fibers, giving it tremendous flexibility. The ears of most vertebrate animals contain this cartilage as do portions of the larynx, or voice box. Fibrocartilage contains a large amount of collagen fibers, giving the tissue tremendous strength.

Fibrocartilage comprises the intervertebral discs in vertebrate animals. Hyaline cartilage found in movable joints such as the knee and shoulder becomes damaged as a result of age or trauma. Damaged hyaline cartilage is replaced by fibrocartilage and results in the joints becoming "stiff."

Bone

Bone, or osseous tissue, is a connective tissue that has a large amount of two different types of matrix material. The organic matrix is similar to the matrix material found in other connective tissues, including some amount of collagen and elastic fibers. This gives strength and flexibility to the tissue. The inorganic matrix consists of mineral salts—mostly calcium salts—that give the tissue hardness. Without adequate organic material in the matrix, the tissue breaks; without adequate inorganic material in the matrix, the tissue bends.

There are three types of cells in bone: osteoblasts, osteocytes, and osteoclasts. Osteoblasts are active in making bone for growth and remodeling. Osteoblasts deposit bone material into the matrix and, after the matrix surrounds them, they continue to live, but in a reduced metabolic state as osteocytes. Osteocytes are found in lacunae of the bone. Osteoclasts are active in breaking down bone for bone remodeling, and they provide access to calcium stored in tissues. Osteoclasts are usually found on the surface of the tissue.

Bone can be divided into two types: compact and spongy. Compact bone is found in the shaft (or diaphysis) of a long bone and the surface of the flat bones, while spongy bone is found in the end (or epiphysis) of a long bone. Compact bone is organized into subunits called osteons. A blood vessel and a nerve are found in the center of the structure within the Haversian canal, with radiating circles of lacunae around it known as lamellae. The wavy lines seen between the lacunae are microchannels called canaliculi; they connect the lacunae to aid diffusion between the cells. Spongy bone is made of tiny plates called trabeculae these plates serve as struts to give the spongy bone strength. Over time, these plates can break causing the bone to become less resilient. Bone tissue forms the internal skeleton of vertebrate animals, providing structure to the animal and points of attachment for tendons.

Adipose Tissue

Adipose tissue, or fat tissue, is considered a connective tissue even though it does not have fibroblasts or a real matrix and only has a few fibers. Adipose tissue is made up of cells called adipocytes that collect and store fat in the form of triglycerides, for energy metabolism. Adipose tissues additionally serve as insulation to help maintain body temperatures, allowing animals to be endothermic, and they function as cushioning against damage to body organs. Under a microscope, adipose tissue cells appear empty due to the extraction of fat during the processing of the material for viewing. The thin lines in the image are the cell membranes, and the nuclei are the small, black dots at the edges of the cells.

Blood

Blood is considered a connective tissue because it has a matrix, as shown in Fig. 10. The living cell types are red blood cells (RBC), also called erythrocytes, and white blood cells (WBC), also called leukocytes. The fluid portion of whole blood, its matrix, is commonly called plasma.

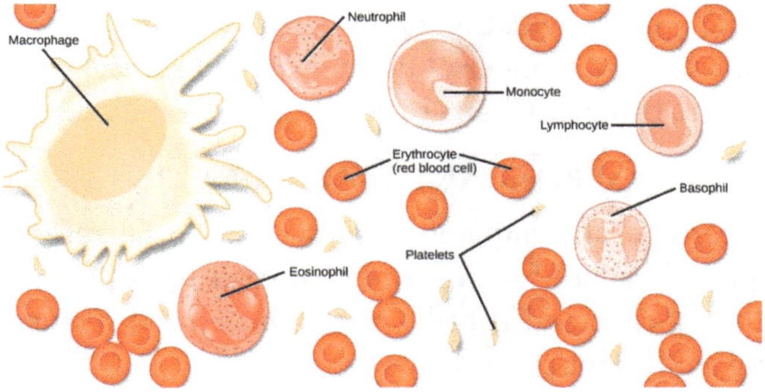

Fig. 10. Blood is a connective tissue that has a fluid matrix, called plasma, and no fibers. Erythrocytes (red blood cells), the predominant cell type, are involved in the transport of oxygen and carbon dioxide. Also present are various leukocytes (white blood cells) involved in immune response.

The cell found in greatest abundance in blood is the erythrocyte. Erythrocytes are counted in millions in a blood sample: the average number of red blood cells in primates is 4.7 to 5.5 million cells per microliter. Erythrocytes are consistently the same size in a species, but vary in size between species. For example, the average diameter of a primate red blood cell is 7.5 µl, a dog is close at 7.0 µl, but a cat's RBC diameter is 5.9 µl. Sheep erythrocytes are even smaller at 4.6 µl. Mammalian erythrocytes lose their nuclei and mitochondria when they are released from the bone marrow where they are made. Fish, amphibian, and avian red blood cells maintain their nuclei and mitochondria throughout the cell's life. The principal job of an erythrocyte is to carry and deliver oxygen to the tissues.

Leukocytes are the predominant white blood cells found in the peripheral blood. Leukocytes are counted in the thousands in the blood with measurements expressed as ranges: primate counts range from 4,800 to 10,800 cells per µl, dogs from 5,600 to 19,200 cells per µl, cats from 8,000 to 25,000 cells per µl, cattle from 4,000 to 12,000 cells per µl, and pigs from 11,000 to 22,000 cells per µl.

Lymphocytes function primarily in the immune response to foreign antigens or material. Different types of lymphocytes make antibodies tailored to the foreign antigens and control the production of those antibodies. Neutrophils are phagocytic cells and they participate in one of the early lines of defense against microbial invaders, aiding in the removal of bacteria that has entered the body. Another leukocyte that is found in the peripheral blood is the monocyte. Monocytes give rise to phagocytic macrophages that clean up dead and damaged cells in the body, whether they are foreign or from the host animal. Two additional leukocytes in the blood are eosinophils and basophils—both help to facilitate the inflammatory response.

The slightly granular material among the cells is a cytoplasmic fragment of a cell in the bone marrow. This is called a platelet or thrombocyte. Platelets participate in the stages leading up to coagulation of the blood to stop bleeding through damaged blood vessels. Blood has a number of functions, but primarily it transports material through the body to bring nutrients to cells and remove waste material from them.

SECONDARY LYMPHOID TISSUE

Secondary (or peripheral) lymphoid tissues can also be referred to as lymphoid organs. They provide a site for immune responses to occur and are populated by relatively mature T cells and B cells, macrophages and dendritic cells with each tissue providing a different environment.

Secondary Lymphoid Organs are the locations of the Immune System, where Lymphocytes are functionally specialized by allowing them to come into contact with different antigens. Such Organs therefore form an array of filters in order to collect antigens, which always track the contents of the extraCellular fluid including the blood, Tissue fluid, and lymph. Some examples of Secondary Lymphoid Organs are lymph nodes, tonsils, spleen, Peyer's patches, mucosa - associated Lymphoid Tissue (MALT), etc.

In addition, about 100 - 200 lymph nodes are present in the body, encapsulating the Lymphoid Tissue. We are mostly concentrated in the back, thorax, abdomen, and pelvis. They have Lymphocytes T and B, as well as antigen-capture macrophages. MALT is also responsible for filtering the fluid in Tissues. The Tissue is about 1 mm tiny in diameter. This exists in the digestive tract, oral passage, nasopharyngeal tract, thyroid, breast, lung, salivary glands, hair, and skin. Often, three different MALT cases are tonsils, Peyer's spots, and appendix. Significantly, all of the above Secondary Lymphoid Organs contain T and B Lymphocytes as well as antigen-capture macrophages.

Bronchial structure

The bronchial wall is microscopically composed of the following five sections: mucosa, muscle, submucosa, cartilage, and peribronchial connective tissue (adventitia)

The epithelial and lamina propria layers constitute the bronchial mucosa layer, which has the characteristics of the respiratory mucosa. The initial part of the bronchi exhibits a similar structure to that of the trachea, which is a pathway responsible for the transmission of air taken from the external environment into the lungs. The structure of the bronchial wall changes histologically at the point where it enters the lungs and transforms into intrapulmonary bronchi. In the beginning, the bronchial mucosa comprises a layer of respiratory epithelium with the same cellular composition as the trachea. The height of the cells of this ciliated layer, also known as the pseudostratified columnar epithelium, decreases in proportion to the diameter of the bronchus. The prominent cell types in the epithelium are ciliated cells, goblet cells, basal cells, brush cells, and neuroendocrine cells. The epithelial layer is separated from other mucosal layers by a basement membrane.

The basement membrane is prominent in the primary bronchi; however, it rapidly decreases in thickness and disappears as a separate structure in the secondary bronchi. The lamina propria layer is similar to the trachea, but it decreases in proportion to the diameter of the bronchi. The lamina propria layer, which appears as a typical loose connective tissue with abundant elastic and collagen threads, is rich in cellular structures. In addition to the cell types such as plasma cells, mast cells, eosinophils, and fibroblasts, it comprises a large number of lymphocyte cells. The lymphocytes in this layer gather in the form of infiltrates at some places and lymph follicles at some.

The muscularis layer, which comprises multiple rows of circular smooth muscle cells, is a continuous layer of smooth muscles in the large bronchi. However, in the small bronchi, it is weakly and loosely organized because it may appear discontinuous due to its spiral route. This layer is responsible for determining the appropriate airway diameter for airflow regulation. In the large bronchi, the loose connective tissue submucosa layer is evident, whereas in the small bronchi, it is only observed as a narrow patch.

In addition to the venous plexus and lymph follicles, bronchial glands known as GI. bronchioles are quite common in this layer. These glands, similar to salivary gland tissue, comprise a mixture of serous and mucinous cells and decrease in quantity as the diameter of the bronchi decreases.

he cartilage layer is observed as a whole in the trachea, whereas it is irregularly present at the beginning of the bronchi in the form of hyaline cartilage. As the diameter of the bronchus decreases, the fragmented cartilage layer becomes smaller and appears as elastic cartilage. On the other hand, the peribronchial connective tissue (adventitia) layer is dense that limits the bronchi from the alveoli and is rich in nerve and elastic fibers in addition to large blood and lymph vessels

Bronchi immunology

The lower respiratory tract is constantly exposed to a wide variety of airborne foreign bodies because it is in direct communication with the external environment for gas exchange. Both the trachea and bronchi function as filters against this exposure due to some of their structural features. The bronchial epithelium has a similar histological structure to the trachea and can capture foreign bodies through the smear of the mucus film secreted by the goblet cells to the kinocilium at the apical ends of the prismatic cells present in its structure. These bodies are captured and removed from the lungs by the movement of the kinocilium toward the larynx. Mechanical filtering of inhaled air is thus ensured due to this primary defense mechanism.

The lower respiratory tract is constantly exposed to allergens, antigens, bacteria, and viruses during gas exchange. This is a very sensitive area for various types of pathogen invasions, such as influenza virus, measles virus, and *Mycobacterium tuberculosis*. Producing rapid and specific adaptive immune responses against these factors are important for survival. At the initial stage of an adaptive immune response, naive T cells migrate through the endothelial venules of blood vessels to secondary lymphoid tissues, where they are stimulated by antigen-bearing cells.

This is critical for the development of appropriate adaptive immunity. This migration therefore leads to the generation of antigen-specific effector and memory T and B cells released from the secondary lymphoid tissue into the bloodstream. In the effector stage of the adaptive immune response, some memory T and B cells migrate from blood vessels to non-lymphoid tissues containing cognate antigens or pathogens. Bronchial lymphoid tissue and lymphatic nodes, two types of secondary lymphoid tissue found in the bronchial mucosa of the lower respiratory tract, are important in this regard. These secondary lymphoid tissues play a key role in the development of bronchopulmonary immune responses. Therefore, the bronchopulmonary adaptive immune system plays an important role in maintaining health as well as in the development of lower respiratory tract diseases. The tracheobronchial tree, which is considered as an immunological organ, is important for the defense mechanism of microorganisms reaching the lungs through inhaled air as well as for hypersensitive reactions that occur through respiration. The lymphoid tissue of the tracheobronchial system contains specialized diffuse, clustered, and solitary lymphatic nodules known as bronchus-associated lymphoid tissue. This secondary lymphoid tissue is a representative of the mucosal immune system in the bronchial wall, which is common in different parts of the body. It forms the immunoglobulins as a result of the immune defense reaction, thus forming a special protective mechanism of the lower respiratory system.

Mucosa-associated lymphoid tissue (MALT)

The immune system can recognize a wide range of unknown antigens and elicit an appropriate respond due to the lymphocytes that have a wide variety of antigen receptors. This system has evolved into a system of secondary lymphoid organs such as the spleen, lymph nodes, Peyer's patches, and other MALT, in line with the defense targets. Highly organized secondary lymphoid organs contain architectural domains that facilitate sequential cellular interactions between antigen-presenting cells and lymphocytes and efficiently promote the activation, selection, and differentiation of B and T cells. Therefore, the immunological response becomes more effective.

MALT can function independently of the systemic immune system and therefore encompasses the mucosal immune system, which is a crucial part of immunopathology.

It plays an important role in immunological defense by eliciting immune responses against specific antigens encountered along the surfaces of all mucosal tissues.

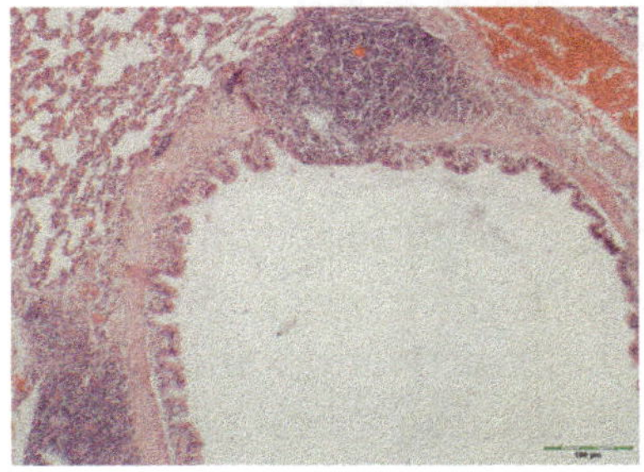

Fig. 11. Light microscopic view of the BALT structure, rat lung (H-E). Red star: BALT formation.

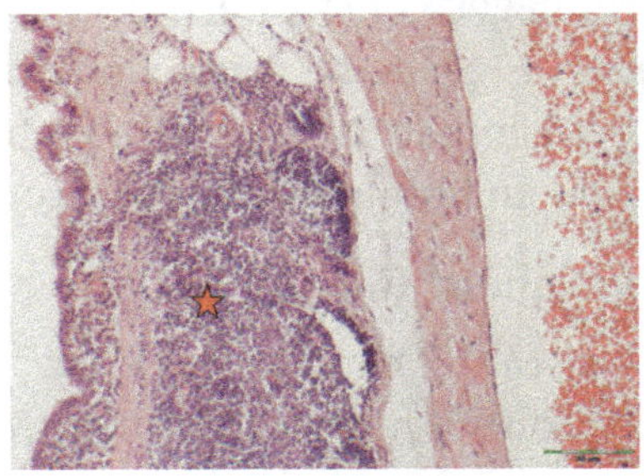

Fig. 12. A higher power light microscopic view of the BALT structure, rat lung (H-E). Red star: BALT formation.

Although MALT is anatomically divided into regions, these regions are functionally interconnected under the name of the common mucosal immune system. In this way, events such as antigen presentation and B-cell activation in a mucosal region can trigger the secretion of immunoglobulin A (IgA) in the mucosal regions of different organs. Due to MALT, which mainly functions to produce and secrete IgA along the mucosal surfaces in antigen-specific, T helper 2-dependent reactions, T helper 1 and cytotoxic T-cell-mediated reactions can occur. This may then result in immunotolerance.

The best-known representatives of MALT, which contains approximately half of the lymphocytes of the immune system, are gut-associated lymphoid tissue (GALT), nasal-associated lymphoid tissue (NALT), and BALT. However, structures such as conjunctival-associated lymphoid tissue (CALT), larynx-associated lymphoid tissue, and duct-associated lymphoid tissue (DALT) are other MALT representatives.

MALT is divided into the two following functional parts: inducer sites and effector sites. Inducer sites include secondary lymphoid tissues, where the clonal expansion of B cells and IgA class transition occur in response to antigen-specific T-cell activation. GALT, BALT, NALT, and CALT in mice, dogs, and baboons and DALT in cynomolgus macaques constitute these inducing sites.

These sites are known as secondary immune tissues where antigen sampling occurs, and immune responses are initiated. Although there are many differences between inducing sites in various organs, they all contain the same functional segments as follows: lymphoid follicles, interfollicular zones, subepithelial dome zones, and follicle-associated epithelium or lymphoepithelium containing microfold (M) cells.

Effector sites distributed as diffuse lymphoid tissue throughout the lamina propria layer on all mucosal surfaces are known as the transport sites of IgA along the mucosal epithelium. After activation and IgA class transition, T- and B cells migrate from inducing sites to these sites .

CD^{4+} and CD^{8+} T cells, IgA, IgG- and IgM-plasma cells, B cells, antigen-presenting dendritic cells, and macrophages constitute the cellular content of these effector regions where secreted IgA (S-IgA) is secreted along the mucosal epithelium. Mast cells and eosinophils can occasionally be seen in the interfollicular area. Thus, all the cell types required to initiate an immune response are present here.

Bronchus-associated lymphoid tissue (BALT)

BALT, an important part of MALT, is classically used to refer to intrapulmonary lymphoid tissue in connection with the pulmonary vessels and adventitia of the bronchi. Researchers named this lymphoid tissue in 1955 as 'sumps' or 'pulmonary tonsils' in which dust and organisms are retained. Subsequently, and identified these formations as subepithelial follicular lymphoid aggregates, primarily composed of lymphocytes, organized in the bronchial mucosa in contact with the surface epithelium, and coined the term BALT to describe them.

Although BALT, a secondary lymphoid tissue that plays an important role in the maintenance and regulation of lung mucosal immune homeostasis, was initially claimed to resemble Peyer's patches in the small intestine; it was later revealed that it was quite different from these formations. Compared to GALT where in the founder Peyer's patches are located, it is accepted that BALT is not regularly present during fetal life due to embryonic preprogramming; however, it occurs with antigenic stimulation during the postnatal period. In other words, it is claimed that there is a relatively special lymphoid tissue in the development of BALT. However, studies have shown that BALT exhibits great differences between species.

BALT, which was first identified in the bronchial wall of rabbits by researchers, is frequently detected in these animals and has the highest number of regions. In terms of the presence and distribution of BALT, rats and guinea pigs follow rabbits, whereas germ-free pigs, cats, dogs, and Syrian hamsters do not have this lymphoid tissue. BALT is frequently present in poultry, particularly hens. In mice and humans, the situation with BALT is a little more contradictory. Some scientists suggest that BALT is present in germ-free mice when antigenic stimulation is absent, whereas others report that it is not. Besides the differing viewpoints on the presence of BALT in mice, it is assumed that it is only observed infrequently after the neonatal period.

Further, it is claimed that BALT is not present in structurally healthy humans because the features similar to BALT in mice are also found in humans. BALT, in particular, is detectable if it is induced in adults; however, it is only observed in 40% healthy children and adolescents. Factors inducing the presence and distribution of BALT in these adults include infection, pathogen exposure, chronic pulmonary inflammation or autoimmune disease, etc. Moreover, it is suggested that the formation, size, and amount of BALT depend on the type and duration of exposure. Therefore, it is concluded that BALT varies in different species as well as indifferent physiological states of the same species.

Inducible BALT (IBALT)

Most of the secondary lymphoid organs found in mice and humans develop embryonically in the absence of microbial stimulation or environmental antigens. Furthermore, the structure and function of several secondary lymphoid organs, particularly those on the mucosal surfaces, are dramatically altered upon exposure to foreign antigens and commensal organisms. Peyer's patches of MALT demonstrate a striking increase in size and complexity following the colonization of commensals.

Similarly, in rodents, NALT is not completely developed until the postnatal period; however, microbial exposure accelerates this process. On the other hand, the appendix tissue of rabbits has the characteristics of the primary and secondary lymphoid tissues in terms of being functionally dependent on microbial colonization. However, some lymphoid tissues, known as tertiary lymphoid tissues, develop only after environmental exposure to microbes, pathogens, or inflammatory stimulations. Interestingly, although the lungs of mice and humans normally lack organized lymphoid tissue, tertiary lymphoid structures are frequently observed in lung tissue.

BALT is recognized as an inducible tertiary or ectopic lymphoid tissue, unlike the related secondary lymphoid organs. BALT develops during the postnatal period and at anatomically non-lymphoid sites. In terms of disease states characterized by chronic inflammation, infection, or autoimmunity, BALT formation can be induced, and these areas are then known as iBALT. iBALT is a classic example of tertiary lymphoid tissue because it does not develop on a preprogrammed basis; its creation, size, and number in the lungs depend on the type and duration of antigenic exposure.

iBALT regions are best characterized in the lungs of rodents and humans. They are observed in the lungs of mammals and birds as well as in possibly all air-breathing vertebrates. The emerging arguments confirm the role of infectious agents, such as isolated lymphoid follicles in the gut, indicating that iBALT may develop in response to microbial exposure. In contrast, BALT is said to have been discovered in germ-free rats and mice as well.

Unlike the classical BALT structure, iBALT does not always have an overlying lymphoepithelium, is not associated with a continuous airway, and can be located adjacent to small pulmonary arteries in the lung parenchyma. However, as both BALT and iBALT have the same function, both tissue types are called BALT.

Microscopic structure of BALT

Microscopically, BALT is defined as a densely packed cluster of lymphocytes with follicular structures enveloped in a network of reticular stromal cells beneath a specialized airway epithelium devoid of cilium. These structures are claimed to be located along the main bronchial airways embedded in the airway wall with extensive lymphocytic infiltration of the epithelial layer forming a classical dome epithelium (Figures 11 and 12).

Further, it is stated that BALT is present in bronchial tree bifurcations to capture respiratory antigens. In species, BALT develops in response to various stimulations rather than being constitutively present in the lung, whereas iBALT does not always have such a defined structure or precise localization in the lung.

As a part of the integrated mucosal system including GALT, NALT, and other secondary lymphoid tissue representatives, BALT is known to contain cell types that are responsible for eliciting an appropriate immune response. BALT is mainly defined as an organized structure comprising T- and B-cell domains, dendritic cells (DCs), stromal cells, and high endothelial venules (HEVs) in the T-cell region. Furthermore, it is stated that most of its cellular component consists of B cells expressing IgM^{lo} IgD^{hi}; however, depending on the nature of the microbe and/or antigen to which the cells respond, IgG-, IgA-, and even IgE-positive plasma cells may also be present.

Moreover, in BALT, the most prominent structure is follicular-like lymphocyte accumulation, which is the common microscopic appearance of secondary lymphoid tissues, forming a classical germinal center (active site). In this structure, surrounded by more mature, small lymphocytes, most of the germinal center comprises antigen-presenting macrophages. Lymphocytes leave the blood and migrate to BALT in the walls of HEVs, which are present at the periphery of the tissue. As there are no afferent lymphatics, these HEVs are thought to be the only entry site where lymphocytes migrate to BALT. In addition, the expression of chemokines in HEVs ensures accurate targeting of lymphocytes to lymphoid tissues.

However, in the direction of the bronchial epithelium, a dome-like protrusion similar to Peyer's patches toward the bronchial lumen is sometimes clearly observed. The B-cell follicle, which is the most noticeable characteristic in classic BALT tissues with dome epithelium, is positioned below the epithelium. CD^{4+} T cells are abundant in B-cell follicles, especially in reactive follicles with germinal centers, and CD^{8+} T cells are uncommon. Moreover, BALT is covered by a lymphoepithelium, which contains M cells that are similar to the M cells present in the dome epithelium of Peyer's patches in some species. M cells are thought to transport antigens from the mucosal lumen to DCs that are in close contact with the dome epithelium. Rabbits, the first and important representative of BALT, have fewer ciliated cells, few goblet cells, and many lymphocytes between epithelial and M cells. Although this basic structure appears to be valid for all species, there are some differences in details.

Another cell type that makes up the cellular component of BALT is follicular DCs (FDCs). These cells depend on the lymphotoxin signaling pathway to differentiate into conventional lymphoid tissues and BALT. Located at the center of B-cell follicles, these cells present antigen to B cells and provide costimulatory signals that increase B-cell activation and proliferation in germinal centers. FDCs in mice are characterized by their ability to bind to antibodies against CD_{21}/CD_{35}, $FDCM_1$, or $FDCM_2$ and to sequester their immune complexes. In addition, FDCs are responsible for the organization of the follicle and expression of $CXCL_{13}$, which is responsible for the recruitment of B cells and some T cells in the B-cell area. DCs located at the highest concentration in the T-cell areas of BALT are reportedly capable of preserving the BALT architecture as well as their antigen-presenting ability.

BALT is induced to produce IgA^+ cells that secrete polymeric IgA, mainly due to its role in immunity. When polymeric IgA is transported into the lumen, it induces the formation of S-IgA, which has considerable immunological importance. Thus, when BALT is identified as part of the integrated mucosal immune system, the term should be restricted to structures tightly associated with an epithelium infiltrated by lymphocytes. In the integrated mucosal immune system, specific antigen uptake and antigen presentation by M cells occur and immune reactions are initiated, including IgA responses.

Immunohistological studies in humans show a preferential central localization of B cells mixed with some CD^{4+} lymphocytes and macrophages. CD^{4+} lymphocytes are also present in the area around the HEV, at the edge resembling a crown, and in the epithelium. In addition to the few proliferative cells positive for Ki67 observed in the follicles, many cells positive for the human leukocyte antigen-DR isotype, which is associated with various autoimmune conditions, disease susceptibility, and disease resistance, are evenly distributed in the follicle. This basic structural distribution of lymphoid and non-lymphoid cells has also been noted in BALT in pathological conditions such as rheumatoid arthritis, hypersensitivity pneumonia, or diffuse panbronchiolitis. Therefore, it is reasonable to conclude that BALT plays an important role in many respiratory system-related pathologies.

ROLE OF BALT IN VARIOUS PATHOLOGIES

BALT plays an important role in pulmonary immunity such as regulating microbial homeostasis, inducing immune tolerance, inhibiting inflammation, and supporting immune clearance. Therefore, BALT frequently encounters many pathologies associated with infectious disease agents, allergens, environmental antigens, airborne particles, autoimmune disease agents, and factors causing malignancy. As these pathological conditions have a broad spectrum, it is not possible to discuss all the roles of BALT; therefore, only a few have been addressed.

Role of BALT in resistance to infectious diseases

The respiratory tract is a typical entry site for viruses. This makes it difficult for the immune system to effectively eliminate viruses and virus-infected cells without causing much damage and inflammation, which jeopardizes the lung's structural and functional integrity. The balance between eliciting an immune response to effectively eliminate viruses and virus-infected cells and to cause less damage and inflammation is maintained by a complex network of innate and adaptive immune mechanisms as well as immunomodulatory and anti-inflammatory mechanisms. Accordingly, BALT could be one of the mechanisms that facilitates viral clearance by eliciting immune responses and decreasing inflammatory responses. BALT reportedly initiates pulmonary immune responses that are faster and more protective than those initiated at systemic sites. It has been proposed that once generated, BALT could play a key role in combating successive rounds of the same infection as well as assisting in establishing local immunity against unrelated viruses or pathogens.

For example, it has been suggested that *Lta*-/- mice without lymph nodes and Peyer's patches are more susceptible to the influenza virus and although they elicit immune responses, both B- and T-cell responses are delayed. Based on flow cytometric identification of germinal center B cells in the lung to question where immune responses might be initiated, it was concluded that both B- and T-cell responses are probably produced in the lungs. BALT is suggested to be formed in the lungs of *Lta*-/- mice and locally initiates immune responses against influenza because the germinal center is present only in secondary lymphoid tissues.

Another study reported that, in addition to germinal centers, plasma cells specific to influenza nucleoprotein were detected in BALT after influenza infection. However, B-cell responses to influenza are accelerated in mice with pre-existing BALT, and morbidity and mortality rates are markedly reduced in response to a variety of viruses, including influenza, severe acute respiratory syndrome coronavirus, and mouse pneumovirus.

Mycobacterium tuberculosis (Mtb) infection is one of the serious health threats worldwide and is typically confined to the lungs. Although local immune mechanisms are primarily responsible for keeping Mtb infection under control, once the infection has settled in the lungs, immune mechanisms alone do not appear to be capable of eliminating these bacteria. In humans, Mtb is localized to the granulomas comprising a central nucleus surrounded by macrophages, multinucleated giant cells, and lymphocytes. The lymphocyte clusters surrounding these granulomas are B cells that form structures similar to BALT.

These BALT areas associated with granuloma have B-cell follicles, and T-cell areas are present at the outer edge of the follicles. Similar BALT domains, for example, have been discovered in murine models of Mtb infection, where B-cell clusters surrounding the granuloma were observed. Well-defined B-cell domains with FDCs are formed as early as day 42 after pulmonary infection and are protected from infection until at least day 90. Considering the link between B follicular structures surrounding the granuloma and Mtb uptake, another study showed that B-cell follicles formed around Mtb lesions in mice developed large germinal centers, and the B cells responded to the antigen. Therefore, it is indicated that BALT initiates local pulmonary immune responses against Mtb infection via B cells.

Role of BALT in pulmonary responses to allergens and environmental antigens

Endotoxin, known as lipopolysaccharide (LPS), is a component of the gram-negative bacteria that is commonly present in the environment. The development or exacerbation of asthma, bronchitis, and chronic obstructive pulmonary disease is linked to considerable LPS exposure. LPS, a classical T-cell-independent B-cell antigen, and mitogen are thought to bind to TLR_4 signaling pathway, triggering B-cell activation, proliferation, and differentiation into antibody-secreting cells. TLR_4 signaling activates macrophages and DCs, epithelial cells, and even fibroblasts, causing them to produce inflammatory cytokines and chemokines.

Experimentally, pulmonary exposure of rats to endotoxin has been found to cause increases in pre-existing BALT and pulmonary plasma cells, ultimately leading to the formation of germinal centers. Sustained dosing of LPS prior to pulmonary inflammation in BALT-deficient mice appeared to result in BALT development in the major airways with an accumulation of B cells, T cells, and macrophages in the lungs, and even in BALT-deficient areas. Thus, environmental exposures to LPS, often with additional antigenic or inflammatory components, cause BALT reactivity and pulmonary physiology alterations.

Considering the importance of pulmonary inflammation in asthma, a correlation between BALT development and asthma is likely. However, some believe that the presence of BALT is not always associated with asthma, but that the reactivity of BALT in patients with asthma is elevated.

Further, there is evidence that specific allergens, such as *Aspergillus fumigatus*, might cause pulmonary allergies that are similar to asthma. In allergic bronchopulmonary aspergillosis, large BALT regions characterized by diffuse and IgE-stained germinal centers have been found. Thus, it is suggested that BALT can potentially contribute to allergic reactions by producing IgE locally in response to *A. fumigatus*.

Hypersensitivity pneumonia is defined as an inflammatory disease of the alveoli induced by hypersensitivity to inhaled organic antigens. In contrast to asthma, which affects the airways, this condition affects the alveoli. An occupational exposure often is the cause of hypersensitivity pneumonia; it can occur particularly when farmers are exposed to mold and fungi in barns. Considering that hypersensitivity pneumonia results from chronic pulmonary exposure to the antigen, the emergence of well-developed BALT areas with vast germinal centers and FDC networks is not surprising for researchers.

Role of BALT in response to particles

The lungs are exposed to a wide range of particles, many of which are naturally inflammatory because they cannot be metabolized and persist in phagocytes or because their components bind to specific receptors that trigger an inflammatory response.

Silicosis, for example, is a chronic diffuse parenchymal lung disease caused by prolonged exposure to inhaled crystalline silica particles. Pulmonary silica exposure reportedly results in nodules of mononuclear cell infiltration at the location of silica deposition, leading to pulmonary fibrosis. It has been proposed that pulmonary exposure of rats to silica causes silica-loaded alveolar macrophages to migrate across the epithelium and accumulate in BALT. This is analogous to the kinetic observation of virus-activated DCs in the airways migrating from the epithelium to BALT .

Role of BALT in autoimmune diseases

Rheumatoid arthritis (RA) and Sjögren's syndrome (SS) are autoimmune disorders characterized by the formation of ectopic lymphoid follicles in target tissues. Ectopic lymphoid follicles in the joints are common in patients with RA; whereas ectopic follicles in the salivary and lacrimal glands are common in those with SS. These follicles are hypothesized to contain separate B- and T-cell domains, germinal centers, FDCs, and HEVs, and they contribute toautoimmunity by generating high-affinity autoreactive B cells and sparing autoreactive effector T cells. BALT areas are observed in lung biopsies from a subset of patients with RA and SS who develop lung disease. It has been suggested to range from very small isolated lymphoid follicles to large, highly organized clusters of B-cell follicles.

Role of BALT in pulmonary malignancy

BALT formation is frequently linked to lung inflammation and exposure to a variety of inflammatory stimuli. Therefore, it is not surprising that experimental exposure to an inflammatory agent via the pulmonary route results in BALT hyperplasia in rats. However, it is possible that an inflammatory agent, which has been linked to tumorigenesis, could also cause pulmonary adenocarcinoma. Therefore, inflammatory responses in the lung can promote BALT and neoplasia at the same time. Indeed, considering the links between chronic inflammation and cancer development, it seems probable that BALT formation precedes tumorigenesis in such cases. Local immune responses to pulmonary pathogens and antigens are clearly associated with BALT formation; thus, it is predicted that BALT development adjacent to pulmonary malignancies would also be beneficial for antitumor immune responses. A study demonstrated tertiary lymphoid tissue neogenesis induced by lymphotoxin: antitumor antibody fusion protein with the accumulations of CD^{4+} and CD^{8+} T cells, B cells, and PNAd-expressing HEVs.

Thus, it was hypothesized that the immune response necessary for tumor eradication was produced locally in tertiary lymphoid tissues. Therefore, it is concluded that local BALT induction surrounding pulmonary metastases may be beneficial in inducing antitumor immunity and tumor regression.

In addition, it is suggested that the development of a lymphoid environment surrounding tumors may trigger antitumor immunity or immunological tolerance due to some unknown factors. Further, some studies indicate that lymphoid-like stromal elements surrounding tumors can impair antitumor immunity and lead to tolerance. Despite the discrepancies and gaps in the literature, the ability of BALT to be spontaneously developed as a clear response to the development of pulmonary tumors or metastasis of other tumors to the lung as well as to boost immunity against lung tumors is an intriguing and research-worthy topic.

CELLS OF THE IMMUNE SYSTEM

The cellular participants of the immune response can be categorized as either migratory cells or fixed cells. Lymphocytes are the principal migratory cells that are free to move anywhere in the body. Recirculation through the lymph or blood is a prominent feature of these leukocytes, ensuring effective surveillance of the tissues. The fixed cells are either mesenchymal or epithelial cells that form a scaffold for the stromal matrix in lymphatic tissue. These cells create a supportive framework that sustains the lymphocytes during different phases of development and function. The remarkable diversity of both migratory and fixed cells creates the unique character of lymphatic tissue.

Lymphocytes

Lymphocytes are migratory cells of the immune system that control adaptive immunity by initiating a specific response after encountering antigens. Antigens are molecular components of exogenous agents, such as bacteria, viruses, protozoa, or toxins, and endogenous agents, such as tumor cells and virus-infected cells. The lymphocytic lineage gives rise to two major cell types: B cells (bone marrow–dependent) and T cells (thymus-dependent). B cells and T cells and their subpopulations are distinguished by different surface molecules that recognize antigens (i.e., antigen receptors [Fig. 13]) and are involved in signal transduction and cell cooperation (e.g., major histocompatibility markers). B and T cells cannot be identified using standard histologic stains such as hematoxylin and eosin.

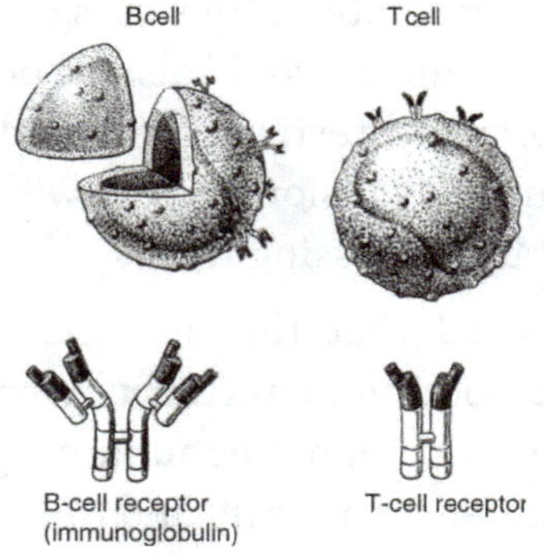

Fig. 13. Schematic drawing of lymphocyte surface antigen receptors. The B-cell receptor is an immunoglobulin (antibody) molecule that has two antigen-binding sites (dark segments), whereas the T-cell receptor has a single antigen-binding site.

B cells and T cells also differ in the way that they effect an immune response. After antigen stimulation, both lymphocyte types undergo proliferation and differentiation to become either memory cells or effector cells. Memory cells are long-lived cells that have the ability to mount an enhanced response upon a reencounter with antigen. Effector B-cell function is mediated by the secreted antigen receptor (immunoglobulin, also known as antibodies).

In their active secretory phase, B effector cells typically are manifest as plasma cells. Since antibodies circulate in the extracellular fluids ("humors"), B cells are said to be responsible for the humoral immune response. Antigen with attached antibody is more easily recognized by phagocytes and eliminated. The antigen–antibody complex also triggers a collection of plasma proteins, called the complement system. The complement system is an important component of innate defense with wide-ranging effects that include the ability to kill microorganisms.

Effector T cells, on the other hand, act more directly on adjacent cells within tissues. The two major subsets of effector T cells mediate their effects in different ways. T helper cells act through the secretion of soluble, local-acting molecules called cytokines, whereas the T cytotoxic cells attach to antigens on target cells to kill them (Fig. 14). Since these cell-killing actions require close cell-to-cell contact, T cells are said to be responsible for the cell-mediated immune response.

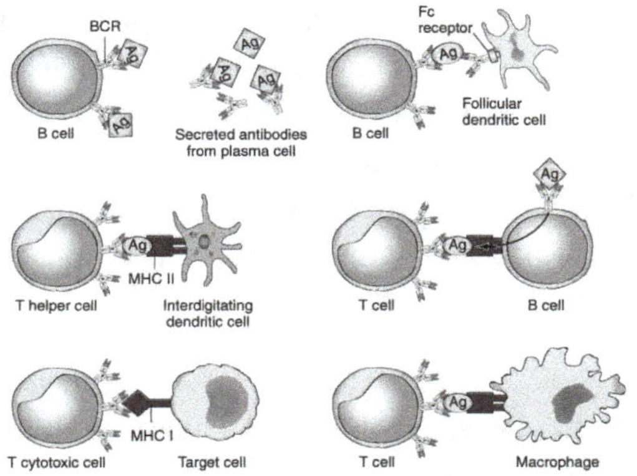

Fig. 14. Schematic drawing of antigen–antigen receptor interaction. The B-cell receptor (BCR) can interact directly with native antigen (Ag), either while bound to the plasma membrane of a B cell or as secreted antibody. The B-cell receptor also recognizes antigen presented by the follicular dendritic cell. The T-cell receptor recognizes processed antigen presented by a major histocompatibility complex (MHC-II) molecule on the surface of the interdigitating dendritic cell. The B cell can present antigen to T cells by binding the antigen, processing it, and presenting it in the context of MHC II (black arrow). Macrophages are also capable of presenting antigen to T cells.

A third category of lymphocyte, the natural killer (NK) cell, lacks an antigen receptor that is typical for either B or T cells. NK cells appear to rely on an antigen recognition system that is less specific than that used by B cells and T cells; however, cell-mediated killing by NK cells is similar to the mechanism of T cyto-toxic cells. NK cells participate in the elimination of tumors and virus-infected cells or other cells that show altered expression of "self" molecules. In some species, these cells appear as large granular lymphocytes.

Lymphocytes circulate continuously from the blood through lymphatic and nonlymphatic tissues and subsequently return to the blood either directly or via the lymph. This process, called lymphocyte recirculation, facilitates the dissemination of an immune response throughout the body and enables effective immune surveillance for foreign invaders and alterations in the body's own cells.

Most lymphocytes enter organs such as the lungs, liver, and bone marrow and return to the blood via venules, whereas some lymphocytes leave these organs via the lymph and drain to lymph nodes via afferent lymph vessels. Tissue fluid from large peripheral areas also drains into regional lymph nodes, further enhancing the likelihood of an encounter between a lymphocyte and its target antigen. A proportion of lymphocytes migrates from blood directly into lymphatic tissues through specialized postcapillary venules called high endothelial venules (Fig. 14). High endothelial venules have lining cells that are cuboidal, in contrast to the flattened endothelial cells of other blood vessels.

These specialized venules are abundant in lymphatic tissue and serve as the sites of entry for both T cells and B cells from the blood circulation. The spleen is an exception, because it does not possess specialized postcapillary venules or afferent lymphatics. Lymphocytes migrate into the spleen via blood capillaries in the marginal zone. Normally, relatively few lymphocytes migrate into organs such as the skin, synovia, muscle, and brain; however, during acute and chronic inflammation, an influx of large numbers of lymphocytes can occur.

Stromal Cells

Stromal cells are fixed cells of the lymphatic system that form a tissue reticulum and support the immune response. Either mesenchymal reticular cells or epithelial reticular cells form a supportive mesh or stroma for the lymphocytes that constitute the parenchyma of lymphatic organs.

Reticular Cells

Reticular cells of mesenchymal origin and fibroblastlike structure form a reticulum in all lymphatic organs except the thymus and cloacal bursa. Because of their numerous long and branching processes, reticular cells have a stellate appearance. These cells synthesize reticular fibers that are closely associated with or invaginated into their cell surface.

Epithelial Reticular Cells

In the thymus and cloacal bursa, stellate epithelial reticular cells form a reticulum that supports developing lymphocytes and macrophages. Unlike reticular cells, epithelial reticular cells do not produce reticular fibers.

Antigen-Presenting Cells

For antigen recognition and the initiation of an immune response to occur, B cells recognize antigen either directly or as complexes presented by an antigen-presenting cell such as the follicular dendritic cell (Fig. 14). T cells require antigen to be presented on the surface of an antigen-presenting cell, such as the inter-digitating dendritic cell, in association with a major histo-compatibility complex (MHC) molecule.

Dendritic Cells

Most dendritic cells (DCs), including the interstitial dendritic cell, interdigitating dendritic cell, veiled cell, and intraepidermal macrophage, are derived from hematopoietic stem cells. The origin of follicular dendritic cells is unclear. Typical dendriticcells have numerous long cytoplasmic processes (Fig. 14). Functionally, dendritic cells bind antigens and cluster lymphocytes on their surface in tissues throughout the body. Once antigens are bound and processed, the dendritic cell then becomes an antigen-presenting cell. In the stratified squamous epithelia, dendritic cells localize in the upper spinous layer and are termed intra-epidermal macrophages (Langerhans cells). When they are in lymph and blood, dendritic cells possess prominent surface folds and have been called veiled cells. Interstitial dendritic cells are located in the heart, kidney, gut and lung. Follicular dendritic cells and interdigitating dendritic cells are found in lymphatic tissues.

Follicular dendritic cells

Follicular dendritic cells are specialized stromal cells localized within the B-cell areas of lymphatic tissue. Receptors on the follicular dendritic cell surface bind to antigen and present it to B cells that induce a humoral immune response (Fig.14). In contrast to other dendritic cells, follicular dendritic cells can trap and maintain antigen in a complex for long periods of time. Follicular dendritic cells lack the MHC-II surface molecules found in interdigitating dendritic cells.

Interdigitating dendritic cells

Interdigitating dendritic cells are found in lymph nodes, thymic medulla, and spleen. Cytoplasmic granules are characteristic features of these dendritic cells, which also have numerous MHC-II molecules on their surface that are associated with antigen presentation (Fig. 14). The interdigitating dendritic cell presents antigen to T lymphocytes (helper cells), which induce a cellular immune response.

Macrophages

Macrophages, also known as mononuclear phagocytes, exist in various tissues and are active in the phagocytosis and degradation of foreign substances. The processing of foreign substances into short peptides is essential for presentation of antigen to T cells in the peptide-binding groove of the MHC-II molecule (Fig. 14).

B Cells

B cells express MHC-II molecules and are very efficient in the presentation of antigen to T helper cells. In contrast to macrophages, which will ingest most foreign substances, B cells bind a specific single antigen through surface immunoglobulin. The bound molecule is then endocytosed, fragmented, and presented by MHC-II molecules.

Mucosal Architecture, Immunophenotype, and Molecular Clonality

Lymphoma is the most common hemopoietic neoplasm in the cat, and the incidence is reported to be the highest for any species. Since the decline (in the United States) in the incidence of feline leukemia virus (FeLV) infection, which is highly lymphomagenic, the incidence of feline lymphoma has actually increased. This increase has mainly been in gastrointestinal lymphomas. Gastrointestinal lymphomas, especially mucosal T-cell lymphomas of the small intestine, have been underreported prior to the advent of T-cell receptor gene rearrangement analysis. Hence, the increased incidence of feline gastrointestinal lymphoma in recent years is likely to be of far greater magnitude.

The gastrointestinal tract harbors the largest population of lymphoid and accessory immune cells in the body. Not surprisingly, it is often a target for lymphoma. The diffuse, mucosal-associated lymphoid tissue (MALT) of the small intestine, which consists of lamina proprial compartments (LPC) and intraepithelial compartments (IEC), is populated largely by $CD3^+$ T cells in normal cats.[12,23] Less than 10% of villous lamina proprial lymphocytes (LPLs) are B cells, and even fewer are found in the IEC.

Intraepithelial lymphocytes (IEL) are almost exclusively T cells. The inductive environment for adaptive immune responses is concentrated in the distal small intestine and ileo–ceco–colic junction, where Peyer patches and solitary lympho-follicular structures are most prominent. Antigen-stimulated B cells are induced to class switch to immunoglobulin A and home to the lamina propria adjacent to intestinal crypts, and are most numerous below the crypt–villous junction. Naive T cells in Peyer patches and mesenteric lymph nodes are induced by interactions with migratory antigen-bearing mucosal dendritic cells (DCs) to express cell surface molecules, such as β7 integrins (α4β7 and αEβ7) and chemokine receptors (especially CCR9), that enable them to traffic to the diffuse MALT and enter the LPC and IEC of the small intestine.

Historically, pathologists have relied on the mucosal effacement and transmural invasion by cytologically atypical lymphocytes to confidently diagnose intestinal lymphoma. However, these morphologic criteria are less relevant when examining endoscopic biopsy specimens, which consist of mucosal and scant submucosal tissue with random orientation. Furthermore, lymphoma manifests in the intestinal mucosa long before transmural progression. T-cell lymphomas of diffuse MALT of the small intestine are the most predominant gastrointestinal lymphomas, which often coexist with lymphoplasmacytic inflammatory bowel disease (IBD) or occur following a clinical history of IBD.

Immunohistochemistry and molecular clonality assays are valuable adjuncts to morphological assessment in diagnosis of lymphoma. Immunophenotypic assessment is most useful in lymphocyte lineage assignment, although it can also highlight distinctive lymphocyte infiltration patterns such as epithelial colonization, which are important in assessing the likelihood of lymphoma.[3,18,23]

Lymphocyte antigen receptor gene rearrangement analysis has become an important method to establish the presence of clonal lymphocyte expansion in lymphoproliferative disease. In a recent article, we characterized the expressed feline T-cell receptor-γ (TCRG) repertoire. Multiple sequence alignment of TCRG variable (V) and joining (J) segments revealed highly conserved regions, which enabled development of primers for polymerase chain reaction (PCR) amplification of the CDR3 region for detection of the clonality status of T cells in feline intestinal lymphoma. In a companion article, we also characterized the expressed feline immunoglobulin heavy chain (IGH) repertoire and established its usefulness in the diagnosis of B-cell neoplasia.

Study Population

A total of 120 cats were included in the study. The majority of cats (*n* = 98) were presented to the Veterinary Medical Teaching Hospital, UC Davis, for clinical evaluation during the period 1995–2006. Tissues from another cohort of cats (*n* = 22) were accessed from a local private pathology laboratory (VDx, Davis, California) during the study period. The cases included in the study were limited to those in which a specialist review (P.F.M.) was requested. Tissues were collected by surgical biopsy (*n* = 47), by endoscopic biopsy (*n* = 35), and at necropsy (*n* = 38).

Immunohistochemistry

Expression of leukocyte antigens was assessed in formalin-fixed, paraffin-embedded (FFPE) tissue sections by a labelled avidin–biotin immunohistochemical technique and heat-based antigen retrieval. Gastrointestinal tissue from all cats was assessed for the expression of CD3 (clone CD3-12, Serotec Inc, Oxford, UK) and CD79a (clone HM57, Dako Inc, Carpinteria, California). Transmural T-cell lymphomas of large granular lymphocyte type (LGL) (*n* = 9) were evaluated for expression of granzyme B by immunohistochemistry with a rabbit polyclonal antibody, which is specific for a conserved human granzyme B-peptide sequence (Fig. 15) (Spring Bioscience, Pleasanton, California).

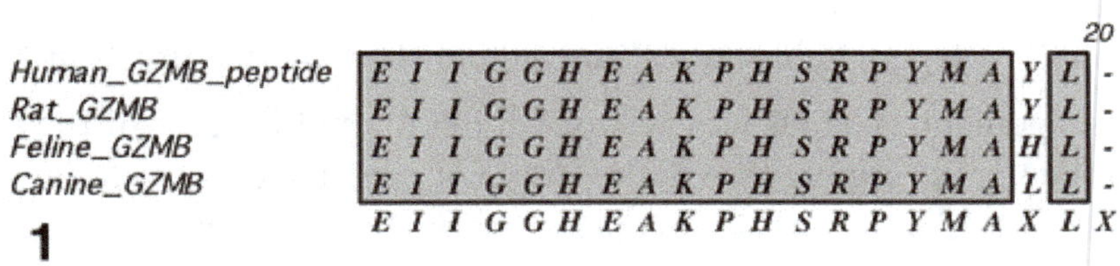

Fig. 15. Multiple-species amino acid sequence alignment of the granzyme B-peptide immunogen (human) demonstrates the highly conserved sequence used to generate the polyclonal antibody to granzyme B.

Lymphoma Classification

Lymphomas were classified as B-cell, T-cell, or non-B, non-T cell lymphoma lymphoma by immunohistochemistry to detect expression of CD3 and CD79a. The lymphomas were further classified as mucosal lymphoma (infiltrate confined to the epithelium and lamina propria with minimal extension into the submucosa) or transmural lymphoma (infiltrate extending markedly into the submucosa and muscularis propria). Endoscopic biopsy specimens, although diagnostically adequate, did not include tissue below the muscularis mucosa. Hence, transmural spread was impossible to assess, resulting in a default diagnosis of mucosal lymphoma. The diagnosis of lymphoma was based on the cytomorphology of the infiltrate, the degree of epitheliotropism (if present), and the pattern of lamina proprial infiltration; the specific criteria are fully described and illustrated below. The infiltration patterns were then compared with the World Health Organization (WHO) classification of tumors of the hematopoietic and lymphoid tissues to further classify B- and T-cell neoplasia into clinicopathologic entities.

Statistical Methods

Survival data were obtained for 54 of the 84 cats with mucosal T-cell lymphoma and for 13 of the 19 cats with transmural T-cell lymphoma. Insufficient survival data were obtained for cats with B-cell lymphoma. The effect of cell size and tumor location on survival time was evaluated using the Kaplan-Meier method of survival function estimation and Cox proportional hazards regression. Regression results are reported as hazard ratios (HRs, ie, the ratio of 2 conditional mortality rates) and 95% confidence intervals (95% CIs). Interaction between model covariates was evaluated with a likelihood ratio test. STATA 10.1 (StataCorp LP, College Station, Texas) was used for all calculations.

LYMPHOCYTE ANTIGEN RECEPTOR GENE REARRANGEMENT ANALYSIS

Clonality of lymphocyte antigen receptor genes (TRG and/or IGH) was performed on tissues from 119 of 120 cats as previously described. Briefly, DNA extraction was performed on 25-μm tissue sections that were cut from FFPE blocks using the DNeasy Extraction Kit (Qiagen, Valencia, California) per the manufacturer's instructions.

Rearrangement of TCRG was assessed by PCR amplification of the CDR3 region between the V and J segments. Briefly, 100 ng of genomic DNA from each sample was amplified in a 50-μl reaction using a consensus primer derived from the TCRG V segment (52 -AAGAGCGAYGAGGGMGTGT-32 —20 pmol) in conjunction with a consensus primer derived from the TCRG J segments (52 -CTGAGCAGTGTGCCAGSACC-32 —10 pmol) of the feline TCRG cDNA transcripts. Specific amplicon size was expected to occur within a target range of about 80–120 base pairs. Amplification conditions used a 2-step, modified touchdown protocol to increase specificity of the reactions. All PCR reactions were run in duplicate.

Rearrangement of IGH was assessed by amplification of the CDR3 region, which encompasses the junction of V, diversity (D), and J segments. Briefly, 100 ng of genomic DNA from each sample was amplified in a 50-μl reaction using consensus primers derived from the IGH V segment framework 2 (FR2) and framework 3 (FR3) (FR2: 52 -CCAGGCTCCAGGGAAGGG-32 —10 pmol, and FR3: 52 -TCCAGAGACAACGCCAAGAAC-32 —10 pmol) in conjunction with consensus primers derived from IGH J segments (J2: 52 -TGAGGACAC TGTGACTATGGTTCC-32 —10 pmol, and JD: 52 -GGACACCGTCACYAKGVY TCC-32 —100 pmol). Amplification conditions used a 2-step, modified touchdown protocol to increase specificity of the reactions. All PCR reactions were run in duplicate.

PCR products were separated by polyacrylamide gel electrophoresis (PAGE) of both native and denatured 15-μl samples of each PCR reaction. Polyacrylamide gels (Criterion Precast gels, Bio-Rad, Hercules, California), which contained both native and denatured PCR products, were run on ice in Tris-borate-EDTA (TBE) buffer at 150 V for 2 hours. Duplicate PCR samples were always run side by side. Gels were then stained for 30 minutes with Gel Star (BioWhitaker Molecular Applications, Rockland, Maine) and visualized with a UV transilluminator (Fisher Scientific, Pittsburgh, Pennsylvania). Samples that produced appropriately and same sized 1 or 2 sharp bands in duplicate were classified as clonal (monoallelic or biallelic rearrangement, respectively). Samples exhibiting 3–5 reproducible bands in duplicate analyses were classified as oligoclonal. Duplicate PCR reactions were used to help distinguish true clonal samples from pseudoclonal samples. Pseudoclonal samples contained 1 or 2 bands of disparate size in duplicate analysis. Samples that produced a broad band, smear, or ladder of bands covering a range of product sizes were classified as a polyclonal.

Signalment

Cats with mucosal lymphoma (n = 86) consisted of 51 males and 35 females; the mean age at the time of diagnosis was 12.6 years (SD 3.4 years; range, 2-20 years). Mucosal T-cell lymphoma predominated (n = 84); non-B- and non-T-cell lymphoma occurred in only 2 cats. Cats with transmural T-cell lymphoma (n = 19) consisted of 7 males and 12 females; the mean age was 13.5 years (SD 2.6 years; range, 7–18 years). Cats with B-cell lymphoma (n = 19) consisted of 11 males and 8 females; the mean age was 12.2 years (SD 4.0 years; range, 2-18 years). There were 120 cats included in the study; 4 cats (cat Nos. 103, 115, 116, and 117) had concurrent B-cell lymphoma and mucosal T-cell lymphoma. Only 3 cats were serologically positive for feline immunodeficiency virus (FIV) (cat Nos. 24, 39, and 120), and none tested positive for FeLV.

Survival

Survival data were available for 54 of the 84 cats with mucosal T-cell lymphoma; 13 of the 19 cats with transmural T-cell lymphoma; and only 6 cats with B-cell lymphoma. Median time to death in the mucosal T-cell lymphoma group (n = 54) was 29 months, in contrast to the transmural T-cell lymphoma group (n = 13), in which it was 1.5

months. The median time to death in the small-cell, T-cell lymphoma group (*n* = 54) was 28 months, in contrast to the large-cell, T-cell lymphoma group (*n* = 13), in which it was 1.5 months. The mucosal T-cell lymphoma group largely consisted of small-cell type (*n* = 50/54), whereas the transmural T-cell lymphoma group was mostly of large-cell type (*n* = 9/13), with most of these (*n* = 8/9) being LGL lymphomas. A multivariate model examining the joint effects of cell size and location found a higher rate of death in the large-cell versus small-cell group (HR = 3.7; 95% CI, 1.2–10.9; *P* = .019) and in the transmural versus mucosal location group (HR = 3.4; 95% CI, 1.3–8.7; *P* = .010). Limited survival data (*n* = 6) were available for the B-cell lymphoma group; the median time to death was 3.5 months. Similarly, limited survival data (*n* = 4) were available for the transmural, small-cell, T-cell lymphoma cats, with a range of survival encompassing 3 days to 28 months.

Topographical Features

Feline intestinal lymphoma in our case series was most frequently of T-cell phenotype and occurred predominately in the diffuse MALT of the small intestine as mucosal (*n* = 84) and transmural lesions (*n* = 19) (Figs. 16, 17).

The jejunum was the most common intestinal segment affected in both mucosal and transmural T-cell lymphoma. However, lesions frequently involved more than 1 intestinal segment (Figs. 16, 17). Endoscopic biopsies were excluded from the topographical analysis, because they only sample the duodenum. Extension of mucosal T-cell lymphoma to the stomach and large bowel occurred with markedly lower frequency. Transmural T-cell lymphoma only occurred in the small intestine.

B-cell lymphomas were often multiple and occurred simultaneously in multiple locations in 9 of 19 cats (47%), for example, in the stomach and at the ileo-cecal-colic junction (Fig. 18). We did not encounter B-cell lymphomas that involved the duodenum except in 1 instance (cat No. 114) in which there was direct extension from lymphoma infiltrating the gastric pylorus. B-cell lymphomas occurred in the distal half of the small intestine from midjejunum to the ileum.

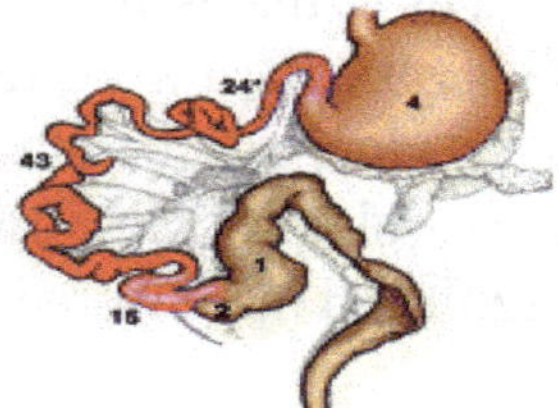

Fig. 16. Frequency of involvement of gastrointestinal segments in mucosal T-cell lymphoma.

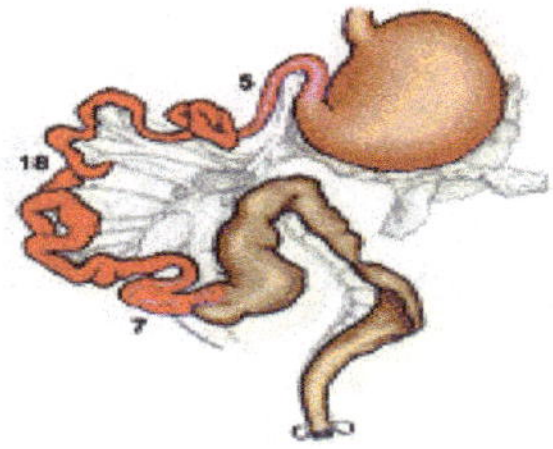

Fig. 17. Frequency of involvement of intestinal segments in transmural T-cell lymphoma.

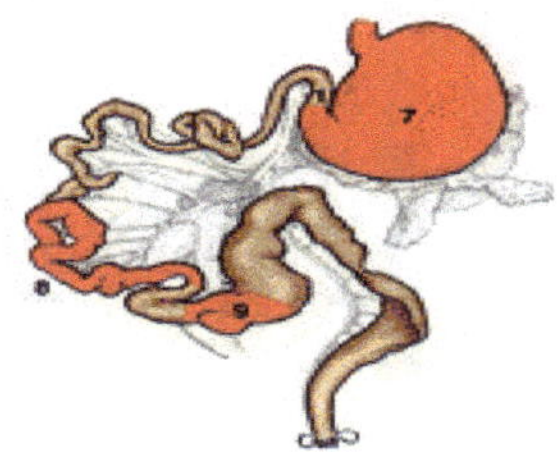

Fig. 18. Frequency of involvement of gastrointestinal segments in B-cell lymphoma.

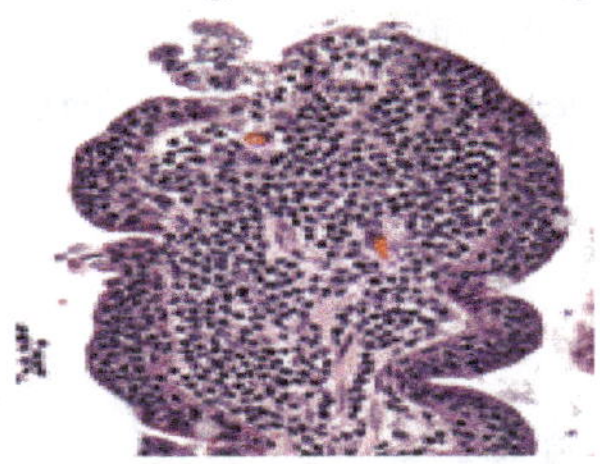

Fig. 19. Duodenum; cat No. 58; mucosal T-cell lymphoma. Patterns of epitheliotropism. There is diffuse lymphocytic infiltration of the villous epithelium and adjacent lamina propria. Lymphocytes are intermediate-sized and have moderately dispersed chromatin. Adjacen. villi were uninvolved (not shown). Hematoxylin and eosin

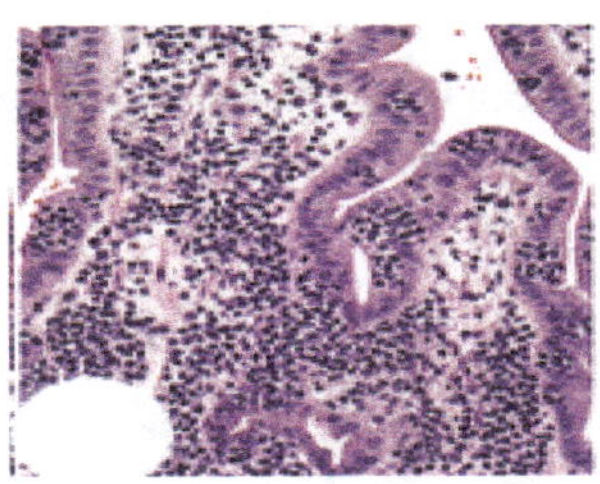

Fig. 20. Jejunum; cat No. 98; mucosal T-cell lymphoma proximal to a transmural lymphoma segment. Patterns of epitheliotropism. Clusters of lymphocytes are found within the villous epithelium. There is patchy lymphocytic infiltration of the adjacent lamina propria.

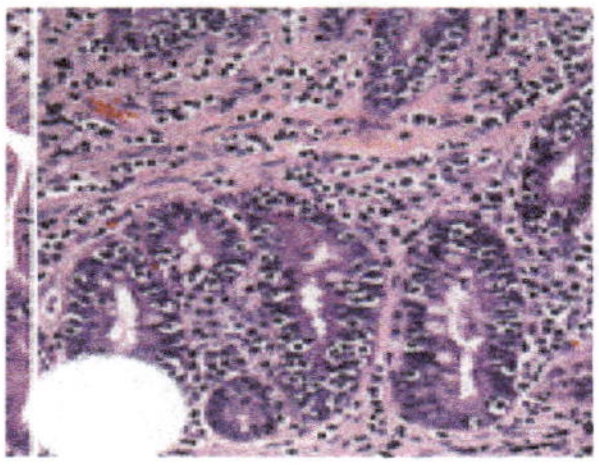

Fig. 21 Jejunum; cat No. 47; mucosal T-cell lymphoma. Patterns of epitheliotropism. There is diffuse lymphocytic infiltration of the crypt epithelium; the villous epithelium was also diffusely infiltrated (not shown).

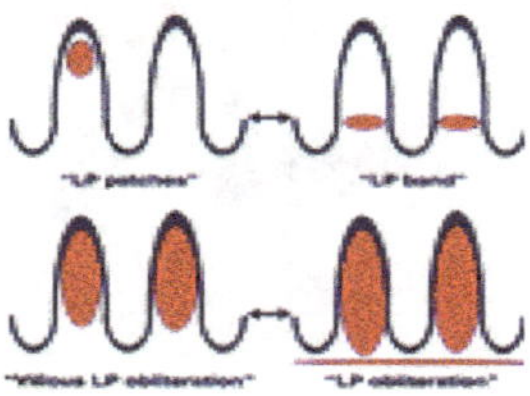

Fig. 22. Patterns of lamina proprial (LP) infiltration in mucosal T-cell lymphoma that are recognizable in endoscopic and surgical biopsy specimens of small intestine. Arrows indicate the level of the crypt–villous junction.

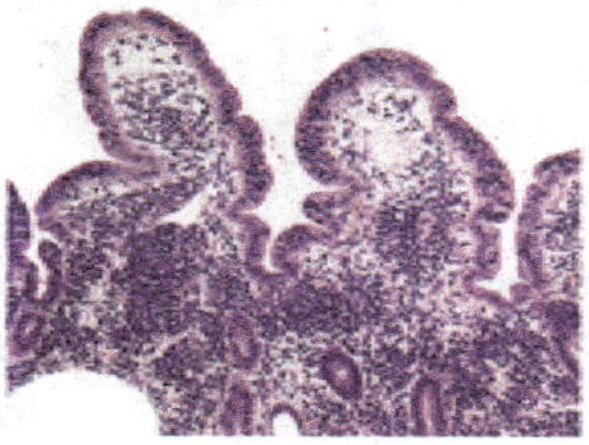

Fig. 23. Jejunum; cat No. 98; mucosal T-cell lymphoma proximal to a transmural lymphoma segment (not shown). Patterns of lamina proprial infiltration. There is a patchy lymphocytic infiltrate in the villous and cryptal lamina propria.

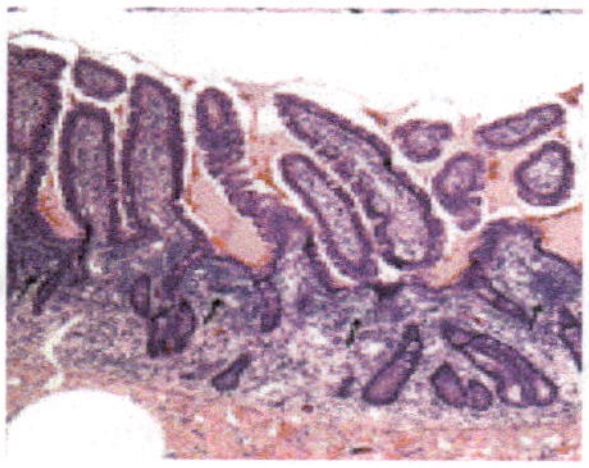

Fig. 24. Jejunum; cat No. 80; mucosal T-cell lymphoma. Patterns of lamina proprial infiltration. There is a band-like lymphocytic infiltrate in the lamina propria spanning the cryptvillous junction (arrows).

Mucosal Architecture in T-Cell Lymphoma

T-cell lymphomas were defined by CD3 expression and characteristic morphological features and initially arose in the diffuse MALT of the intestine. T-cell lymphomas arose in the IEC and the LPC.

Epitheliotropism was a dominant feature of T-cell lymphoma. Two patterns of T-cell epitheliotropism were encountered: diffuse lymphocytic infiltration of the IEC and discrete clusters of lymphocytes within the IEC (Figs. 19–21). Lymphocyte epitheliotropism occurred most commonly in the villous epithelium and less commonly in the crypt epithelium (Fig. 21). Epitheliotropic lymphocytic infiltrates, which exceeded normal IEL density, occurred in 52 of the 84 cats (62%) with mucosal T-cell lymphoma and in 11 of the 19 cats (58%) with transmural T-cell lymphoma. The recognition of IELs was significantly enhanced in sections stained for CD3 expression.

Mucosal T-cell lymphomas, with and without marked epitheliotropism, involved the lamina propria of the small intestine in a variety of patterns, ranging from discrete, patchy, lymphocytic infiltrates to total effacement of the lamina propria (Fig. 22). In the least severe lesions, discrete regions of increased lymphocyte density occurred within the villous lamina propria; adjacent villi were often uninvolved (Fig. 23). Alternatively, infiltration occurred as a band of increased lymphocyte density that spanned the crypt–villous junction (Fig. 24). In more advanced lesions, dense lymphocytic infiltrates expanded the villous lamina propria (Fig. 25). The most severe lesions were associated with complete lymphocytic infiltration of the villous and crypt lamina propria with the formation of a lymphocytic band beneath the crypt epithelium but above the muscularis mucosae (Fig. 26). In the latter instances, marked mucosal changes, such as villous blunting, villous fusion, and crypt effacement, were evident (Fig. 26).

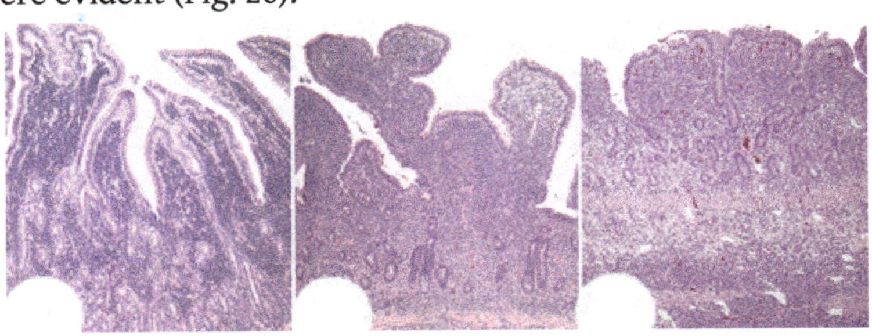

Fig. 25. Jejunum; cat No. 94; mucosal T-cell lymphoma. Patterns of lamina proprial infiltration. There is dense monomorphous, lymphocytic infiltration of the villous lamina propria. HE.

Fig. 26. Jejunum; cat No. 47; mucosal T-cell lymphoma. Patterns of lamina proprial infiltration. There is dense monomorphous, lymphocytic infiltration of the villous and cryptal lamina propria. The infiltrate extends beneath the crypts but above the muscularis mucosa. The mucosal architecture is markedly altered by villous blunting and fusion and crypt obliteration. HE.

Fig. 27. Jejunum; cat No. 98; transmural T-cell lymphoma. Dense monomorphous, lymphocytic infiltration of the lamina propria, submucosa, and muscularis propria is associated with villous blunting and fusion.

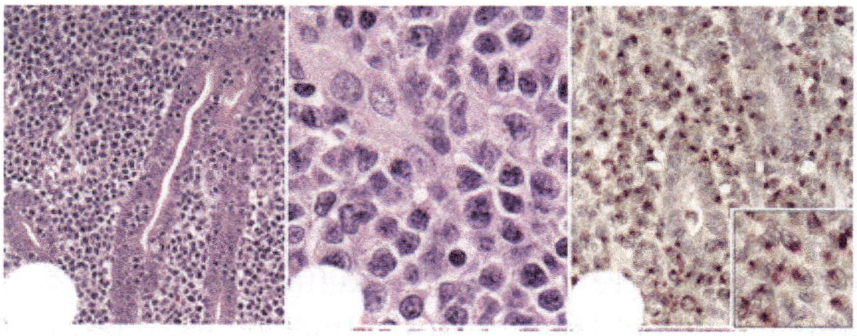

Fig. 28. Jejunum; cat No. 98; transmural T-cell lymphoma. Large lymphocytes infiltrate the lamina propria and form clusters in the crypt epithelium. HE.

Fig. 29. Jejunum; cat No. 98; transmural T-cell lymphoma. The lymphoid infiltrate is pleomorphic; the nuclei are large and frequently cleaved. Juxtanuclear, eosinophilic, cytoplasmic granules are visible in many lymphocytes. HE.

Fig. 30. Jejunum; cat No. 98; transmural T-cell lymphoma. Granzyme B expression is manifest as juxtanuclear, intracytoplasmic, aggregated granules. Inset: higher magnification. immunoperoxidase stain with Vector red substrate; hematoxylin counterstain.

The lymphoid infiltrates in mucosal T-cell lymphoma were composed of small to intermediate-sized lymphocytes (nuclear diameter <2 red cell diameters) in 80 of 84 cats (Figs. 19, 20). In 2 instances each, the infiltrates consisted of large lymphocytes or large lymphocytes with eosinophilic cytoplasmic granules (LGL) (nuclear diameter >2 red cell diameters). Based on the above array of features, mucosal T-cell lymphoma closely matched the WHO entity enteropathy-associated T-cell lymphoma (EATCL) type II.

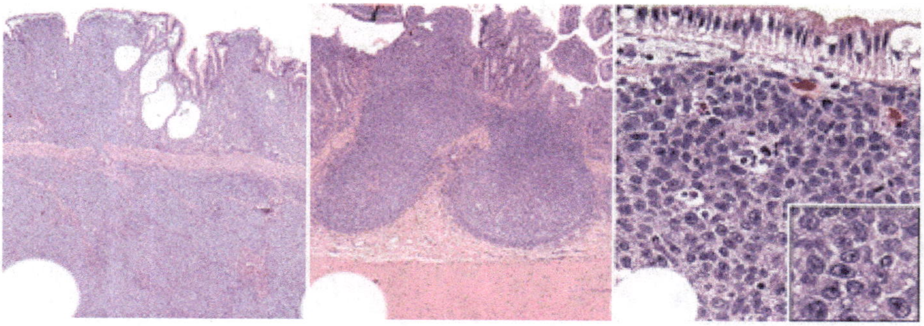

Fig. 31. Stomach; cat No. 116; transmural B-cell lymphoma. Dense, monomorphous lymphocytic infiltrate has effaced the gastric mucosa, leaving sparse, dilated glands. The infiltrate extends into and effaces the muscularis propria.

Fig. 32. Distal ileum; cat No. 116; B-cell lymphoma. There is diffuse infiltration of a Peyer patch by large lymphocytes. Follicular germinal centers have been effaced and the infiltrates extend into the mucosa above.

Fig. 33. Stomach; cat No. 116; transmural B-cell lymphoma. The infiltrate consists of large lymphocytes with pleomorphic nuclear morphology. Inset: most possess a single, large, central nucleolus (immunoblastic morphology); others have multiple, peripherally located, small nucleoli (centroblastic morphology).

Transmural T-cell lymphomas of the small intestine occurred both focally and multifocally. Characteristically, the mucosal lamina propria was effaced and the submucosa was heavily infiltrated (Fig. 27). In the least severe transmural lesions, the lymphocytic infiltrate traversed the muscularis propria (tunica muscularis) perivascularly, leading to a trabecular pattern of involvement. In advanced lesions, coalescence of the lymphocytic infiltrate obliterated the muscularis propria and spilled into the serosa and adjacent mesentery. This often resulted in mass formation, intestinal obstruction, and even perforation with peritonitis. Mucosal changes such as villous blunting, villous fusion, and crypt effacement were most severe in transmural lymphomas (Fig. 27). Intestinal segments proximal and distal to transmural foci almost invariably manifested with mucosal lymphoma (Fig. 23).

The lymphoid infiltrates in transmural T-cell lymphoma were composed of large lymphocytes in 11 of 19 cats (Fig. 28, 29); the infiltrate was composed of small to intermediate-sized lymphocytes in the remainder. In 9 of 11 cats, the lymphoid infiltrate was characterized by the presence of eosinophilic cytoplasmic granules (Fig. 29), which are a feature of LGL. All 9 transmural LGL T-cell lymphomas expressed the cytotoxic granule protein, granzyme B (Fig. 30). Based on the above array of features, transmural T-cell lymphomas closely matched the WHO entity EATCL type I.

Mucosal Architecture in B-Cell Lymphoma

Gastric and intestinal B-cell lymphomas occurred as transmural lesions in 18 of 19 cats (95%). Neoplastic B cells expressed CD79a in all cases.

In the gastric mucosa, B-cell lymphomas often infiltrated the lamina propria without clear association with preexisting lymphoid follicles (Fig. 31). However, in the small intestine, cecum, and colon, B-cell lymphomas were often clearly associated with mucosal lymphoid follicles (Fig. 32). This association was obscured as foci of proliferation expanded, coalesced, and traversed the muscularis propria to manifest as transmural, diffuse, large B-cell lymphoma in both stomach and intestinal sites (Fig. 31). Incursion of neoplastic B cells into the overlying mucosal epithelium was an infrequent occurrence (cat No. 113). B-cell lymphomas were classified as the WHO entity diffuse large B-cell lymphoma. Cytologically, B-cell lymphomas most commonly had centroblastic nuclear morphology, in which multiple nucleoli were visible, often adjacent to the nuclear membrane. B-cell lymphomas of immunoblastic type occurred in only 2 of 19 cats (11%); single large central nucleoli predominated in these instances (Fig. 33).

Concurrent Lymphomas

We encountered cats that had more than 1 lymphoma in the gastrointestinal tract. Four cats (cat Nos. 103, 115, 116, and 117) had diffuse large B-cell lymphoma in the stomach and/or the cecum and colon. Additionally, these cats had small T-cell lymphoma of the diffuse MALT of the small intestine, which was confirmed by TCRG gene rearrangement analysis. One of these cats (cat No. 103) also had T-cell lymphoma in the stomach and large intestine adjacent to the foci of B-cell lymphoma (collision tumor). The existence of concurrent T-cell lymphomas originating from distinct T-cell clones was documented in 2 cats (cat Nos. 24 and 38). In each instance, a different T-cell clone (based on PCR product size) was found in the lamina propria of the stomach and the duodenum by analysis of TCRG gene rearrangement in both sites.

Molecular Clonality

Molecular clonality assessment of mucosal T-cell lymphoma revealed clonal rearrangement of TCRG in 66 of 84 cats (78%). Oligoclonal rearrangements were detected in 11 cats (13%). Polyclonal TCRG rearrangements were detected in the remaining 7 cats. Clonality assessment was particularly sensitive in the least severe lesions; only 1 of 21 cats returned a polyclonal result.

Molecular clonality assessment of transmural T-cell lymphoma revealed clonal rearrangement of TCRG in 15 of 19 cats (79%). Oligoclonal rearrangements were detected in 2 cats (11%). Polyclonal TCRG rearrangements were detected in the remaining 2 cats.

Molecular clonality assessment of gastrointestinal B-cell lymphoma revealed clonal rearrangement of IGH in 9 of 18 cats tested (50%). Pseudoclonality was detected in 7 of 18 cats (39%); this occurred when the primers failed to amplify tumor target DNA and, instead, randomly amplified target DNA from scant normal residual B cells. Pseudoclonality was only detectable with duplicate PCR reactions. Polyclonal IGH rearrangements were detected in the remaining 2 cats.

Transmural lymphomas (B- or T-cell type) were readily diagnosed by morphological features alone. Immunohistochemistry to detect specific antigen receptor–associated membrane proteins, CD3 and CD79a, was only necessary to determine lineage. Transmural T-cell lymphoma, large-cell type, corresponded closely to human EATCL type I. Together, mucosal and transmural T-cell lymphomas accounted for 83% of all gastrointestinal lymphomas (lymphomas). In previous studies, the true incidence of feline gastrointestinal T-cell lymphoma was likely underestimated because of difficulty in distinguishing mucosal T-cell lymphoma from lymphoplasmacytic IBD before widespread availability of molecular clonality assays. Indications that T-cell lymphomas may be more common in the small intestine of cats than previously realized have also been reported. However, the dominance of T-cell lymphoma in the small intestine of cats was recently confirmed in studies in which T-cell antigen receptor rearrangement analysis was used.18,35 Furthermore, the common occurrence of epitheliotropism in small intestinal T-cell lymphoma of cats has also been described. In a recent report, the low-grade nature of T-cell lymphoma of small-cell type and its association with prolonged survival (median 18.9 months) were highlighted.

T-cell lymphomas (mucosal and transmural) were almost exclusively localized to the small intestine, especially the jejunum. There were only 7 instances (7%) of T-cell lymphoma involving the stomach or large intestine. Trafficking of T cells to the intestinal mucosa is precisely regulated and is dependent in part upon T-cell expression of a4b7 (a mucosal homing integrin). Small intestinal T-cell homing, in particular, is largely dependent upon the additional expression of CCR9. CCL25, the ligand of CCR9, is almost exclusively expressed in the epithelium of the small intestine. Entry of T cells into the epithelium is dependent on CCR9/CCL25 interaction. Epitheliotropism is associated with upregulation of CD103 (aE), which associates with b7 (aEb7). E-cadherin, which is expressed by enterocytes, is a ligand of CD103 and may contribute to tethering of IELs within the IEC. We have documented the expression of CD103 in IELs of feline small intestine and in epitheliotropic T-cell LGL lymphoma of the small intestine. Hence, expression of mucosal b7 integrins, especially a4 and CD103, and CCR9 in mucosal T-cell lymphoma would be expected to lead to localization within the lamina propria and IEC of the small intestine preferentially.

Epitheliotropism of T cells is a normal feature in the small intestine of many species including cats, and IELs are an important first line of defense of the intestinal mucosa. IELs are also involved in immunoregulatory functions and serve to limit inflammation in an environment shared with many commensal microorganisms. The density of IELs has often been expressed as a percentage of enterocytes (i.e. number of IELs per 100 enterocytes). The density of IELs in normal cats as reported covers a wide range. In one study from the United Kingdom, feline IELs ranged from 40 to 80 per 100 villous enterocytes depending on the intestinal segment. This range far exceeded the density of IELs (18 per 100 villous enterocytes) reported in a second study conducted in the United States. A similar study from the United Kingdom conducted in dogs reported an average of 20 IELs per 100 villous enterocytes. The reasons for these marked differences in the 2 feline studies are unknown but likely include the source of the "normal" cats, diet, and environmental factors. The distribution of IELs also differs markedly between villous and crypt epithelium. IEL counts in normal small intestine of cats and dogs were 4- to 10-fold higher in villous epithelium than in crypt epithelium.

The normal IEL distribution pattern was echoed in T-cell lymphoma with prominent epitheliotropism, which occurred in about 60% of T-cell lymphoma cases (mucosal and transmural). Epitheliotropism was more frequent in villous epithelium and less in crypt epithelium. However, prominent crypt epitheliotrop-ism by IELs was distinctly abnormal and readily recognizable, and it increased the likelihood that the disease process was epitheliotropic T-cell lymphoma. Epitheliotropism was manifest as discrete clusters of IELs or as a diffuse infiltrate of the villous and/or crypt epithelium. Clusters of IELs in villous or crypt epithelium were readily recognizable and increased the likelihood of lymphoma. The significance of intraepithelial lymphocyte clusters in establishing a diagnosis of intestinal lymphoma in cats has been previously emphasized.

However, recognition that epitheliotropic lymphocytes were of T-cell lineage relied on studies that used immunohistochemical and immunofluorescence techniques. Diffuse villous epitheliotropism is more difficult to assess, and interobserver variability is high. However, if the number of IELs exceeds 40 per 100 enterocytes, there is higher likelihood of lymphoma. Importantly, IELs are often underrecognized in HE-stained sections and definitely appear more numerous in CD3 stained sections; this has been previously noticed by others.

Epitheliotropism was not a prominent feature in about 40% of T-cell lymphoma cases. However, in both epitheliotropic and nonepitheliotropic T-cell lymphomas, we recognized distinctive patterns of lymphocytic infiltration of the lamina propria by small to intermediate-sized lymphocytes. These patterns were highly correlated with the presence of mucosal T-cell lymphoma and hence were diagnostically important. A characteristic of the least severe T-cell lymphoma (commonly referred to as "emerging") was patchy infiltration of the lamina propria (and epithelium), such that some villi were infiltrated whereas adjacent villi were spared.

In some instances, a band-like lymphocytic infiltration of the lamina propria, which spanned the crypt–villous junction, was observed in early mucosal T-cell lymphoma. These 2 patterns of lamina proprial infiltration have been portrayed as representing early or emerging intestinal lymphoma in cats, although formal proof of this concept would be difficult to achieve in a clinical setting. Heavy monomorphous lymphoid infiltrates of small to intermediate-sized cells were readily recognized as mucosal T-cell lymphoma when they effaced the villous lamina propria or the entire mucosa. Associated mucosal architectural alterations such as villous blunting and fusion and crypt effacement were only observed in advanced mucosal T-cell lymphoma. It is highly likely that continued expression of mucosal homing molecules by neoplastic T cells would reinforce these mucosal infiltrative patterns and result in an extended sojourn within the mucosal environment without spread to extraintestinal sites.

Analysis of TCRG rearrangement proved to be highly sensitive for detection of mucosal T-cell lymphoma regardless of the severity of the lesion. If clonal and oligoclonal results were combined, the sensitivity was 91%. In transmural T-cell lymphoma, the combined sensitivity (clonal plus oligoclonal results) was 90%. Failure to detect clonality (polyclonal result) can occur if gene segments, which are unaccounted for by the TCRG V and J primers, are used in the rearrangement process. Identification of all TCRG gene segments will only be possible once the feline genome is assembled.

The interpretation of TCRG oligoclonality is complex. Oligoclonality is consistent with markedly reduced TCRG repertoire diversity in a chronic inflammatory background or emerging lymphoma with multiple neoplastic clones.2 The latter is the more likely reason for an oligoclonal result in a lesion that is morphologically consistent with lymphoma. The presence of 2 neoplastic T-cell clones in topologically distinct sites in the gut of a single cat has been reported and also occurred in this series in 2 cats that had concurrent, distinct T-cell lymphomas in different locations.18 If these clones occurred in the same site, an oligoclonal TCRG rearrangement could be observed in the event of biallelic rearrangement. An alternative explanation for apparent TCRG oligoclonality is the presence of multiple TCRG rearrangements on a single chromosome as occurs in the dog (manuscript in preparation).

This is facilitated by the complex genomic structure of the canine TCRG locus, which is organized into 8 V–J–C cassettes, many of which are capable of independent rearrangement.17 However, until the genomic structure of the feline TCRG locus is known, the likelihood of multiple rearrangements on a single chromosome is unknown.

Cats with mucosal T-cell lymphoma had a median survival of 29 months (n = 54). The vast majority of these cats (n = 50) had small-cell lymphoma (median survival 28 months). The favorable survival of cats with T-cell lymphoma of small-cell type has also been reported by others. Cats with transmural T-cell lymphoma (n = 13) had a much shorter median survival (1.5 months). The majority of these cats (n = 9) had large-cell lymphoma, especially of LGL type (n = 8). Transmural T-cell lymphoma of small-cell type occurred with low frequency (n = 4) and a wide survival range (3 days to 28 months); meaningful median survival data were not obtained for this group of cats. The poor median survival of cats with transmural LGL lymphoma is reinforced by the findings of our previous work in which the median survival of cats with LGL lymphoma and secondary leukemia was only 19 days. Clearly, the presence of secondary leukemia had a markedly adverse effect on prognosis. Survival time may be influenced by choice of treatment; we did not attempt to correlate treatment regimens with survival time, because these data were not readily available for many of the cats, which were commonly treated by the referring veterinarian (remotely).

Feline gastrointestinal B-cell lymphomas were exclusively classified as diffuse, large B-cell lymphomas. Evidence for progression from an initial mucosal marginal zone lymphoma was lacking. Mucosal marginal zone lymphomas in humans characteristically originate as perifollicular B cell expansions with prominent epitheliotropism; the latter was only observed in a single cat in the absence of perifollicular growth. B-cell lymphomas occurred with higher frequency in the stomach and ileo–ceco–colic junction of cats. The latter sites are enriched for organized lymphoid tissues (mucosal lymphofollicular structures), and evidence of B-cell lymphoma could be found in lymphoid follicles adjacent to transmural lesions. Further indication of postgerminal center origin of gastrointestinal B-cell lymphoma was evident in the results of molecular clonality determination. Analysis of IGH rearrangement in feline gastrointestinal B-cell lymphoma was relatively insensitive (50%). This was likely attributable to somatic hypermutation of IGH V segments that occurs normally in B cells, which pass through follicular germinal centers and are subjected to affinity maturation of the immunoglobulin response to antigen. However, B-cell lymphomas in the stomach did not clearly originate in mucosal lymphofollicular structures, although it is possible that rapid transmural extension may have obscured these relationships.

CHAPTER 7

THE MAJOR HISTOCOMPATIBILITY COMPLEX

INTRODUCTION

The major histocompatibility complex (MHC) (also called human leukocyte antigens, HLAs) is the mechanism by which the immune system is able to differentiate between self and nonself cells. The MHC is a collection of glycoproteins (proteins with a carbohydrate) that exist on the plasma membranes of nearly all body cells. The proteins of a single individual are unique, originating from 20 genes, with more than 50 variations per gene between individuals. Thus, it is extremely unlikely that two people, except for identical twins, will possess cells with the same set of MHC molecules.

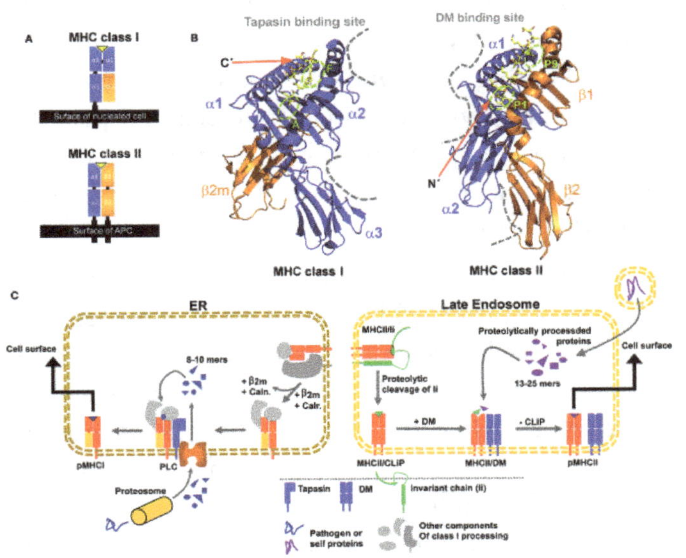

Fig. 1. Structural Characteristics Of Major Histocompatibility Complex (MHC) Class I and MHC Class II proteins and their compartment-dependent loading with processed peptides. (A) Domain topology of a pMHC class I and pMHC class II complex. (B) Structure of HLAA68 in complex with an HIV-derived peptide (PDB: 4HWZ, left) and HLA

The immune system is able to identify nonself cells by aberrations in the MHC displayed on the plasma membrane. There are two groups of MHC molecules, and each group generates different markings on the plasma membrane:

- MHC I glycoproteins are produced by all body cells (except red blood cells). When a cell becomes cancerous or is invaded by a virus, unfamiliar proteins are synthesized in the cell. These proteins are endogenous antigens—that is, antigens produced inside the cell. Portions of these antigens are combined with MHC I glycoproteins and, when displayed on the plasma membrane, indicate a nonself cell.
- MHC II glycoproteins are produced only by antigen presenting cells (APCs)—mostly macrophages and B cells. APCs actively ingest exogenous antigens—antigens that originate outside the cell. Exogenous antigens include viruses, toxins, pollen, or bacteria that are circulating in the blood, lymph, or body fluids. APCs break down the antigens and incorporate pieces of them with MHC II glycoproteins. This aberrant display of MHC markers is recognized as nonself.

Major histocompatibility complex class I and class II share an overall similar fold. The binding platform is composed of two domains, originating from a single heavy α-chain (HC) in the case of MHC class I and from two chains in the case of MHC class II (α-chain and β-chain) (Fig. 1A). The two domains evolved to form a slightly curved β-sheet as a base and two α-helices on top, which are far enough apart to accommodate a peptide chain in-between. Two membrane-proximal immunoglobulin (Ig) domains support the peptide-binding unit. One Ig domain is present in each chain of MHC class II, while the second Ig-type domain of MHC class I is provided by non-covalent association of the invariant light chain beta-2 microglobulin (β_2m) with the HC. Transmembrane helices anchor the HC of MHC class I and both chains of MHC class II in the membrane (Fig. 1A).

The groove in-between the two helices accommodates peptides based on (i) the formation of a set of conserved hydrogen bonds between the side-chains of the MHC molecule and the backbone of the peptide and (ii) the occupation of defined pockets by peptide side chains (anchor residues P2 or P5/6 and PÙ in MHC class I and P1, P4, P6, and P9 in MHC class II) (1–4). The type of interactions of individual peptide side-chains with the MHC depend on the geometry, charge distribution, and hydrophobicity of the binding groove. Predicting the affinity of these distinct MHC–antigen interactions for individual allotypes has been a long-standing goal in the community. While good progress has been made in developing and optimizing bioinformatic algorithms to estimate peptide binding to MHC proteins, these *in silico* predictions, however, still yield false positives, and often fail in predicting immunodominance. We argue that understanding the relevance of transient or energetically excited protein conformations that are visited during the equilibrium fluctuations of the molecular structure is important for making good predictions.

In MHC class I, the binding groove is closed at both ends by conserved tyrosine residues leading to a size restriction of the bound peptides to usually 8–10 residues with its C-terminal end docking into the F-pocket. In contrast, MHC class II proteins usually accommodate peptides of 13-25 residues in length in their open binding groove, with the peptide N-terminus usually extruding from the P1 pocket. It has been reported that the interactions at the F pocket region in MHC class I and the P1 region (including the P2 site) in MHC class II appear to have a dominant effect on the presentation of stable pMHC complexes and on the immunodominance of certain peptidic epitopes. Interestingly, these pockets are located at opposite ends of the binding groove of the respective MHC class I and MHC class II structures (Fig. 1B).

The most polymorphic human MHC class I and class II proteins (human leukocyte antigens, HLAs) are each expressed from three gene regions (MHC class I: HLA-A, -B, -C; MHC class II: HLA-DR, -DP, -DQ), which are all highly polymorphic. This allelic variation mainly affects the nature and composition of the peptide-binding groove and thus modulates the peptide repertoire that is presented on the surface by MHC class I or MHC class II proteins for CD8+ or CD4+ T cell recognition, respectively. A good match of the peptide and the MHC binding groove is an important, but certainly not the sole determinant of its presentation.

In fact, the formation of a pMHC complex depends on its peptide-loading pathway, in which the selection of peptides is influenced by several factors, such as antigen availability, protease activity, or the availability of chaperones. In addition, for each MHC class, a "catalyst" is available to enhance peptide exchange for certain peptides: tapasin for MHC class I and HLA-DM for MHC class II. These molecules edit the presented peptide repertoire and bias the exchange reaction toward the presentation of thermodynamically stable complexes. Tapasin and HLA-DM thus act similar to typical enzymes by reducing the energy barrier for peptide exchange. However, in the case of HLA-DM and tapasin, no covalent bonds are formed or cleaved during the exchange reaction.

The MHC class I HC folds and assembles with β_2m in the lumen of the endoplasmic reticulum (ER). The partially folded heterodimer is then incorporated into the peptide-loading complex (PLC) for peptide binding and exchange. In the PLC, tapasin is a protein that catalyzes, together with other chaperones, the loading of high-affinity peptides derived from proteolysis of endogenously expressed proteins (Fig. 1C, left panel). In the absence of tapasin, some class I allotypes (such as HLA-B*44:02) are retained in the ER (tapasin-dependent), whereas other class I proteins (tapasin-independent, such as HLA-B*44:05 and HLA-B*27:09) can bind peptides and travel to the cell surface. There is no crystal structure of the MHC class I/tapasin complex, but several structural models and mutational studies suggested that tapasin binds two regions in the HC of MHC class I, a loop in the α_3 domain (residues 229–222), and a region of the α_2 domain (residues 137–128) adjacent to the F-pocket (Fig. 1B).

Major histocompatibility complex class II proteins fold in the ER in complex with a protein called invariant chain (Ii) (30) and are then transported to late endosomal compartments (also coined MHC class II compartment, MIIC). There, Ii is cleaved by cathepsin proteases and a short fragment remains bound to the peptide-binding groove of MHC class II proteins, termed class II-associated invariant chain peptide (CLIP). This placeholder peptide is then normally exchanged against higher affinity peptides, which are derived from proteolytically degraded proteins available in endocytic compartments (Fig. 1C, right panel).

HLA-DM accelerates peptide exchange, with different allelic variants being more or less susceptible to catalysis. HLA-DM has a highly similar structural fold compared to classical MHC class II proteins, but its closed-up binding groove prevents peptide binding. Crystal structures of HLA-DM in complex with the MHC class II protein HLA-DR1 and in complex with the competitive inhibitor HLA-DO revealed that HLA-DM mainly contacts the α_1-domain of MHC class II proteins close to the P1 pocket and additionally the membrane-proximal β2-domain, in line with previous mutational analyses (Fig. 1B).

Despite the structural differences between tapasin and HLA-DM as well as their presumably opposite sites of interaction with regard to the orientation of the binding groove, a similar mode of action has been suggested, hinting at a possible convergent evolution of the two exchange catalysts (Fig. 1B). A common feature seems to be that both catalysts target regions in the vicinity of those pockets in the peptide-binding groove that are of great relevance for the stability of the respective pMHC complex. Furthermore, in both cases, the binding of a high-affinity peptide is able to release the interaction with tapasin/DM and allows for transport of stable pMHC complexes to the cell surface.

While the general hallmarks of antigen processing and editing have been established, the discussion is now moving toward the dynamics of the system, both at the cellular and molecular level. The mechanistic questions relate to a description of how exactly peptides are selected for presentation and how tapasin and HLA-DM catalyze this reaction in an allele-specific manner.

GRAFT REJECTION

Although the immune response first attracted the attention of scientists because of the body's ability to fight infections, the observation that animals reject foreign organ grafts led to a much broader view of the immune system in that it indicated that the immune system had a surveillance function. The rejection of a foreign organ graft simply reflects the role of the immune system in identifying and destroying "abnormal" cells.

Grafting of Organs

Advances in surgery have permitted the transfer of many tissues or organs between different parts of the body or between different individuals. When moved to a different part of an animal's own body, such transplants do not trigger an immune response. This type of graft within an individual is called an autograft (Fig. 2). Examples of autografting include the use of skin to cover a burn in plastic surgery and the use of a segment of vein to bypass blocked cardiac arteries. Since autografts do not express foreign antigens, they do not trigger an immune response.

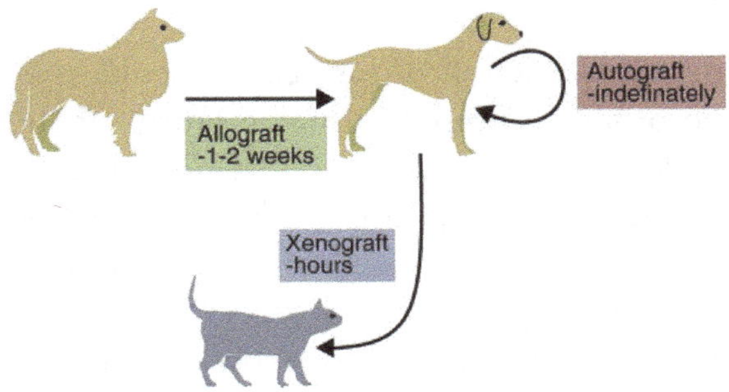

Fig. 2 The differences among autografts, allografts, and xenografts.

Isografts are grafts transplanted between two genetically identical individuals. Thus a graft between identical (monozygotic) twins is an isograft. Similarly, grafts between two inbred mice of the same strain are isografts and present no immunological difficulties. Since the animals are identical, the immune system of the recipient does not differentiate between the graft and normal body cells.

Allografts are transplanted between genetically different members of the same species. Most grafts performed on animals or humans for therapeutic reasons are of this type because tissues are obtained from a donor who is usually unrelated to the graft recipient. Because the major histocompatibility complex (MHC) and blood group molecules on the allograft are different from those of their host, allografts induce a strong immune response that causes graft rejection. This rejection process must be suppressed if the grafted organ is to survive.

Xenografts are organ grafts transplanted between animals of different species. Thus, the transplant of a baboon heart into a human infant is a xenograft. Xenografted tissues differ from their host both biochemically and immunologically. As a result, they can provoke a rapid, intense rejection response that is very difficult to suppress.

Clinical grafting in domestic animals is a recent procedure. However, renal allografting is now routine in dogs and cats, and bone marrow allografts promise to be very useful in some forms of tumor therapy. It is unlikely that cadaveric allografting will become important in veterinary medicine. Most current organ grafts are obtained from healthy donor animals. This raises significant ethical issues as to whether it is appropriate to subject a donor animal to major surgery in order to provide an organ for another animal. Although the benefits of allografting to the recipient are obvious, it is unclear how the donor animal might benefit. Unlike human donors driven by altruism, an animal donor is given no choice in the matter. It is possible, however, to justify organ donation if thereby an animal would be saved from inevitable euthanasia and if the donor could be provided with a good home. For this reason, many animal transplantation centers require that the donor animal be adopted and cared for by the owner of the recipient animal.

Allograft Rejection

The identification and destruction of foreign molecules are central to the body's defense. Allografted organs represent a major source of these foreign molecules. They include not only antigens such as the foreign blood group glycoproteins and MHC molecules expressed on the grafted cells, but also any endogenous antigens presented on the MHC class I molecules of these same cells. The mechanisms of allograft rejection are basically the same irrespective of the organ grafted, and both antibodies and T cells participate in the rejection of allografts.

Histocompatibility Antigens

When an organ is transplanted into a genetically dissimilar animal, the recipient will mount an immune response against many different antigens in and on the cells of the allograft. These are called histocompatibility antigens. Three types of histocompatibility antigens are of major importance in stimulating graft rejection. These are the MHC class I molecules, the MHC class II molecules, and the major blood group molecules. All are expressed on the surface of the graft cells, but their distribution varies. MHC class I antigens are found on almost all nucleated cells. The major blood group antigens are found both on red cells and nucleated cells. MHC class II antigens, in contrast, have a restricted distribution that varies among mammals. For example, in rats and mice, MHC class II molecules are expressed only on the professional antigen-presenting cells (APCs): macrophages, dendritic cells, and B cells. In other species, such as humans and pigs, MHC class II molecules are also expressed on the endothelium of renal arteries and glomeruli, the sites where host cells first make contact with the graft. These MHC class II molecules are recognized as foreign and trigger the rejection process. It is interesting to note that, as a result of these differences, it is much easier to prolong renal allograft survival in laboratory rodents than in humans or pigs.

As would be expected, grafts that differ minimally from the recipient will generally survive longer than grafts that are highly incompatible. When blood group

A-O-compatible pigs are given renal allografts, median survival is about 12 days for MHC-unmatched grafts, 25 days for grafts compatible for MHC class I alone, 32 days for grafts compatible for MHC class II alone, and 80 days for grafts compatible for both class I and class II (Fig. 3). When dogs are given MHC-unmatched renal allografts, the grafts survive for about 10 days. Completely matched allografts in dogs survive for about 40 days. A more impressive result is obtained with canine liver grafts, which survive for about 8 days in unmatched animals and for 200 to 300 days in DLA-matched recipients.

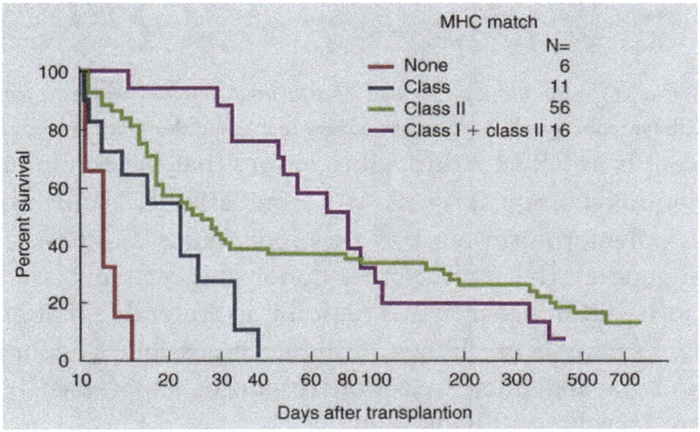

Fig. 3 Survival time of organ allografts between SLA-incompatible minipigs clearly depends on the degree of MHC compatibility between donor and host

The failure of MHC and blood group-compatible grafts to survive indefinitely is a result of the cumulative effects of many other minor antigenic differences. For example, skin grafts from male donors placed on histocompatible females are usually rejected, although the reverse is not the case. This is because male cells carry an antigen coded for by genes on the Y chromosome called the H-Y antigen.

During the acute rejection process, the grafted tissue gradually becomes infiltrated with cytotoxic T cells, which cause progressive damage to the endothelial cells lining small blood vessels (Fig. 4). The T cells roll along the endothelial surface and bind using leukocyte function-associated antigen-1 (LFA-1). T cell-mediated damage releases chemokines that attract more T cells into the graft. Cellular destruction, stoppage of blood flow, hemorrhage, and death of the grafted organ follow thrombosis of these vessels. The blood vessels of second organ grafts become blocked even more rapidly as a result of the action of antibodies and complement on the vascular endothelium. This secondary reaction is specific for any graft from the original donor or from a donor syngeneic with the first. It is not restricted to any particular site or to any specific organ since MHC and blood group molecules are present on most nucleated cells.

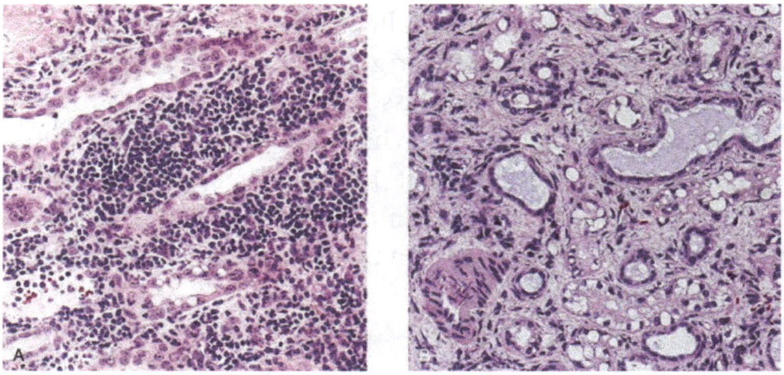

Fig. 4 A, Section of a canine kidney that had been acutely rejected and as a consequence is densely infiltrated with lymphocytes. B, Section of a kidney that has undergone chronic allograft rejection.

In practice it is usually not difficult to ensure that the donor and recipient have identical major blood group antigens. MHC compatibility is much harder to achieve because MHC polymorphism ensures that individuals differ widely in their MHC haplotype. In general, the more closely donor and recipient are related, the less will be their MHC difference. For this reason it is preferable that grafts be obtained from a recipient's parents or siblings. If this is not possible, a donor must be selected at random and the inevitable rejection responses suppressed by drugs such as cyclosporine or tacrolimus (Chapter 39).

Renal Allografts

Clinical Allograft Rejection

Renal allograft rejection is of major clinical importance in humans and has been widely studied in animals. It therefore serves as a good example of the allograft response. Rejection may occur at any time after transplantation. In humans, in whom a great deal of experience with transplantation has been gained, four distinct clinical rejection syndromes are recognized. *Hyperacute rejection* occurs within 48 hours after grafting. Rejection occurring up to 7 days after grafting is called *accelerated rejection.* Rejection after 7 days is called *acute rejection. Chronic rejection* develops several months after grafting. It is unclear whether a similar classification is useful in animals.

When kidneys are allografted, the blood supply to the transplanted kidney is established at the time of transplantation. The graft and host cells come into contact almost immediately. In an unsensitized host, a primary immune response is mounted, and renal allografts are only rejected after at least 10 days and possibly much longer. In sensitized animals in which the immune system is already primed, hyperacute rejection occurs, and the graft is destroyed within days or even hours without ever becoming functional. Acute rejection should be suspected when the recipient shows a rapidly rising blood creatinine associated with an enlarged, painful kidney accompanied by signs of depression, anorexia, vomiting, proteinuria, hematuria, and ultrasonography showing an enlarged, hypoechoic kidney. In contrast, chronic rejection should be suspected if the creatinine and urea levels rise gradually, and this is associated with proteinuria, microscopic hematuria, and a small, hyperechoic kidney. It is also associated with a slow loss of renal function and tends to be related to with interstitial fibrosis and proliferation of vascular endothelium. Renal biopsy is necessary to confirm rejection.

Pathogenesis of Allograft Rejection

The allograft rejection process is directed against the dominant antigens on the cells of the graft. The MHC molecules tend to trigger a T cell-mediated rejection response, whereas the blood group antigens tend to trigger antibody formation. The rejection process may be divided into two stages. First, the host's lymphocytes encounter the antigens of the graft and trigger a response. Second, cytotoxic T cells and antibodies from the host enter the graft and destroy graft cells (Fig. 5).

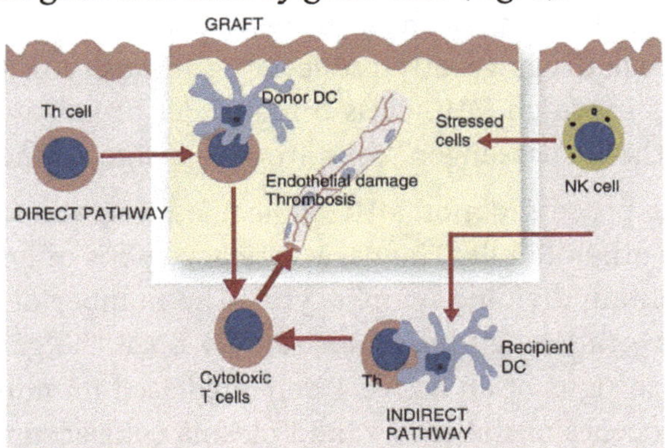

Fig. 5. Some of the mechanisms involved in the rejection of an allograft

Innate Mechanisms

Damage to the graft as a result of surgical trauma and ischemia followed by reperfusion upregulates MHC expression and generates cytokines and inflammatory mediators that attract neutrophils and macrophages into the graft. If large quantities of damage-associated molecular patterns (DAMPs) such as high mobility group box protein-1 (HMGB1) are generated, they will activate toll-like receptors and other pattern-recognition receptors. An increase in expression of MICA molecules on graft endothelial cells can activate natural killer (NK) cells. Complement components such as C5a and C3a may also activate APCs within the graft.

Adaptive Mechanisms

Donor antigens are presented to the T cells of the recipient by APCs. The graft recipients may be sensitized by a direct pathway in which recipient T cells circulating through the graft encounter antigens presented by donor APCs. These donor APCs may also carry antigens to draining lymph nodes and the spleen. Alternatively, recipients may be sensitized when their own APCs circulate through the graft and encounter and process donor antigens (the indirect pathway). The direct pathway operates early in the rejection process but is replaced by the indirect pathway once donor APCs have been destroyed.

In humans, the direct pathway is responsible for the vigorous immune response that occurs in acute rejection, whereas the indirect pathway is more important in chronic rejection. Although macrophages and dendritic cells are important APCs, donor B cells and tubular epithelial and endothelial cells can also process antigen, and they can migrate to lymphoid organs where they activate recipient T cells.

In laboratory rodents, MHC class II molecules are expressed on professional APCs. In these species the intensity of graft rejection is related to the number of donor B cells, macrophages, and dendritic cells transplanted within the graft. Removal of these cells by careful flushing of the graft before surgery or by pretreatment of the donor with cytotoxic drugs greatly reduces the intensity of the rejection process. In other mammals in which MHC class II molecules are also expressed on vascular endothelial cells, these "passenger" cells are of less significance.

The APCs that process donor MHC molecules migrate to the draining lymph node and activate other T cells. The paracortical regions of lymph nodes draining a graft therefore contain dividing lymphocytes. The number of these cells is greatest about 6 days after grafting and declines rapidly once the graft has been rejected. In addition to these signs of an active T cell–mediated immune response, germinal center formation occurs in the cortex, and plasma cells accumulate in the medulla, indicating that antibody formation is also occurring. In a conventional immune response, only one cell in 10^5 to 10^6 T cells can respond to a specific antigen. In graft rejection, however, there may be %1 to %10 of responding T cells since these cells have low activation thresholds for foreign MHC molecules.

The activated Th1 cells produce interleukin-2 (IL-2) and interferon-ã (IFN-ã) and so activate cytotoxic T cells and NK cells. The NK cells produce more IFN-ã and tumor necrosis factor-α (TNF-α) that activates macrophages and additional NK cells. The cytotoxic CD8+ T cells recognize the foreign peptides bound to recipient MHC class I molecules and kill any target cell they encounter. Donor MHC class II molecules trigger an immune response in two ways. First, because they are foreign proteins, they are processed as endogenous antigens. Second, they may directly bind to recipient T cell receptors (TCRs) and trigger cytotoxicity.

IL-2 and IFN-ã not only promote cytotoxic T cell activity but also enhance the expression of MHC molecules on the cells of the graft. During allograft rejection, therefore, MHC expression is increased, and the graft becomes an even more attractive target for cytotoxic T cells.

Although cytotoxic T cells are of major importance in acute allograft rejection, B cells, eosinophils, and macrophages also play a significant role in hyperacute and chronic rejection (Fig. 6). Hyperacute rejection occurs when the recipient has preexisting antibodies to graft MHC or blood groups. These bind to graft vascular endothelial cells, activate complement by the classical pathway, and cause endothelial cell lysis. The damaged endothelial cells trigger platelet deposition as well as multiple chemokines and cytokines, especially IL-1β, CXCL8, and CCL2. These attract leukocytes as well, and the damage results in thrombosis and infarction. Anti-MHC antibodies also play a major role in secondary rejection, in which they activate the classical complement pathway and mediate antibody-dependent cytotoxic cell activity.

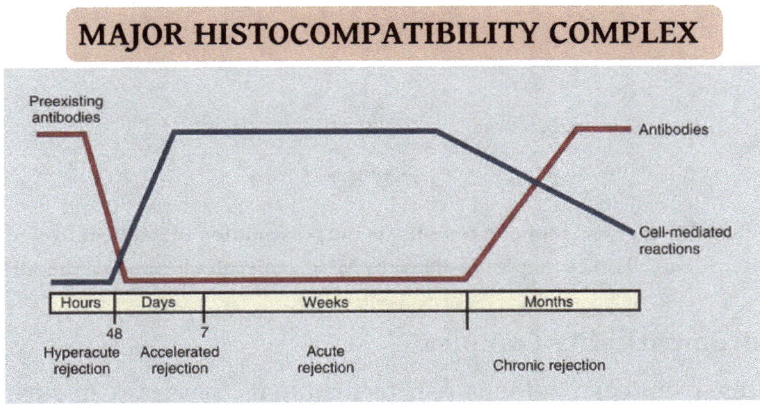

Fig. 6 Role of antibodies and cell-mediated immunity in different allograft rejection syndromes.

In order to trigger an adaptive immune response, antigen molecules must be broken up inside cells, and the fragments generated must then be bound to appropriate antigen-presenting receptors (Fig. 7). These antigen-presenting receptors are glycoproteins encoded by genes located in a large gene cluster called the major histocompatibility complex (MHC). The receptors are therefore called MHC molecules. Antigen fragments can trigger an immune response only after they have bound to MHC molecules, and these antigen-MHC complexes have bound to T cell antigen receptors. Since the MHC molecules serve as specific antigen receptors, MHC genes determine which antigens can trigger adaptive immunity. Thus the MHC can be considered an organized cluster of genes that control antigen presentation and so determine an animal's susceptibility to infectious or autoimmune diseases.

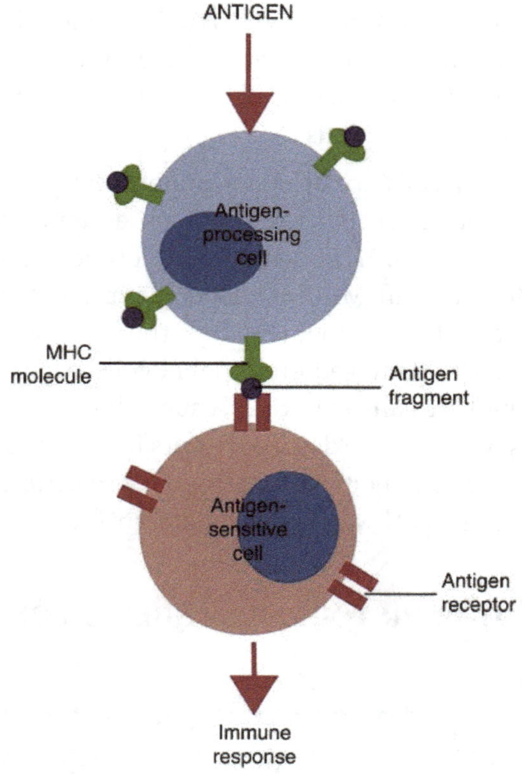

Fig. 7 The key initial step in any immune response is the presentation of antigens by antigen-processing cells to antigen-sensitive cells. This step is mediated by MHC molecules located on the surface of antigen-processing cells.

Major Histocompatibility Complex

All vertebrates, from cartilaginous fish to mammals, possess cell-surface proteins coded for by genes clustered within an MHC. Each MHC has a fairly consistent structure consisting of about 200 expressed genes distributed over about 3 mb of DNA and divided into three regions containing different classes of MHC gene loci (I, II, and III) (Fig. 8). Classical class I loci code for the MHC molecules expressed on most nucleated cells. Class I genes can be subdivided into those that are highly polymorphic (class Ia genes) and those that show very little polymorphism (class Ib, Ic, or Id genes). (Polymorphism refers to structural variations between proteins.) Class Id genes are located outside the MHC on a different chromosome. Genes in class II loci, on the other hand, encode polymorphic MHC molecules mainly restricted to professional antigen-presenting cells (dendritic cells, macrophages, and B cells) (Table 1). Genes in the class III region code for a diverse mixture of proteins, many of which are linked to innate immunity, such as complement proteins. Although each MHC contains all three gene regions, their gene content, and arrangement vary between species.

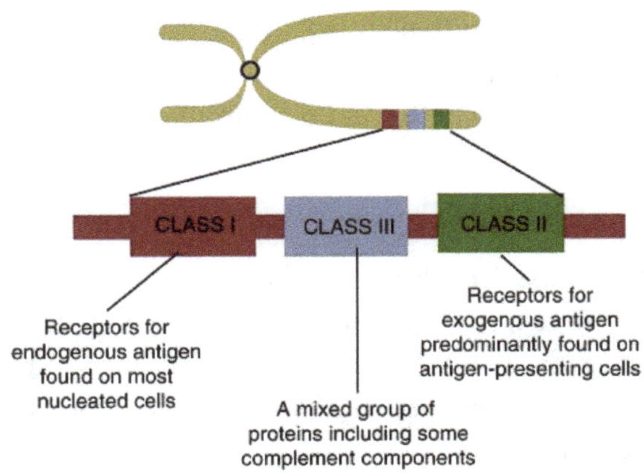

Fig. 8 The three major classes of genes located within the major histocompatibility complex are grouped together in regions: their distribution and functions.

Table 1 Comparison of MHC Class I and Class I Structure

	CLASS I	CLASS II
Loci include	Typically A, B, and C	DP, DQ, and DR,
Distribution	Most nucleated cells	B cells, macrophages, and dendritic cells
Function	Present antigen to cytotoxic T cells	Present antigen to T helper cells
Result	T-cell–mediated toxicity	T-cell–mediated help

The collective name given to the proteins encoded by MHC genes depends on the species. In humans these molecules are called human leukocyte antigen (HLA); in dogs they are called DLA; in rabbits, RLA; in cattle (bovines), BoLA; in horses, ELA; in swine, SLA; and so forth. In some species, MHC molecules were identified as transplantation antigens before their true function was recognized. In these cases, the nomenclature is anomalous. Thus, in the mouse the MHC is called H-2, and in chickens it is called B. The complete set of alleles found within an individual animal's MHC is called its MHC haplotype.

MHC Class Ia Molecules

Class Ia molecules are expressed on most nucleated cells. In pigs, for example, class I molecules have been detected on lymphocytes, platelets, granulocytes, hepatocytes, kidney cells, and sperm. They are not usually found on mammalian red cells, gametes, neurons, or trophoblast cells. Some cells, such as myocardium and skeletal muscle, may express very few class Ia molecules.

Structure

Class Ia molecules consist of two linked glycoprotein chains. An α chain (45 kDa) is associated with a much smaller chain called β_2-microglobulin (β_2M) (12 kDa). The α chain is inserted in the cell membrane (Fig. 9). It consists of five domains:

three extracellular domains called α_1, α_2, and α_3, each about 100 amino acids long; a transmembrane domain; and a cytoplasmic domain. The antigen-binding site on these molecules is formed by the α_1 and α_2 domains. β_2M consists of a single domain and serves to stabilize the structure.

Gene Arrangement

The size of the MHC class I region varies among mammals. Humans and rodents have the largest, and pigs have the smallest. The chicken class I region is very much smaller than in mammals. The MHC class I region has a common framework of non-MHC genes, and size differences are mainly due to variations in the size and number of these framework genes.

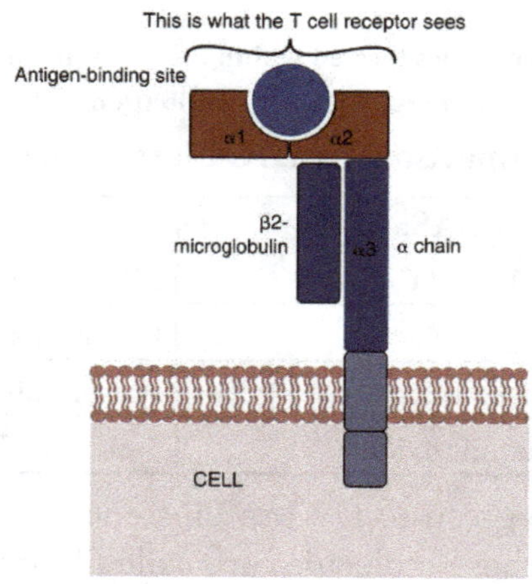

Fig. 9 The structure of a class Ia MHC molecule on a cell membrane. Its antigenbinding site is formed by the folding of both its a1 and a2 domains.

The number of class Ia gene loci varies between mammals. For example, rats have more than 60, mice have about 30, humans have 20, cattle have 13 to 15, and pigs have 11. Not all these genes are functional. For example, in mice, only two or three class I genes are expressed. The remainder are pseudogenes (defective genes that cannot be expressed). In humans the functional polymorphic genes are called *A*, *B*, and *C*. In mice they are called *K* and *D* (and in some strains, *L*) (Fig. 10). In other species they are usually numbered.

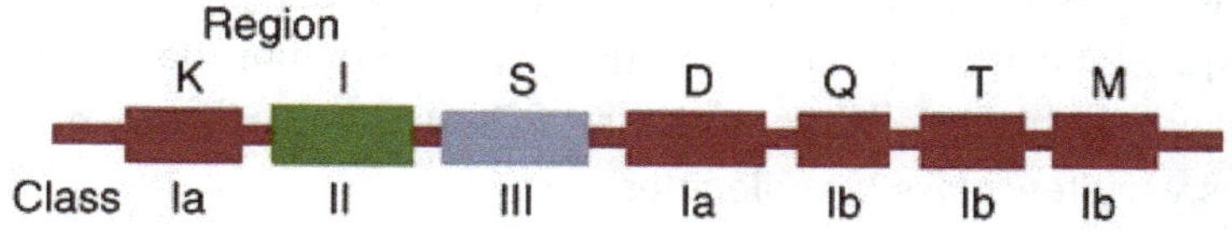

Fig. 10. Arrangement of major loci within the MHC of the mouse - a typical mammalian MHC

Polymorphism

Some class Ia loci encode proteins with very large numbers of alleles. These allelic differences cause variations in the amino acid sequences of the α_1 and α_2 domains.

This variation is called polymorphism. The most extreme polymorphism is restricted to three to four small regions located within the α_1 and α_2 domains. In these variable regions, two or three different amino acids may occur at each position. The other domains of MHC class Ia molecules show little variation.

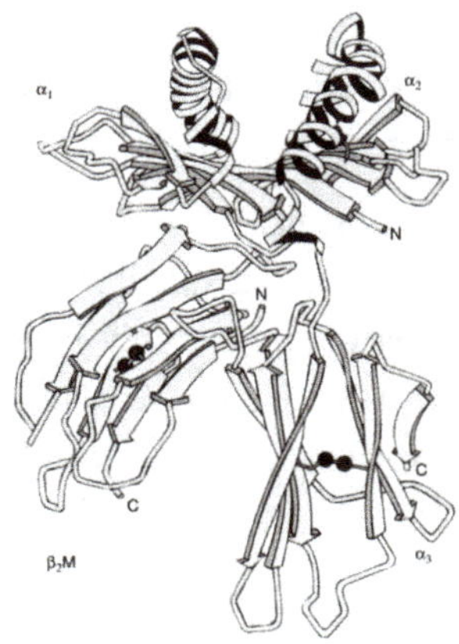

Fig. 11 Schematic three-dimensional view of the complete structure of HLA-A2 derived by xray crystallography. The antigen-binding groove at the top is formed by the a1 and a2 domains, whereas the a3 domain binds to the cell membrane. The b chain (b2- microglobulin) has no direct role in antigen binding

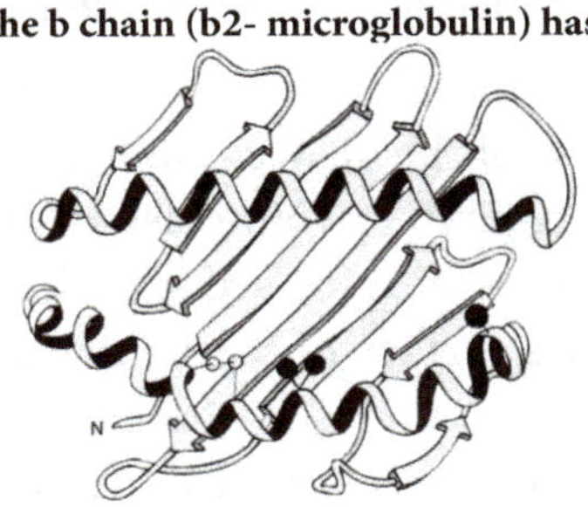

Fig. 12. A view (from above) of the antigen-binding groove on an MHC class I molecule. The floor of the groove is formed by an extensive b-pleated sheet. The walls of the groove are formed by two parallel a helices. This structure is formed by the folding of the a1 and a2 domain of the a chain.

The α_1 and α_2 domains of MHC class I molecules fold together to form an open-ended groove (Fig. 11). A flat β sheet forms the floor of this groove, and its walls are formed by two α helices (Fig. 12). This groove binds antigenic peptides, 8 to 10 amino acids in size. The variable regions located along the walls of this groove determine its shape. The shape of the groove in turn determines which peptides can be bound and thus trigger immune responses.

The amino acid variability in the α_1 and α_2 domains results from variations in the nucleotide sequences between MHC alleles. These nucleotide variations result from point mutations, reciprocal recombination, and gene conversion. Point mutations are simply changes in individual nucleotides. Reciprocal recombination involves crossing over between two chromosomes.

In gene conversion, small blocks of DNA are exchanged between different class I genes in a nonreciprocal fashion. The donated DNA blocks may come from nearby nonpolymorphic class I genes, from nonfunctional pseudogenes, or from other polymorphic class I genes. Class I MHC genes have the highest mutation rate of any germline genes yet studied (10^{-3} mutations per gene per generation in mice). This high mutation rate implies that there are significant advantages to be gained by having very polymorphic MHC genes.

Mammals use two distinct strategies for maintaining high levels of MHC class I diversity. Mice and humans simply use a small number of highly polymorphic genes. In other primates and rats, however, diversity is generated by varying the number and combinations of many different genes. Cattle use both strategies by employing various combinations of six or more classical class I genes, but three of these are also highly polymorphic.

Nonpolymorphic MHC Class I Molecules

Mammalian cells also express many nonpolymorphic class I molecules. Some are encoded by genes within the MHC class I region, others by genes on other chromosomes. They are classified according to their evolutionary origin.

Class Ib molecules show reduced expression and tissue distribution compared with class Ia molecules but are part of the MHC complex. They have limited polymorphism and their genes probably originated from class Ia precursors by gene duplication. For example, the class Ib genes in mice are found in three loci called *Q*, *T*, and *M*. They code for proteins on the surface of regulatory and immature lymphocytes and on hematopoietic cells. These also consist of a membrane-bound α chain associated with β_2-microglobulin, so their overall shape and antigen-binding groove are similar to those in MHC class Ia molecules. Since they are not polymorphic, MHC class Ib molecules bind a limited range of ligands. Thus they are receptors for commonly encountered, microbial pathogen-associated molecular patterns (PAMPs).

Class Ic genes have limited polymorphism and are found within the MHC but probably originated before the radiation of the placental mammals. Their products include MICA and MICB, specialized proteins that are involved in signaling to natural killer (NK) cells but do not bind antigenic peptides.

Class Id genes are nonpolymorphic class I–related genes not located on the MHC chromosome. Many of their products contribute to innate immunity since they bind PAMPs. For example, CD1 molecules bind bacterial lipids. FcRn is a class Id MHC molecule that serves as an antibody (Fc) receptor on epithelial cells. It is expressed on mammary gland epithelium and on the enterocytes of newborn mammals.

MHC Class II Molecules

Mammals differ in their expression of MHC class II molecules. In rodents, they are restricted to the professional antigen-presenting cells (dendritic cells, macrophages, and B cells) but can be induced on T cells, keratinocytes, and vascular endothelial cells. Resting mouse T cells do not express MHC class II molecules, but in pigs, dogs, cats, mink, and horses, the MHC class II molecules are constitutively expressed on nearly all resting adult T cells.

In cattle, most MHC class II molecules are expressed only on B cells and activated T cells. In pigs, resting T cells express MHC class II molecules at about the same level as macrophages. In humans and pigs, MHC class II molecules are expressed on renal vascular endothelium and glomeruli—a fact of significance in kidney graft rejection. The expression of class II molecules is enhanced in rapidly dividing cells and in cells treated with interferon-γ (IFN-γ).

Structure

MHC class II molecules consist of two chains called α and β. Each chain has two extracellular domains (one constant and one variable), a connecting peptide, a transmembrane domain, and a cytoplasmic domain (Fig. 13).

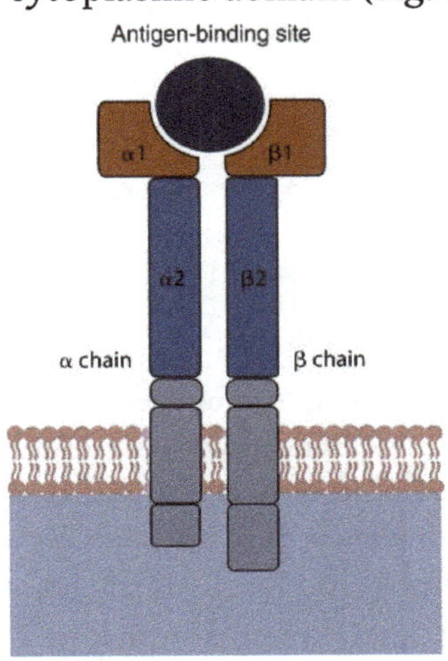

Fig. 13 Diagram showing the structure of a MHC class II antigen located on a cell surface. Note that the antigen-binding site is formed by the variable domains from both peptide chains.

Inheritance of Major Histocompatibility Complex

Most of the current knowledge about these molecules arose from pioneer studies on the rejection of normal and malignant transplanted tissues in mice and rabbits. The evidence produced by these studies indicated that the destruction of the grafted tissue was determined upon the existence of inherited antigenic differences between transplant and host, leading to the discovery of the mMHC and, later on, their genetic complexity.

The mMHCs have different domain organizations but similar structure. The variations are concentrated in three to four discrete hypervariable regions in the extracellular domains, while the rest of the molecule is highly conserved. The X ray crystallography of the proteins demonstrated that the class I mMHC is a heterodimer consisting of a transmembrane α chain non covalently linked to a small non transmembrane chain, called β2 microglobulin (β2m). Besides a transmembrane and an intracellular region, the α chain has three extracellular globular domains (α1, α2, and α3). The α1 and α2 domains of the α chain form a groove that accommodates an 8 to 10 mer antigenic peptide. The class II mMHC is a heterodimer composed of an α and a β chain, both with an intracellular, a transmembrane, and two extracellular domains (Fig. 14A). The pairing of the α1 and β1 domains form an antigen binding groove with open ends, allowing the allocation for a larger peptide (14 mer or more) extending out of both sides of the groove (Fig. 14B).

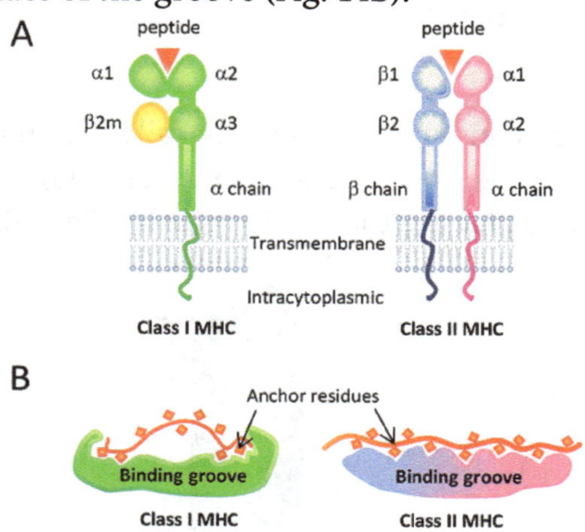

Fig. 14. Structure of MHC molecules and its binding sites. Panel A: schematic representation of class I and class II mMHCs. Panel B. MHC peptide binding sites. Amino acid positioning within the peptide binding grooves of class I and class II MHC proteins is shown. Squares represent individual amino acids of the antigenic peptides binding in the groove of each class I and class II mMHC.

The polygenic and polymorphic features of the MHC grant these molecules with an enormous capability for antigen presentation. A single individual co expresses several mMHCs from a large pool of alleles within a population. Moreover, each mMHC molecule can associate with a great amount of similar peptides, expanding even more the breadth of MHC regulated immune responses to pathogens. The polymorphic residues in the mMHC antigen binding groove are responsible for the different peptide specificities of the different alleles.

The class I molecules require an allele specific peptide length and a defined peptide motif that includes two anchor amino acids or residues with closely related side chains, which interact with both ends of the antigen binding site of that particular mMHC. The class II mMHCs have less stringency for size but also have allele specific peptide motifs (or anchor residues) that reach into pockets within and on the sides of the groove of the class II mMHC (Fig. 14B). Moreover, conserved residues within the class II peptide binding groove induce a conformational change, forcing bound peptides into a twisted configuration and exposing sites for external interactions.

Organization of the Major Histocompatibility Complex

Since its first description in mice and humans, the study of the MHC genetic architecture has expanded substantially, with the discovery and characterization of many class I and class II genes in different vertebrate species, except for jawless fish. The collective name given to the proteins encoded by MHC genes depends on the species, except for mice and chickens, in which they were first described as transplantation antigens and maintain their original nomenclature H2 and B, respectively. Hence, in humans, they are called human leukocyte antigen (HLA); in swine, SLA; in ovine, OLA; in equine, ELA; in dogs, DLA; in bovine, BoLA; and so on. The genetic structure of the MHC is best known for HLA and is relatively conserved among other mammalian species.

The HLA complex covers about 4 Mb of the short arm of chromosome 6 and contains three major regions with the confirmed presence of more than 260 loci, including over 160 protein coding genes.

The HLA locus is divided into three closely linked regions: class I, class II, and class III. The first two regions contain genes that control the specific immune response (so called "classical" MHC genes), and the class III region, enclosing about 75 genes, encodes a variety of different proteins, some related to the innate immunity.

The class I region contains three classical genes, *HLA A*, *HLA B*, and *HLA C*, and three nonclassical genes: *HLA E*, *HLA F*, and *HLA G*. Each of the classical HLA is a single functional gene, encoding a class I mMHC α chain. The gene coding for the β2m is located outside the MHC, on chromosome 15. *HLA H*, *HLA J*, *HLA K*, and *HLA L* are nonfunctional pseudogenes, closely related in nucleotide sequence to the class I functional genes.

The class II HLA cluster comprises three classical class II genes: *HLA DP*, *HLA DQ*, and *HLA DR*, each encoding one α and one or two β chains; three nonclassical, non polymorphic class II genes; *HLA DM*, *HLA DN*, and *HLA DO*; and some pseudogenes. These nonclassical class II genes are not expressed on the cell surface, but form heterotetrameric complexes involved in catalytic peptide exchange and loading onto classical class II molecules.

The class III region is located between the class I and class II regions and contains genes coding for molecules with diverse function. Among the most prominent are the complement factor genes coding for factors C2, C4, and B; genes coding for cytokines belonging to the tumor necrosis factor (TNF) superfamily, TNF-α, lymphotoxin α and lymphotoxin β, which are involved in various inflammatory pathways; heat shock protein genes; and many other genes encoding proteins not related to the immune system.

The major histocompatibility complex in cattle

In cattle, the first evidence for the existence of a MHC system was found by lymphocyte immunizations and by the generation of monospecific antilymphocyte antisera against skin grafts, followed by studies on the inheritance of the antigens they detected. As in the human, the *BoLA* locus is highly complex and contains about 154 predicted functional genes spanning about 4 centimorgan on chromosome 23. Compared to the HLA system, the BoLA system differs in gene arrangement without compromising its functions. Class I genes are clustered in two regions: *BoLA A* and *BoLA B*. Only the *A* locus seems to be functional with at least six putative classical class I genes, named *genes 1–6*. To date, 96 *BoLA A* alleles are listed on the Immuno Polymorphism Database (IPD) MHC database, and 29 different haplotypes have been identified, expressing between one and three combinations of these classical class I genes. The nonclassical BoLA class I genes include *NC1*, *NC2*, and *NC3*, encoding molecules with a relevant role during reproduction in dairy cows.

The main difference between BoLA and HLA gene organization is that in cattle the class II gene cluster is divided into two subregions, separated about 15 cM apart from each other: the class IIa, located near the class I/III regions, and the class IIb, resulting from a transposition, located close to the centromere on autosome 23. This feature is shared by various ruminant species.

The subregion IIa incorporates the gene clusters *DR* and *DQ* but lack a *DP* gene. This subregion expresses one DR molecule and one or two DQ molecules per haplotype. Bovines have one monomorphic *DRA* gene. By contrast, there are three genes that encode for the β chain of the DR (*DRB*) molecule of which *DRB1* is a pseudogene and *DRB2* is poorly expressed, leaving the *DRB3* locus as the most polymorphic and strongly expressed gene from this group. To date, 130 alleles have been identified using different approaches in various breeds of cattle.

The *DQ* cluster comprises five *DQA* (*DQA 1–5*) and five *DQB* (*DQB 1–5*) genes, which have arisen from gene duplication. From this cluster, at least 61 *BoLA DQA* and 81 *BoLA DQB* alleles have been described and listed in the IPD MHC database, and 56 different haplotypes were described in Japanese Black and Holstein cattle. The high number of different alleles, both on the *DR* and *DQ* loci, suggests that DR and DQ molecules complement each other for the presentation of a broad spectrum of antigens in cattle.

The BoLA class IIb locus is divided into two regions. The region known as "extended class II" region contains some genes involved in antigen processing and transport, i.e., LMP complex (low molecular mass polypeptide, *LMP2*, *LMP7*) and *TAP* genes (transporter associated with antigen processing: TAP2.1, TAP1, and TAP2) and also some non MHC genes like *H2B* (histone H2B like), among others.The second region is known as "classical class II" region and encloses genes of unknown function and unique to ruminants: *DSB (DRβ like)*, *DYA*, and *DYB*. The *DYA* and *DYB* genes encode for proteins of 253 and 259 amino acids, respectively. DY molecule has been shown to be expressed by a subpopulation of afferent lymph dendritic cells, suggesting its involvement in the prominent antigen processing and presentation capability of these cells.

Association of the major histocompatibility complex to disease susceptibility and resistance

Although age, stress, and physiologic status are important factors influencing the outcome of infection, evidence for genetic control has been observed in many animal species. Based on data registered in the Domestic Animal Diversity Information System (DAD IS) 2015 report, 483 mammalian breed populations are recorded as having resistance or tolerance to specific diseases or parasites, among which 236 correspond to breeds of cattle, 94 breeds of sheep, 56 breeds of chicken, 54 breeds of goats, and 36 breeds of pigs.

Not unexpectedly, the high degree of genetic polymorphism in the MHC has been associated with health status, vaccine responsiveness, and production traits in cattle. Examples of some studies for which there is documented evidence of MHC association with resistance or susceptibility to disease include mastitis in cattle and sheep, tick borne disease, dermatophilosis in cattle, enzootic bovine leucosis in cattle and sheep, neosporosis in cattle, theileriosis in cattle, gastrointestinal parasites in sheep, diarrhea in pigs, Marek's disease in chicken, coccidiosis in chicken, and coronavirus resistance in chickens, among others.

MAJOR HISTOCOMPATIBILITY COMPLEX DISEASE ASSOCIATIONS

The Major Histocompatibility Complex (MHC) gene products are critical for the regulation of the immune responses in all higher animals. They are fundamental for explaining variation in susceptibility to infections, immune response to vaccines, the development of auto-immunity and also for transplantation survival.

The canine MHC which is known as DLA (for Dog Leukocyte Antigen) has been extensively studied and shown to be very variable. Various DLA alleles and haplotypes have been shown to be associated with several immune mediated diseases, severity of infection in Leishmaniasis and response to rabies vaccination.[11]

Hypothesis

Many human immune mediated diseases have been shown to have MHC associations. Dogs have similar spontaneously occurring diseases, and if such diseases are also

MHC associated, this would provide good evidence that the canine diseases were homologues of the human diseases.

The Canine MHC

The canine MHC comprises three regions of genes which are called class I, class II and class III. The class I region contains several genes, one of which is very polymorphic. This gene is called DLA-88 and there are currently 51 official alleles, although we have identified at least another ten. The class II region has three polymorphic genes, called DLA-DRB1, DLA-DQA1 and DLA-DQB1. The class III region contains genes such as TNFalpha, and has been less well characterised.

DLA class II alleles can be identified using sequence based typing (SBT). Each locus is amplified using locus specific primers. The PCR product is sequenced and the homozygous or heterozygous sequence can be decoded using specialist software programs that compare the sequence to libraries of known alleles. Alleles can be assigned to haplotypes based on previously identified haplotypes. New haplotypes are identified in homozygous animals.

DLA Variation

We have now characterised over 7,000 dogs for their DLA class II alleles and haplotypes for three class II loci. These include dogs from over 150 different breeds with numbers per breed ranging from 1-500. We can see that most breeds have four to five major haplotypes with frequencies greater than 10%. Breeds with large populations, such as Labrador retrievers, tend to have more haplotypes, while breeds which have been through population bottlenecks, such as the Clumber spaniel have fewer haplotypes.

We have typed over 600 dogs from many multi-generation families, and shown that DLA alleles and haplotypes are inherited as expected.

DLA Disease Associations

Clear associations have been shown for several immune mediated diseases. These include diabetes, immune mediated haemolytic anaemia, hypothyroid disease, anal furunculosis and polyarthritis, It is clear that different breeds can have different DLA associations for the same disease.

Susceptibility to Leishmania infection has been shown to be associated with one DLA-DRB1 allele.

We have also shown that there is variation of response to rabies vaccination that can be attributed to the breed of the dog, which is presumably genetic. Unpublished data indicates that there is an effect of DLA on this vaccine response.

Additional Detail

The Major Histocompatibility Complex (MHC) gene products are critical for the regulation of the immune responses in all higher animals. They provide the basis for self-recognition and are fundamental for explaining variation in susceptibility to infections, immune response to vaccines, the development of auto-immunity and also to allotransplantation and rejection. They are also involved in immune surveillance and tumor immunology. Both MHC class I and II cell surface molecules are responsible for presenting antigens to the T cell receptor. Class I molecules present endogenously derived antigen (e.g. viral) to CD8 positive T cells, while class II molecules present exogenously derived antigens (e.g. bacterial) to CD4 positive T cells. Variability within the amino acid sequence of such MHC molecules influences the repertoire and affinity of peptide antigen binding and this is likely to influence the efficiency of acquired immunity to specific antigens. MHC sequence variability is thus under strong selective evolutionary pressure and consequently, in higher animals, these have become the most polymorphic genes observed at a population level.

When bottlenecks occur in the history of a population, such as those due to catastrophic events, or the establishment of new populations from a relatively small number of founders, major differences in the frequency distribution and extent of alleles can be seen between different populations. This is certainly the case in humans where HLA allele distribution can differ markedly between different populations across the world. Similarly differences are seen where closed selective line breeding has occurred, and this is the situation observed in a wide range of domestic dog breeds.

The canine Major Histocompatibility Complex (MHC), which is known as DLA (for Dog Leukocyte Antigen) has been shown to be very variable. As more breeds have been studied, more alleles have been identified. The grey wolf is the ancestor of the domestic dog and we have also investigated the DLA profile of grey wolves from Alaska and Northern Canada.[21]

The dog population is composed of around 400 purebred breeds; each one can be considered to be a genetic isolate with unique characteristics resulting from continuous selection for specific attributes (e.g. short legs, floppy ears or curly coat), from genetic drift or inbreeding. Dogs tend to suffer from the same range of diseases as humans but the genetic complexity of these diseases within a breed is reduced as a consequence of the genetic drift and due to long-range linkage disequilibrium.

It is therefore easier to look for genetic markers for disease in dogs than humans, since fewer cases are needed to give the same power for a study.

CHAPTER

ANTIGEN PRESENTATION AND CYTOKINE

8

INTRODUCTION

Antigen presentation in an organism is accomplished by antigen-presenting cells (APC). Antigen-presenting cells are a kind of cells capable of processing antigens and presenting antigen peptides to T cells in the form of antigen peptide-MHC molecular complexes, and play an important role in immune recognition, immune response and immune regulation of the body.

The process of antigen processing and presentation mainly involves two processes. The first is antigen processing, which means that APC degrades and processes the exogenous antigen or the endogenous antigen produced by cytoplasm itself to a polypeptide fragment of a certain size, so that the antigen peptide is suitable for binding to the MHC molecule, and the complex is combined. Finally, the complex can be transported to the cell surface. The process is called antigen processing. Followed by antigen presentation, the antigen peptide-MHC molecular complex expressed on the surface of APC is recognized by T cells, thereby presenting antigen peptides to T cells and inducing T cell activation. Since T cells can only recognize antigenic peptides presented by APC, antigen processing and presentation play an important role in immune responses, especially cellular immunity.

CLASSES AND FUNCTION

Antigen-presenting cells (APC)

Depending on the source of the presented antigen and MHC molecule, antigen-presenting cells can be divided into two categories: 1. APCs present exogenous antigens by MHC class II molecules. 2. APCs present endogenous antigens by MHC class II molecules. The former APC can take up, process exogenous antigens and present antigen peptides to $CD4^+$ T cells in the form of antigen peptide-MHC class II molecular complexes. Both dendritic cells and monocytes/macrophages can express multiple receptors to recognize pathogenic microorganisms or antigen-antibody complexes, and take up antigenic substances through pinocytosis, phagocytosis and receptor-mediated endocytosis. B cells take up antigen mainly by B cell receptors concentrate and internalize antigen or pinocytosis. DC will present the antigen to the initial T cells, promoting T cell activation, proliferation and differentiation.

Monocytes/macrophages and B cells present antigens to T helper cells (Th), and T helper cells further activate macrophages and B cells, and improve cellular and humoral immunity. According to its cellular function, it can be divided into professional APC and non-professional APC. The former includes dendritic cells (DC), monocytes/macrophages, and B lymphocytes. They constitutively express MHC class II molecules, costimulatory molecules and adhesion molecules, and have the function of directly ingesting, processing and presenting antigens. Non-professional APCs mainly include endothelial cells, epithelial cells and fibroblasts. In non-professional APCs, MHC class II molecules are generally not expressed or under-expressed, but can be induced by inflammation or certain cytokines, and their ability to process and present antigens is weak.

For APCs, endogenous antigens are presented by MHC class I molecules, which degrade and process the endogenous antigen, and then present the antigen peptides to CD8$^+$ T cells in the form of antigen peptide-MHCI type molecular complexes. The endogenous antigen is mainly derived from an intracellular parasitic pathogen or mutational protein.

THE PROCESS OF ANTIGEN PROCESSING AND PRESENTATION

Depending on the nature and source of the antigen, APC processes and presents antigens through four pathways: the MHC class I molecular pathway, the MHC class II molecular pathway, the non-canonical antigen presentation pathway, and the CD1 molecular pathway of lipid antigens. The MHC class I molecular pathway is an endogenous antigen presenting pathway. Endogenous antigens bind to transporter associated with antigen processing (TAP) after ubiquitinated endogenous antigens are degraded by the proteasome. TAP selectively transports 8-12 amino acid antigen peptides to the endoplasmic reticulum (ER). The antigen polypeptide binds to the antigen-binding peptide groove of the MHC class I molecule assembled by the endoplasmic reticulum to form an antigen peptide-MHC I -like molecular complex.

The complex is then transported to the cell membrane via the Golgi apparatus for recognition by CD8$^+$ T cells, thereby completing antigen presentation process; the MHC class II molecular pathway is an exogenous antigen presenting pathway. The exogenous antigen are recognized and taken up by APC, and then APC will form endosomes or phagocytose lysosomes. After the endosomes or phagocytose lysosomes fuse with MHC class II compartment (M II C), the antigen is degraded into a polypeptide. MIIC is the nonamer of MHC II/Ii, in which the Ii chain is degraded in MIIC, leaving class II -associated invariant chain peptide(CLIP) in the antigenic peptide binding groove of MHC class II molecules. Under the action of HLA-DM, the CLIP of the antigen peptide binding groove is replaced by the antigen peptide to form a stable antigen peptide-MHC class II molecular complex, which is then transported to the surface of the APC membrane for recognition by $CD4^+$ T cells, thereby completing the antigen presentation process. Cross-presentation means that APC can uptake and process exogenous antigens to $CD8^+$ T cells via MHC class I molecular pathways or present endogenous antigens to $CD4^+$ T cells via MHC class II molecular pathways. The CD1 molecular pathway for lipid antigens is a pathway that specifically targets lipid antigens, mainly through the CD1 molecule on the surface of APC.

DENDRITIC CELLS AND ANTIGEN PROCESSING

The innate immune defenses have evolved to destroy microbes as soon as they enter the body. Most invaders, especially if they are of low virulence, are rapidly eliminated. However, in addition to being uncomfortable and damaging, inflammation is not a foolproof process. If the body is to be defended effectively, an animal must have defenses that detect and eliminate all microbial invaders without the damage and discomfort associated with inflammation. This is the task of the adaptive immune system.

In order to trigger adaptive immunity, a sample of foreign material must first be captured, processed, and presented in the correct fashion to cells that can recognize it. This is the responsibility of antigen-processing cells.

Antigen-processing cells are attracted by microbial products and tissue damage and are activated by the same stimuli that trigger inflammation. Indeed, dendritic cells and macrophages are both sentinel cells and antigen-processing cells. As a result, antigen processing can be initiated at the same time as the invader is being eliminated by the innate defenses. Once an invader has been eliminated, the body can proceed to develop adaptive immunity against a second attack by the same organism.

Processing involves breaking large protein molecules into small peptides within a cell. These peptides are then attached to specialized antigen-presenting receptors called major histocompatibility complex (MHC) molecules. The peptides bound to MHC molecules are then carried to the cell surface. Adaptive immunity is triggered when these MHC-bound peptides are recognized by specific receptors on lymphocytes. These lymphocytes (called T cells) bind and respond only to peptides that have been correctly processed and presented. This ensures that adaptive immune responses do not proceed indiscriminately. The organisms that trigger adaptive immune responses are of two general types. One type is typified by the bacteria that invade the body from outside and then grow in the tissues and extracellular fluid. Their antigens are called exogenous antigens, and they are processed by specialized antigen-processing cells. A second type of invading organism is typified by viruses that invade a cell and force it to make viral proteins. These new proteins are called endogenous antigens. Endogenous antigens are processed by the cells in which they are produced. There are two classes of MHC molecules called MHC class I and MHC class II. MHC class I molecules are made by all nucleated cells and bind endogenous antigens. MHC class II molecules, in contrast, are restricted to specialized antigen-processing cells and bind exogenous antigens. The body mainly employs three cell types: dendritic cells, macrophages, and B cells to process exogenous antigens. The most important of these are dendritic cells (Fig. 1).

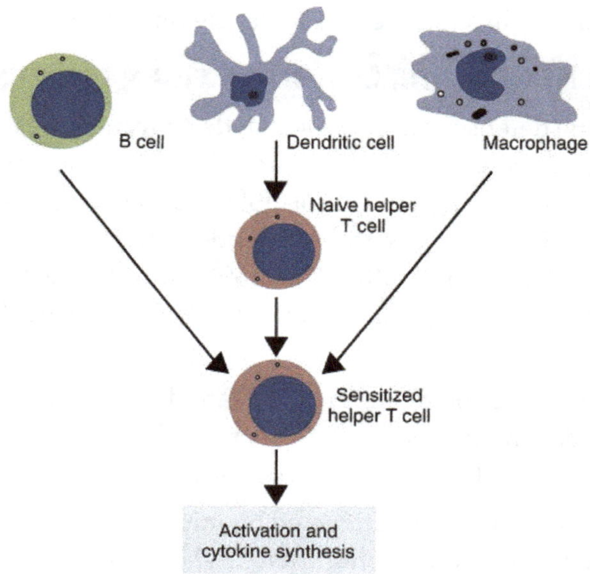

FIG. 1 The three major populations of antigen-presenting cells: B cells, dendritic cells, and macrophages. Of these, only dendritic cells can activate naïve T cells and trigger a primary immune response.

Dendritic Cells

Dendritic cells perform three major functions. First, they serve as sentinel cells and activate innate defenses when they first encounter invaders. Second, they process exogenous antigens and thus initiate adaptive immune responses. Third, they can regulate adaptive immunity by determining whether an antigen will trigger an antibody-mediated or a cell-mediated response. Dendritic cells are at least 100 times more effective antigen-presenting cells than macrophages or B cells. Dendritic cells can take up many different antigens, including dead microorganisms, soluble antigens in tissue fluids, and antigens released by dying cells, and present them to T cells. Dendritic cells are the only antigen-processing cells that can activate those T cells that have never previously encountered an antigen (naïve cells) and therefore are essential for initiating primary immune responses.

Origin

Dendritic cell precursors are derived from myeloid stem cells in the bone marrow. Under the influence of growth factors and cytokines, they differentiate into specialized subpopulations. Immature dendritic cells migrate throughout the body and form networks in virtually every tissue. Monocytes may also develop into dendritic cells when exposed to appropriate cytokines. (The precise relationship between dendritic cells and monocytes is currently being debated. Recent data are in conflict with the long-held belief that dendritic cells are simply specialized monocytes. This will take some time to sort out.) Dendritic cells are found in all organs except the brain, parts of the eye, and the testes. They are especially prominent in lymph nodes, skin, and mucosal surfaces—sites where invading microbes are most likely to be encountered.

Structure

The shape of dendritic cells depends on their state of activation. Typically, however, they are characterized by having a small cell body with many long cytoplasmic processes known as dendrites (Fig. 2). The dendrites increase the efficiency of antigen trapping and maximize contact between dendritic cells and other cells.

Subpopulations

Dendritic cells are a mixture of several different subpopulations. Thus they are divided into myeloid (M-DC) and plasmacytoid (P-DC) dendritic cells (Fig. 3). These two subpopulations differ in morphology, in surface antigens, and in their functions, although they share adhesion molecules, co-stimulatory molecules, and activation markers. Other specialized dendritic cell subpopulations are found in the skin (Langerhans cells) and in lymphoid organs (follicular dendritic cells).

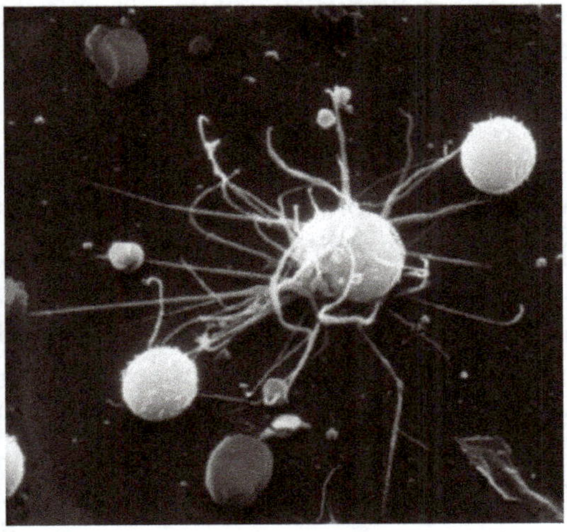

FIG. 2 A scanning electron micrograph of a dendritic cell from a guinea pig lymph node. Note the relatively small cell body and the numerous long dendrites.

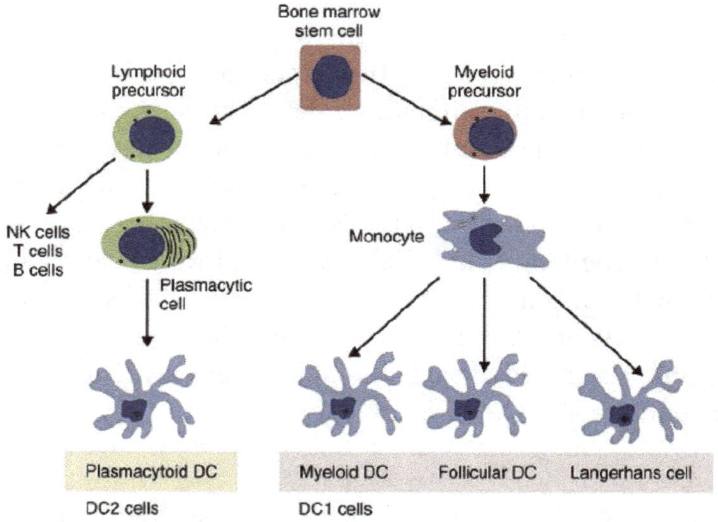

FIG. 3 The origins of dendritic cells. One population, the plasmacytoid dendritic cells, originates from lymphoid precursors. These give rise to DC2-type cells. The second major population arises from myeloid precursors and is closely related to monocytes. These, together with follicular dendritic cells and Langerhans cells, constitute the DC1 type.

As pointed out earlier, the adaptive immune system has two major branches: the antibody-mediated and cell-mediated immune responses. The type of immune response mounted by an animal is determined by the type of helper T (Th) cells triggered in response to an antigen. Thus there are several types of Th cells. One major type, Th1 cells, stimulates cell-mediated immune responses designed to protect animals against intracellular organisms. The other major type, Th2 cells, stimulates antibody-mediated immune responses designed to protect animals against extracellular invaders. Which Th cell type is activated depends on the use of different dendritic cell subpopulations.

Myeloid Dendritic Cells

Blood monocytes are the immediate precursors of both tissue macrophages and M-DCs. Which of these cell types is produced depends on the mixture of cytokines and cells encountered by the monocyte as it differentiates. Each cell type can convert to the other until late in the differentiation process. M-DCs can therefore be considered part of the mononuclear phagocytic system being derived from a common stem cell, respond to the same growth factors, express the same surface markers, and in effect are in no specific way uniquely different from other macrophages. Thus macrophages may consist of a spectrum of cell types ranging from highly effective antigen presenters (dendritic cells) at one extreme to suppressors of T cell activation (M2 cells) at the other. Monocytes exposed to certain T cell cytokines differentiate into M-DCs, and functionally different dendritic cells can be induced according to the local cytokine environment. Bovine peripheral blood monocytes exposed to staphylococcal enterotoxin C1, a superantigen, will convert to dendritic cells.

Plasmacytoid Dendritic Cells

P-DCs are long-lived cells found in blood, bone marrow, and lymphoid organs. They are specialized to respond to viruses by producing massive amounts of the type I interferons (IFN-α and IFN-β). Their numbers increase during infection. It is possible that the P-DCs serve as an early warning system for viral infections since they are rapidly activated by viral nucleic acids. Plasmacytoid dendritic cells have a unique ability to link innate and adaptive immunity. After producing large amounts of type I interferon, they are still able to differentiate into mature DCs that can stimulate naïve T cells. Because P-DCs secrete large amounts of IFN-α, they also activate natural killer (NK) cells.

Langerhans Cells

Several dendritic cell subpopulations are found in skin. Langerhans cells, for example, are specialized, long-lived M-DCs found in the epidermis. Their long dendrites form an extensive network that is ideally situated to capture antigens. These antigens include not only invading microbes but also topically applied antigens, such as the resins of poison ivy, or intradermally injected antigens, such as those in mosquito saliva. Langerhans cells express multiple pattern-recognition receptors (PRRs), including the C-type lectins langerin and DC-SIGN that can bind bacteria, fungi, and some viruses. Langerhans cells influence the development of skin immune responses, such as delayed hypersensitivity and allergic contact dermatitis. Langerhans cells contain characteristic rod- or racquet-shaped cytoplasmic granules called Birbeck granules whose function is unclear. Once antigens are captured, the Langerhans cells migrate to draining lymph nodes, where they present the antigen to T cells.

Follicular Dendritic Cells

Specialized dendritic cells called follicular dendritic cells are found in secondary lymphoid organs. They are a form of M-DC derived from stromal cell precursors. Follicular dendritic cells present antigens to B cells in two different ways. In an animal that has not previously been exposed to the antigen, antigen presentation is a passive process. The dendritic cells simply provide a surface on which antigen can be presented. In contrast, in animals that have previously been exposed to an antigen and possess antibodies, the antigen and antibody combine to form antibody-antigen complexes (also called immune complexes). Follicular dendritic cells take up these immune complexes on their surface and then shed them in membrane vesicles called exosomes. B cells can take up these exosomes and after processing the antigen present it to antigen-sensitive T cells. Follicular dendritic cells can retain antigens on their surface for more than 3 months.

They integrate signals from toll-like receptors (TLRs) and other sources to support effective germinal center responses. Follicular dendritic cells play an important role in promoting immunoglobulin A (IgA) responses in Peyer's patches in the intestinal wall. They respond to lipopolysaccharides, lipopeptides, and retinoic acid from the gut flora and support the recruitment and survival of IgA-producing B cells.

DENDRITIC CELL MATURATION

Although many subpopulations of dendritic cells have been characterized, their most important division is based on their state of maturity. Thus immature dendritic cells are highly specialized and efficient antigen-trapping cells. As they mature, dendritic cells undergo cellular reorganization and become specialized and efficient antigen-presenting cells.

Immature Dendritic Cells

Newly generated M-DCs migrate from the bone marrow through the blood to lymph nodes or tissues. Here they act as "sentinels" whose role is to capture invading microbes. With their short life span, they can be regarded as disposable antigen-trapping cells. If they do not encounter antigens, they die in a few days. If, however, they encounter antigens and are stimulated by tissue damage or inflammation, they become activated and mature rapidly. Immature dendritic cells have receptors that help them carry out their functions. These include cytokine receptors such as interleukin-1 receptor (IL-1R) and tumor necrosis factor receptor (TNFR), chemokine receptors; C-type lectins, Fc receptors (FcγR and FcεR), mannose receptors (CD206), heat-shock protein receptors, and TLRs.

Although the most important functions of dendritic cells are to trap, process, and present antigen to the cells of the immune system, they must also be able to kill any pathogens they encounter. Thus dendritic cells produce NADPH oxidase (NOX) and can kill invaders by mounting a respiratory burst. Activation of TLRs by pathogen-associated molecular patterns (PAMPs) enhances their production of superoxide.

Dendritic cells mature in response to interleukin-1 (IL-1) and tumor necrosis factor-α (TNF-α) as well as to PAMPs and damage-associated molecular patterns (DAMPs). Injured and inflamed tissues release large amounts of soluble heparan sulfate that binds to TLR4 and activates dendritic cells. Breakdown of nucleic acids generates uric acid, another potent dendritic cell activator. One of the most important activators of immature dendritic cells is high mobility group box protein-1 (HMGB1). Immature dendritic cells are attracted to areas of inflammation by chemokines, defensins, and HMGB1.

Immature dendritic cells specialize in capturing antigens and cell fragments by phagocytosis, by pinocytosis (the uptake of fluid droplets—cell drinking), and by interaction with various cell surface receptors. They also capture apoptotic cell bodies. If they ingest bacteria, they can usually kill them. They can distinguish between normal tissue debris and foreign organisms by selectively sampling their environment. This differentiation depends on the ability of the foreign material to bind to TLRs. Activation of TLRs by PAMPs ensures that ingested material is processed in such a way that it triggers adaptive immunity. Material that does not activate TLRs is not processed and will not trigger an adaptive response.

The phagosomal contents of conventional phagocytic cells such as neutrophils and macrophages are very acidic and hence optimized for proteolytic destruction of foreign material. The pH within dendritic cell and B cell phagosomes is in contrast relatively alkaline since these phagosomes do not fuse with lysosomes. Cysteine and aspartyl proteases are inhibited at these high pH levels, and as a result, antigen is not completely degraded but rather is preserved for presentation on MHC class I molecules.

ENDOGENOUS ANTIGEN PRESENTATION

In order to initiate a specific immune response to an infectious agent, the immune system must be able to wade through the sea of molecules that are associated with pathogenic invasion and isolate particular protein products that will sharpen the efforts of host defense. Implicit to this model of counteraction is the processing of an immunogenic peptide epitope (antigen processing) and its presentation on the surface of a team of cells, referred to as APCs (Antigen Presenting Cells) (antigen presentation). The result of these actions is the induction of a T-cell response that recruits and engages the other molecular participants of the immune response.

Antigen processing and presentation refer to the processes that occur within a cell that result in fragmentation (proteolysis) of proteins, association of the fragments with MHC (Major Histocompatibility Complex) molecules, and expression of the peptide-MHC molecules at the cell surface where they can be recognized by the TCR (T-Cell Receptor) on a T-Cell. The TCR can recognize antigen only in the form of a peptide bound to an MHC molecule on a human cell surface. The antigens recognized by T-cells are peptides that arise from the breakdown of macromolecular structures, the unfolding of individual proteins and their cleavage into short fragments through antigen processing. The peptides must be bound by an MHC molecule and presented at the cell surface. At the core of this immune system element is the MHC. Located on human chromosome 6, the MHC is a highly polymorphic set of genes that encode for molecules essential to self/non-self discrimination and antigen processing and presentation. There are two classes of MHC molecules, MHC-I (MHC-Class I) and MHC-II (MHC-Class II). MHC-I and MHC-II molecules are both trans-membrane glycoproteins belonging to the immunoglobulin supergene family. MHC-I molecules are composed of a transmembrane alpha chain associated non-covalently with the Beta2M (Beta2-Microglobulin) chain.

MHC-I molecules are specialized for the presentation of peptides derived from endogenous proteins (intracellular antigens) to the TCR of CD8+ T-cells (CD8-expressing T-cells). MHC-II molecules are composed of two non-covalently linked transmembrane chains, called Alphafn (33 kD) and Betafn(29 kD). They are specialized for the presentation of extracellular antigens to the TCR of CD4+ T-cells (CD4-expressing T-cells).

Endogenous/intracellular antigens are produced by viruses replicating within a nucleated host cell, processed by the proteolytic system acting on host intercellular proteins, and presented by MHC molecules. Intracellular proteins are cut into short peptides in the cell's multifunctional protease complex, the proteasome. The proteasome is a large proteolytic complex that contains many subunits, including two subunits, LMP2 (Large Multifunctional Protease-2) and LMP7 (Large Multifunctional Protease-7), encoded within the MHC locus. Proteins bound for degradation are targeted to the proteasome by covalent linkage with a small protein known as ubiquitin.

The two subunits of the proteasome, LMP2 and LMP7, induce the proteolytic complex to generate peptides that bind especially well to MHC-I molecules. The actual cleaving of protein occurs in the channel of the proteasome molecule. Peptides generated in the cytosol are then transported into the RER (Rough Endoplasmic Reticulum) to enable interaction with MHC molecules. TAP (Transporters Associated with Antigen Processing) is a transmembrane heterodimeric protein that allows for the crucial step of peptide translocation. TAP transports peptides into the ER (Endoplasmic Reticulum) that are ideally suited for binding with MHC-I molecules. The peptides consist of 8–13 amino acids. MHC-I molecules are tethered to the TAP transporter via a novel protein, tapasin. Peptides are then loaded onto the MHC-I molecule and transported to the cell surface for recognition by $CD8^+$ T-cells.

Exogenous/extracellular antigens are internalized by APCs such as macrophages, dendritic cells and B-cells. APCs can phagocytose and/or endocytose antigen, endosomally process it, and present it in association with MHC-II molecules. Internalized antigen is processed within three increasingly acidic endosomal environments: early endosomes (pH 6.0–6.5), late endosomes (pH 5.0–6.0) and lysosomes (pH 4.5–5.0). Acid-dependent hydrolytic enzymes degrade antigen into peptides consisting of 13–18 amino acids. Class-II Alpha and Beta chains associate within the RER. A protein known as the Ii (Invariant Chain) binds to the peptide-binding cleft of the MHC-II molecule and thereby prevents its binding with endogenous antigens meant to be targeted to MHC-I molecules only. The Ii seems to provide other important functions for the MHC-II molecule, too. It is involved in the folding of Alpha and Beta chains, the exit of the complex from the ER, and its targeting to the endocytic compartments. The MHC-II-Ii complex is transported to early endosomes. Ii also functions to transport the Class-II heterodimer to the late endosomal compartments: MIICs (MHC-Class II Compartments) where MHC-II molecules are loaded with peptide. Once in the MIIC, Ii is degraded by proteases (Cathepsins) until only a small fragment called CLIP (Class II-associated Invariant Chain Peptide) remains associated with the peptide-binding cleft to prevent premature interaction with partially-processed antigen. In the lysosome, HLA-DM, a vesicle membrane protein, mediates the removal of CLIP and the binding of antigen to MHC-II. The MHC-II-Antigen complex then moves to the plasma membrane where the neutral environment stabilizes it. At the cell surface, antigen is presented to CD4+ T-cells

ANTIGEN PRESENTATION

Antigens are macromolecules that elicit an immune response in the body. Antigens can be proteins, polysaccharides, conjugates of lipids with proteins (lipoproteins) and polysaccharides (glycolipids). Most of this page will describe how protein antigens are presented to the immune system. The presentation of lipid and polysaccharide antigens will be mentioned at the end. It will be helpful to distinguish between two limiting cases.

Antigens that enter the body from the environment; these would include inhaled macromolecules (e.g., proteins on cat hairs that can trigger an attack of asthma in susceptible people), ingested macromolecules (e.g., shellfish proteins that trigger an allergic response in susceptible people), and molecules that are introduced beneath the skin (e.g., on a splinter or in an injected vaccine). Alternatively, antigens can be generated within the cells of the body; these would include proteins encoded by the genes of viruses that have infected a cell and aberrant proteins that are encoded by mutant genes; such as mutated genes in cancer cells. In all cases, however, the initial immune response to any antigen absolutely requires that the antigen be recognized by a T lymphocyte ("T cell"). The truth of this rule is clearly demonstrated in AIDS: the infections (viral or fungal or bacterial) that so often claim the life of AIDS patients do so when the patient has lost virtually all of his or her $CD4^{+}$ T cells. The two categories of antigens are processed and presented to T cells by quite different mechanisms.

EXOGENOUS ANTIGENS

Exogenous antigens (inhaled, ingested, or injected) are taken up by antigen-presenting cells (APCs). These include phagocytic cells like dendritic cells and macrophages and B lymphocytes ("B cells") which are responsible for producing antibodies against the antigen.

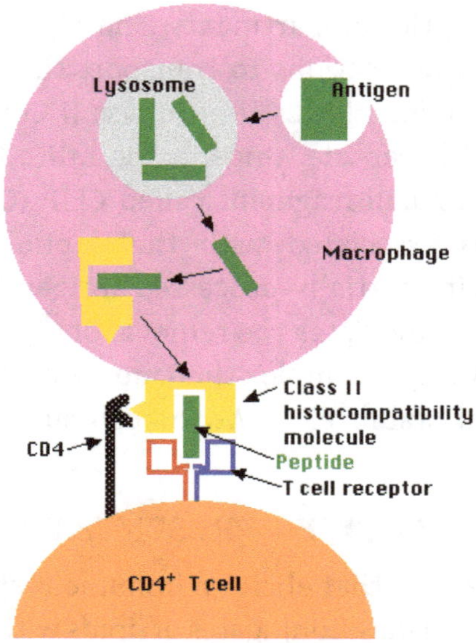

Fig. 4. Class I histocompatibility molecule

Antigen-presenting cells

- engulf the antigen by endocytosis
- endosome fuses with a lysosome where the antigen is degraded into fragments (e.g. short peptides)
- these antigenic peptides are then displayed at the surface of the cell nestled within a class II histocompatibility molecule.
- they may be recognized by CD4+T cells

The Class I Pathway

Class I histocompatibility molecules are transmembrane proteins expressed at the cell surface. Like all transmembrane proteins, they are synthesized by ribosomes on the rough endoplasmic reticulum (RER) and assembled within its lumen. There are three subunits in each class I histocompatibility molecule:

- the transmembrane polypeptide (called the "heavy chain")
- the antigenic peptide
- beta-2 microglobulin

All of these must be present within the lumen of the endoplasmic reticulum if they are to assemble correctly and move through the Golgi apparatus to the cell surface. The Problem: proteins encoded by the genes of an infecting virus are synthesized in the cytosol. How to get them into the endoplasmic reticulum?

The Solution: TAP (= transporter associated with antigen processing).

- Viral proteins in the cytosol are degraded by proteasomes into viral peptides.
- The peptides are picked up by TAP proteins embedded in the membrane of the endoplasmic reticulum.
- Using the energy of ATP, the peptides are pumped into the lumen of the endoplasmic reticulum where they assemble with the transmembrane polypeptide and beta-2 microglobulin.
- This trimolecular complex then moves through the Golgi apparatus and is inserted in the plasma membrane.
- The complex can be bound by a T cell with a receptor (TCR) able to bind the peptide and flanking portions of the histocompatibility molecule (the hot dog in the bun) and CD8 molecules that bind the CD8 receptor (shown above as a gray hemisphere) on the histocompatibility molecule.

The Class II Pathway

Class II histocompatibility molecules consist of two transmembrane polypeptides and a third molecule nestled in the groove they form. All three components of this complex must be present in the endoplasmic reticulum for proper assembly. But antigenic peptides are not transported to the endoplasmic reticulum, so a protein called the invariant chain ("Ii") temporarily occupies the groove.

The steps:

- The two chains of the class II molecule are inserted into the membrane of the endoplasmic reticulum.
- They bind (in their groove) one molecule of invariant chain.
- This trimolecular complex is transported through the Golgi apparatus and into vesicles called lysosomes.

Meanwhile foreign antigenic material is engulfed by endocytosis forming endosomes. These also fuse with lysosomes. Then,

- The antigen is digested into fragments.
- The invariant (Ii) chain is digested.
- This frees the groove for occupancy by the antigenic fragment.
- The vesicles move to the plasma membrane and the complex is displayed at the cell surface.
- The complex can be bound by a T cell with
    - a receptor (TCR) able to bind the peptide and flanking portions of the histocompatibility molecule (the hot dog in the bun) and

- CD4 molecules that bind the CD4 receptor (shown above as a yellow triangle) found on all class II histocompatibility molecules.

Interconnections Between the Class I and Class II Pathways

Cross-Presentation: Transferring Exogenous Antigens to the Class I Pathway

Cross-presentation is the transferring of extracellular antigens like bacteria, some tumor antigens, and antigens in cells infected by viruses into the class I pathway for stimulation of $CD8^+$ cytotoxic T cells (CTL). Only certain "professional" antigen-presenting cells (APCs) like dendritic cells can do this - use the class I as well as the class II pathways of antigen presentation.

Cross-presentation following infection by viruses is important because:

- Most viruses infect cells other than APCs (e.g., liver cells, epithelial cells of the lung) (and, of course, are intracellular in these).
- While viral antigens displayed on the surface of any infected cell can serve as targets for cytotoxic T cells (CTLs),
- the lack of any costimulatory molecules on the cell surface makes them poor stimulants for the development of clones of CTLs in the first place.

However, when an infected cell dies, it can be engulfed by a professional APC, and the antigens within it can enter the class I pathway. One mechanism:

- The dead cell is engulfed by endocytosis.
- The endosome that forms fuses with a lysosome and degradation of the dead cell begins.
- Antigens pass into the cytosol and are degraded in proteasomes.
- The peptides formed are then are picked up by TAP and inserted into class I MHC molecules and displayed at the cell surface — along with the costimulatory molecules needed to start a vigorous clonal expansion of $CD8^+$ cytotoxic T cells.

Diverting Antigens from the Class I to the Class II Pathway

Autophagy provides a mechanism by which cells can transfer endogenous (intracellular) antigens into the class II pathway, for example

- self-proteins so as to be able to delete $CD4^+$ T cells with receptors capable of attacking them and thus potentially capable of causing autoimmunity
- proteins synthesized by an infecting virus. In this way viral infection can generate $CD4^+$ T cells as well as cytotoxic T cells ($CD8^+$)

B LYMPHOCYTES: A SPECIAL CASE

B lymphocytes are both antigen-receiving and antigen-presenting cells. They bind intact antigens (e.g., virus particles, proteins) with their B cell receptor (BCR). They can come in contact with these antigens by encountering them in the surrounding lymph or by being presented them by macrophages or dendritic cells. B lymphocytes process antigen by the class II pathway for presentation to T cells.

The process:

- B cells engulf antigen by receptor-mediated endocytosis
- The B cell receptors for antigen (BCRs) are antibodies anchored in the plasma membrane.
- The affinity of these for an epitope on an antigen may be so high that the B cell can bind and internalize the antigen when it is present in body fluids in concentrations thousands of times smaller than a macrophage would need.
- The remaining steps of antigen processing occur by the same class II pathway described above for macrophages producing
- fragments of antigen displayed at the cell surface nestled in the groove of class II histocompatibility molecules.
- A $CD4^+$ T cell that recognizes the displayed antigen is stimulated to release lymphokines.
- These, in turn, stimulate the B cell to enter the cell cycle.
- Because of the part they play in stimulating B cells, these $CD4^+$ T cells are called Helper T cells ("Th").
- The B cell grows into a clone of cells (called plasma cells)
- These synthesize receptors (BCRs) with the identical binding site for the epitope but without the transmembrane tail.
- These antibodies are secreted into the surroundings.

Lipid and Polysaccharide Antigens

Lipid Antigens

- Lipid antigens are presented to T cells by cell-surface molecules designated CD1 ("cluster of differentiation" 1).
- Antigen-presenting cells express several different forms of CD1 at their surface. Each is probably specialized to bind a particular type of lipid antigen (e.g. lipopeptide vs glycolipid).

- The exposed surface of CD1 molecules forms an antigen-binding groove much like that of MHC molecules except that
- the amino acids in the groove are more hydrophobic than those in MHC molecules.
- Like protein antigens, lipid antigens are also presented as fragments, i.e., as a "hot dog in a bun".

POLYSACCHARIDE ANTIGENS

Some bacterial polysaccharides ingested by APCs

- can be degraded in their lysosomes
- and presented to T cells by MHC class II molecules.

The binding of a T cell to an antigen-presenting cell (APC) is by itself not enough to activate the T cell and turn it into an effector cell: one able to, for examples,

- kill the APC ($CD8^+$ cytotoxic T lymphocytes [CTLs])
- carry out cell-mediated immune reactions ($CD4^+$ Th1 cells)
- provide help to B cells ($CD4^+$ Th2 cells)

In order to become activated, the T cell must not only bind to the epitope (MHC-peptide) with its TCR but also receive a second signal from the APC. The receipt of this second signal is called costimulation. Among the most important of these costimulators are molecules on the APC designated B7 and their ligand on the T cell designated CD28. The binding of CD28 to B7 provides the second signal needed to activate the T cell.

Although T cells may encounter self antigens in body tissues, they will not respond unless they receive a second signal. In fact, binding of their TCR ("signal one") without "signal two" causes them to self-destruct by apoptosis. Most of the time, the cells presenting the body's own antigens either

- fail to provide signal two or
- transmit an as-yet-unidentified second signal that turns the T cell into a regulatory T cell (Treg) that suppresses immune responses.

ANTIGEN PRESENTING BY B CELLS

Introduction

$CD4^+$ T cells are activated by the recognition of peptide in the context of self-MHC class II molecules expressed by professional antigen-presenting cells (APC) such as macrophages, dendritic cells (DC) and B cells. For complete T cell activation, APC also have to express a variety of co-stimulatory molecules, mainly CD40, CD80 and CD86. Although all professional APC can present antigen, it is unclear whether individual subsets of APC have unique properties in certain immune responses or environments. The first *in vivo* evidence that B cells are essential APC in lymph nodes (LN) came from studies using mice that lacked peripheral B cells due to the administration of anti-μ antibodies from birth [μ-suppressed mice (μSM)]. μSM mice showed a severe impairment in CD4⁺ T cell priming when antigen was injected locally in complete Freund's adjuvant (CFA). These mice also had increased susceptibility to viral infections, reduced delayed-type hypersensitivity (DTH) responses, and were resistant to autoimmune diseases like experimental autoimmune encephalomyelitis (EAE) and diabetes (μSM NOD mice), strongly suggesting that in the absence of B cells, $CD4^+$ T cells could not be efficiently primed. All the $CD4^+$ T cell defects observed in μSM could be reversed upon adoptive transfer of B cells prior to antigenic challenge, which pointed to a direct role for B cells as APC and argued against a deleterious effect caused by the prolonged exposure to high levels of anti-μ antibodies.

The role of B cells as important APC *in vivo* became controversial after B cell-deficient mice were generated by gene disruption of the transmembrane domain (μMT) or the J_H segment of the Ig heavy chain (JHD). Although both μSM and μMT mice lack mature peripheral B cells, studies of T cell priming in μMT mice gave conflicting results ranging from near normal to severely impaired responses. T cell proliferative responses to foreign proteins like keyhole limpet hemocyanin (KLH), human γ-globulin or purified protein derivative (PPD) were reported to be similar to normal controls, although at least in the work of researchers control responses were unusually low making it difficult to evaluate differences in responses between control and μMT mice.

In studies employing JHD B cell-deficient mice, Liu *et al.* reported a severe impairment of both T cell proliferation and T cell help to proteins like KLH and ovalbumin. Normal priming of $CD4^+$ T cells could be restored by adoptive transfer of mature B cells before priming. In contrast, Macaulay *et al.* reported that $CD4^+$ T cell proliferative responses to KLH were normal in JHD mice, but that the cytokine profile was skewed such that the primed $CD4^+$ cells were unable to provide B cell help for antibody production.

T cell responses to small peptide antigens (which do not require processing) in B cell-deficient mice were also variable. While researchers reported reduced $CD4^+$ T cell responses to small peptide antigens irrespective of whether the T cells were derived from LN or spleen, researchers reported normal T cell proliferative responses to peptide antigens in μMT mice, but greatly reduced responses to large protein antigens. Differences in responses to whole proteins versus responses to small peptides were also reported in the induction of EAE. μMT mice have been found to be consistently susceptible to EAE induction with peptides in two different mouse strains with similar disease severity and onset as normal controls. In contrast, researchers reported that although µMT mice were susceptible to EAE induction with the MOG35–55 encephalitogenic peptide, the mice were resistant to EAE induction with the whole MOG protein.

In spontaneous autoimmune diseases, an absolute requirement for B cells as APC has been reported for the development of diabetes in NOD mice and autoimmune responses in MRL/*lpr/lpr* mice. µMT.NOD mice do not exhibit the characteristic T cell infiltration in the pancreas and do not develop insulin-dependent diabetes. Furthermore, a direct role for B cells as APC in the development of disease was clearly demonstrated in NOD mice that did not express I-A^{g7} molecules exclusively on B cells (NOD BCIID). Although NOD BCIID mice had normal class II expression in all APC other than B cells, these mice were resistant to autoimmune diabetes. Similarly, when the JHD mutation was backcrossed to the MRL/*lpr/lpr* mouse, the animals did not develop spontaneous autoimmune nephritis and vasculitis with complete absence of the typical T cell infiltrates.

The fact that in order for autoimmunity to develop in the MRL/*lpr/lpr* mice, B cells were required as APC and not as antibody-producing cells, was elegantly demonstrated utilizing transgenic mice that expressed cell-surface IgM but not secreted IgM (Tg mIgM). Tg mIgM on the MRL/*lpr/lpr* background had no serum antibodies and still developed nephritis. Moreover, these mice had T cell infiltrates, similar numbers of memory cells as controls and greater disease-related mortality, phenotypes that were not observed in JHD-MRL/*lpr/lpr* mice.

In order to clarify the requirement for B cells as APC for T cell activation *in vivo*, we analyzed a variety of $CD4^+$ T cell responses in µMT mice of various genetic backgrounds and in µMT $\rightarrow F_1$ chimeras. We also investigated whether antigen-specific B cells are essential for antigen presentation.

Media

For most procedures cells were prepared and manipulated in PBS (Cellgrow, Herdon, VA). For *in vitro* assays cells were grown in T cell media consisting of RPMI 1640 (Cellgrow) supplemented with 10% FCS (HyClone, Pittsburgh, PA), 5×10^{-5}M 2-mercaptoethanol (Sigma, St Louis, MO) and 50 mg/ml of gentamycin (Gibco/BRL, Grand Island, NY).

Antigens

Highly purified KLH and foul ã-globulin (FGG) were obtained from Calbiochem (La Jolla, CA). BSA was obtained from Sigma. Sheep red blood cells (SRBC) were purchased from Colorado Serum (Denver, CO).

T cell proliferation assay

µMT and control mice were injected with 50 µl/footpad of antigen emulsified in CFA containing 1 mg/ml of antigen. Eight days later, draining LN were removed and single-cell suspensions were prepared by using the frosted ends of two glass slides. Total LN cells were plated in -96well plates at a concentration of 10×4^5 cells/well (or at 2×10^5 cells/well in half-area 96-well plates) in T cell media. Cells were cultured for 90–96 h together with increasing doses of the relevant antigen and with 0.5–1 µCi/well of [^{3}H]thymidine during the last 8–12 h. Cells were then harvested and processed for liquid scintillation measurements of radioactivity. Unless otherwise stated, LN preparations tested for T cell proliferation were not supplemented with exogenous APC. In several experiments, B cells were depleted from the normal control LN cells prior to *in vitro* culture with magnetic beads coated with goat-anti mouse IgG (H & L) (BioMag, Framingham, MA) according to the manufacturer's instructions. In experiments where only CD4$^+$ T cells were used, B cells were removed in the same manner, and CD8$^+$ T cells were depleted by antibody and complement treatment. Cell depletions were verified by FACS analysis.

Bone marrow chimeras

Recipient mice (2–3 months old) were lethally irradiated using a ^{137}Cs source, (110 rad/min; Atomic Energy of Canada). C57BL/6 mice were irradiated with 900 rad and CB6F$_1$ mice with 1050 rad at least 2 h before bone marrow transfer. Bone marrow from donor µMT or control mice were obtained from femur and tibia, and depleted of T cells by antibody plus complement using a mixture of J1j, GK1.5 and 3.168 mAb and guinea pig/rabbit complement mixture (Colorado Serum). All recipient mice were injected with $2–8\times10^6$ bone marrow cells and allowed to reconstitute for 2 months. All chimeras were kept on drinking water containing 100,000 U/l of Polymyxin B and 25 mg/l of neomycin sulfate (Pharma-Tek, Hungtington, NY) for 4–6 weeks before returning to regular water

FACS analysis

The absence of peripheral B cells in µMT mice and bone marrow chimeras was determined by staining 1×10^6 LN or spleen cells with anti-CD19 antibodies or anti-IgG antibodies. The samples were processed in an Epics profile analyzer (Coulter, Hialeah, FL). The chimeric status of bone marrow reconstituted mice was analyzed by two-color staining with J1j and 34-4-21S or Y3P for typing of T cells, and with CD19 or RA3.3 plus 34-4-21S or Y3P for typing of B cells. Samples from all mice used in the experiments were FACS analyzed.

Preparation of B cells

For adoptive transfers, B cells were obtained from the spleens of normal or Ig transgenic (IgHelMD4) mice. Spleen cells were depleted of T cells by treatment with J1j and complement for 45 min at 37°C. Cells were washed 4 times and doses of $50\times10^6–1\times10^7$ cells in PBS were injected i.v. into recipient mice 1 week before antigen challenge. Reconstitution of B cells in the recipients was confirmed by FACS analysis.

DTH

Mice were sensitized on day 0 by i.v. injection of 200 µl of 0.01% SRBC in PBS solution. At day 4, sensitized and control animals were challenged in the right hind footpad with 50 µl of a 20% SRBC suspension. At 24 and 48 h later footpad swelling was measured with a micrometer. The magnitude of the response was determined by subtracting measurements of uninjected left footpads from experimental right ones.

T_h assay

Mice that were to be used as a source of B cells for measuring T_h function were injected i.p. with 0.5 ml of a 10% SRBC solution 2–6 months before. B cells were prepared by depleting the spleens of T cells with J1j plus complement lysis. As a source of primed T cells the spleens of mice that had been injected i.v. with 0.5 ml of 10% SRBC 8 days before were used after depletion of B cells with J11d and complement treatment. To measure T_h function *in vivo*, 5×10^6 primed B cells and 5×10^5 primed T cells were transferred together with 100 µl of 5% SRBC to lethally irradiated syngeneic recipient mice. The spleens of recipient mice were removed 6 days later and were assayed for direct (IgM, non-enhanced) and indirect (IgG, enhanced) plaque-forming cells as described.

DIAGNOSTIC ANTIBODIES AND ANTIGENS FOR BOVINES/CATTLE INFECTIOUS AND NON-INFECTIOUS DISEASE TESTING

Cattle diseases cost millions of money losses every year. In addition to death, they cause loss of production and frequently a loss of body condition. Unhealthy animals require more food and take longer time for growth than healthy ones. Generally, animals are born free of diseases or parasites. But they usually acquire these diseases either through contact with diseased animals or due to improper sanitation, feeding, care and management. Knowledge of cattle diseases is necessary from public health point of view also as many diseases can be transmitted to man through milk.

Keeping animals healthy by employing sound principles of sanitation, management and feeding and by judicious use of appropriate and dependable vaccines are the practical and economical ways to avoid losses from the disease. By proper management and feeding, the dairy farmer can, to a great extent, prevent disease out-breaks. Cattle are infected by a community of endemic pathogens with different epidemiological properties that invoke different managerial and governmental responses. Genemedi developed the antigen and antibody to detect the abortion, acute severe metritis, borna disease, borrelia theileri infection, bovine amyloidosis, bovine besnoitiosis, bovine parainfluenza-3 virus (bpi3) infection, bovine respiratory syncytial virus infection, bovine spongiform encephalopathy, bovine viral diarrhea, calf enteritis, chronic endometritis, chronic wasting disease, contagious bovine pleuropneumonia, cystic hydatidosis, cysticercosis, diarrhea, enzootic bovine leukosis, enzootic pneumonia complex, gastrointestinal infections, hormone disorders, hypodermiasis, infectious bovine rhinotracheitis, infectious pustular vulvovaginitis, ketosis, mastitis, arthritis and pneumonia, milk fever, paratuberculosis, respiratory and enteric infections, respiratory syndrome, retained placenta, rotaviral diarrhea, septicemia, severe mastitis, systemic infection in neonates, thromboembolic meningoencepahlitis (teme), transmissible spongiform encephalopathies (tses), tuberculosis/leprosy and so on.

Due to the physiology and structure of bovines, cattle health issues are also unique. With their four-chambered stomachs and a surprising susceptibility to heat, cattle require special care, monitoring and handling to maintain optimum health and longevity. Good grassland management will ensure that cattle have access to plenty of leafy grass that they can readily digest and will provide all of their energy requirements for maintenance and growth. In addition, the diet must also provide small amounts of certain essential chemical elements (trace elements).

Deficiencies of any of these micronutrients can result in ill-thrift. Fortunately, there are a few simple ways to improve your herd's health. Watchful ranchers can detect early signs of the most common cattle health issues, and then take preventative measures to correct potentially detrimental conditions. Genemedi developed the antigen and antibody to detect the non-infectious disease such as immune dysfunction, abortion and teratology, nonbacterial diarrheic disease, Prion associated diseases (Scrapie, Bovine Spongiform Encephalopathy, Chronical Waste Disease), winter dysentery and so on.

DIAGNOSTIC ANTIBODIES AND ANTIGENS FOR OVINES/SHEEP DISEASE TESTING

A sound management program to keep animals healthy is basic to production of both sheep and goats. Producers must observe animals closely to keep individual animals and the whole herd or flock healthy and productive. To recognize clinical signs of diseases common to sheep and goats, it is important to be familiar with what is normal. Producers should assess the herd or flock's general health on a regular basis, including vital signs, body condition, and coat. Correct diagnosis of sheep is most difficult.

Hence, Genemedi developed the antigen and antibody to detect the disease such as campylobacteriosis, caprine arthritis encephalitis, caprine pleuropneumonia, congenital diseases, contagious agalactia, gastroenteritis, leptospirosis, lumpy skin disease, sheeppox and goatpox, maedi visna virus infection, mycoplasma pneumonia, PESTE des petits ruminants, pneumonia, rift valley fever, sexually transmitted infectious disease and so on.

DIAGNOSTIC ANTIBODIES AND ANTIGENS FOR CAPRINE/GOAT DISEASE TESTING

Goats are important domestic animals in many parts of the world. They provide substance in the form of food and clothing. The rising demand for goat meat, milk, and cheese offers commercial goat production opportunities. Goats are also a source of immediate income. The management of goat health is a critical aspect for improving goat production. It is important to understand health and disease of goat. Hence, Genemedi developed the antigen and antibody to detect the disease such as abortions and mortality in neonates, akabane disease, bacteremia, cholangitis, bluetongue disease, caprine pleuropneumonia, chlamydiosis, cholecystitis, congenital diseases, contagious agalactia, gastroenteritis, leptospirosis, maedi visna virus infection, paratuberculosis, Q fever, respiratory syndrome, rift valley fever, schmallenberg disease, septicemic colibacillosis, traveler's diarrhea, trichomoniasis, urinary tract infection (UTI) and so on.

DIAGNOSTIC ANTIBODIES AND ANTIGENS FOR DEER DISEASE TESTING

Managing the deer population is essential to maintaining or improving forest health. It plays a crucial role in the ecosystem, providing food for large predators such as gray wolves (*Canis lupis*), cougars (*Puma concolor*), bobcats (*Lynx rufus*), and coyotes (*Canis latrans*). They feed primarily on grasses, herbaceous plants, fruits, and legumes and are active throughout the year. Their economic importance includes the use of their meat as venison, their skins as soft, strong buckskin, and their antlers as handles for knives. Dears are prone to diseases caused by a long list of environmental pathogens. Those can rapidly spread throughout deer populations and cause outbreaks that cause death and chronic illness. Hence, Genemedi developed the antigen and antibody to detect the disease such as cholecystitis, bacteremia, cholangitis, urinary tract infection (UTI), traveler's diarrhea, septicemic colibacillosis, respiratory syndrome and so on.

DIAGNOSTIC ANTIBODIES AND ANTIGENS FOR DOG/CANINE INFECTIOUS AND NON-INFECTIOUS DISEASE TESTING

Dogs are the best friends, and most human keep pets for its ompanionship. Dogs need a proper space, diet and health care for their healthy life. However, sometimes the dogs are affected by the different infectious diseases such as amyloidosis, anaplasmosis, anemia, intestinal infection, canine cyclic thrombocytopenia, canine herpes, canine infectious tracheobronchitis, canine parvovirus infection, conjunctivitis, croup, dirofilariasis, gastroenteritis, hepatitis, hormone disorders, inflammation, leptospirosis, mediterranean spotted fever, otitis media, pancreatitis, pharyngitis, pneumonia, pregnancy, rabies, rocky mountain spotted fever, spotted fever group rickettsia, tracheobronchitis, visceral leishmaniasis and so on. Genemedi developed the antigen and antibody to detect these diseases at early stages.

Dog is known to be a very intelligent animal that can detect human psychology easily, and even a well-trained dog can be used as a substitute of a qualified person to perform certain specific crucial functions. Further, dogs play a pivotal role to detect crimes and criminals. The common diseases of dogs can be categorized into infectious, non-infectious, and non-specific diseases. Among non-infectious diseases, dogs are mostly prone to fracture, lacerated wound, abortion, dystocia, Cancer, Diabetes and vitamin deficiency and the most frequent non-specific cases are gastroenteritis, otorrhea, dermatitis, and alopecia. A good knowledge of the epidemiology of these diseases of dogs is important for their prevention and control. Genemedi developed the antigen and antibody to detect the various non-infectious disease of dogs.

DIAGNOSTIC ANTIBODIES AND ANTIGENS FOR CAT/FELINE INFECTIOUS AND NON-INFECTIOUS DISEASE TESTING

Cats are credited with promoting socialization among older individuals and physically or mentally disabled people. Research has shown that cats can provide emotional support, improve moods, and contribute to the overall morale of their owners. Although cats are great companions, cat owners should be aware that sometimes cats can carry harmful germs that can cause a variety of illnesses. Since cats are fiercely independent and sometimes mysterious little creatures, it can be difficult for pet parents to tell the difference between a minor issue and a serious health problem. Genemedi developed the antigen and antibody to detect the amyloidosis, anaplasmosis, canine angiostrongylosis, canine brucellosis, cardiac disease, cat HIV, cat scratch disease, feline infectious enteritis, feline infectious peritonitis, feline panleukopenia, feline viral rhinotracheitis, hormone disorders, inflammation of feline conjunctiva, leishmaniasis, leukemia, pancreatitis, respiratory disease, rhinitis and so on.

No one likes to think about their cat getting sick or contracting a disease, but unfortunately there are many diseases affect the cat. It is important to understand signs and symptoms of cat and most importantly to prevent cat diseases. Genemedi developed the antigen and antibody to detect the non-infectious disease such as chronic kidney disease, degenerative joint disease (arthritis), diabetes, hypertension (high blood pressure), hyperthyroidism lower urinary tract disease, obesity and so on.

DIAGNOSTIC ANTIBODIES AND ANTIGENS FOR RABBIT INFECTIOUS DISEASE AND NON-INFECTIOUS TESTING

Rabbits are perhaps the most popular small mammals kept as pets. They make great companions and can live a dozen or more years when they are cared for properly.

However, they do commonly develop a few illnesses and infection that all rabbit owners should be aware to prevent the disease. The most common diseases of rabbits include rabbit hemorrhagic disease and so on have been detected using the antigen and antibody produced by Genemedi.

It's important to know how to care and prevent common types of rabbit illness. Rabbits fed with a suitable diet and kept in a healthy environment can live as long as 10 to 12 years. The most common diseases of rabbits include digestive system problems, respiratory infections, and skin disorders. In addition to the infectious disease testing, Genemedi also developed antigen and antibody to detect the common rabbit illness.

DIAGNOSTIC ANTIBODIES AND ANTIGENS FOR SWINE DISEASE TESTING

Pork accounts for more than one-third of meat produced worldwide and is an important component of global food security, agricultural economies, and trade. Infectious diseases are among the primary constraints to swine production, and the globalization of the swine industry has contributed to the emergence and spread of pathogens. Infectious diseases result in direct losses to livestock production through mortality, loss of productivity, trade restrictions, reduced market value, and often food insecurity. The constant threat of endemic and emerging diseases affecting swine, which in some instances also impact human health, highlight the potential vulnerability of pork production around the world. Indeed, infectious diseases of swine are among the primary constraints to pork production and trade.

Genemedi developed the antigen and antibody to detect the swine disease such as african swine fever, arthritis, aujeszky's disease, bacteremia, brucella suis, chlamydial infections, cholangitis, cholecystitis, classical swine fever, diarrhea, ecephalitis, endocarditis, enzootic pneumonia, erysipelas, gastroenteritis, glässers disease, idiopathic vesicular disease, japanese encephalitis, leptospirosis, meningitis, multisystemic wasting syndrome, nipah virus infection, porcine colonic spirochetosis, porcine diarrhea, porcine enzootic pneumonia, porcine pleuropneumonia, porcine reproductive and respiratory syndrome, proliferative hemorrhagic enteritis, pseudorabies, reproductive disease, respiratory disease, salmonellosis, septicemia, swine brucellosis, swine enteric coronavirus disease (SECD), swine flu, swine pleuropneumonia, swine vesicular disease, traveler's diarrhea, urinary tract infection, viral enteritis, white chick syndrome and so on. Detecting the quantity of marker proteins from different samples may benefit from ELISA, Lateral flow immunoassay (LFIA), colloidal gold immuno-chromatographic assay, Chemiluminescent immunoassay (CLIA), turbidimetric inhibition immuno assay (TINIA), immunonephelometry and POCT.

DIAGNOSTIC ANTIBODIES AND ANTIGENS FOR INFECTIOUS AND NON-INFECTIOUS EQUINE/HORSE DISEASE TESTING

Common health problems and infections are a constant threat to the health and welfare of horses. Several diseases have assumed greater importance as the performance and pleasure horse populations and equine activities have increased and there are new owners who do not understand the implications of equine infectious disease outbreaks to their animals. In addition, emerging diseases have beset the equine species in recent years. Genemedi developed the antigen and antibody to detect the horse herpes myeloencephalopathy, respiratory disease, horse infectious anemia, equine influenza, thrombocytopenia, anaplasmosis, contagious equine metritis, horse viral arteritis, horse piroplasmosis, horse theileriosis, pneumonia; urinary tract infections, respiratory system infections, dermatitis, soft tissue infections, bacteremia, bone and joint infections, gastrointestinal infections, eastern equine/horse encephalitis (EEE), equine/horse morbillivirus pneumonia and so on. Detecting the quantity of marker proteins from different samples may benefit from ELISA, Lateral flow immunoassay (LFIA), colloidal gold immunochromatographic assay, Chemiluminescent immunoassay (CLIA), turbidimetric inhibition immuno assay (TINIA), immunonephelometry and POCT.

Most horses are very resilient animals, yet like all animals, they are subject to their own set of illnesses. They are susceptible to a number of common horse health problems and issues ranging from illness and disease, to injuries. Horse owners are responsible for the supervision of horses should be able to recognize signs of ill health. It is also important that owners/keepers to diagnose or treat any illness, injury or disease. Hence, Genemedi developed the antigen and antibody to detect the Arthritis/Osteoarthritis, laminitis, Equine Cushing's Disease and so on.

DIAGNOSTIC ANTIBODIES AND ANTIGENS FOR AVIAN DISEASE TESTING

Infectious diseases continue to threaten the sustainability, productivity and growth of the poultry industry worldwide and some present a risk to public health. Many are also present in wild bird populations, with the potential to spill over into domestic birds. The avian infectious disease cause huge economic loss in poultry production and are of great significance in public health. However, they are usually not covered in the systems for reporting of animal diseases. Several methods have been employed to develop conventional assays to detect avian disease, Genemedi developed the antigen and antibody to detect the upper respiratory tract infection, newcastle disease, duck hepatitis, derzsy's disease, infectious bursal disease, chlamydiosis, respiratory disease, arthritis, duck plague, avian influenza, cholecystitis, bacteremia, cholangitis, urinary tract infection (UTI), and traveler's diarrhea, respiratory disease, avian metapneumovirus infection, treponeme, encephalomyelitis, infectious bronchitis, mycoplasmosis, nephritis, blackhead disease (histomoniasis), bordetellosis, campylobacteriosis, infectious anemia, chlamydia, duck septicaemia, Goose 'flu, riemerellosis, polyserositis, egg drop syndrome, erysipeloid, fowl cholera, fowl typhoid, pullorum, fowlpox, gastroenteritis, hemorrhagic nephritis, enteritis of geese, hepatitis-splenomegaly syndrome, immunosuppression, inclusion body hepatitis, infectious bronchitis, infectious coryza, infectious laryngotracheitis, infectious synovitis, avian mycoplasmosis, infectious sinusitis, mycoplasma arthritis, lymphoid leukosis, Marek's disease, mycoplasma air sacculitis, mycoplasmosis, ornithobacteriosis, feather disease, psittacosi, pullorum, reticuloendotheliosis, salmonellosis, turkey hepatitis, swollen head syndrome, white chick syndrome, young pigeon disease syndrome and so on.

Detecting the quantity of marker proteins from different samples may benefit from ELISA, Lateral flow immunoassay (LFIA), colloidal gold immuno-chromatographic assay, Chemiluminescent immunoassay (CLIA), turbidimetric inhibition immuno assay (TINIA), immunonephelometry and POCT.

Cytokine

Cytokinesis of animal cells begins during anaphase with the formation of a cleavage furrow at the cell equator, between the separating chromosomes. At the base of this furrow is a "contractile ring" (CR) that exerts force to dramatically reduce the circumference of the cell's plasma membrane and form a midbody ring, which then orchestrates abscission. Pioneering electron microscopy of sea urchin embryos by Schroeder showed that the CR contains circumferential actin filaments. This was quickly followed by studies showing that the CR contains myosin. It was initially thought that the CR might have a muscle sarcomere-like organization and close like a purse-string.

However, the actin filaments of the CR are not organized as in sarcomeres, but are rather organized as a meshwork of filaments in a random order of mixed polarity. An additional class of cytoskeletal filaments, the septins, was discovered as membrane-associated filaments of the budding yeast CR. Septins are conserved components of CRs from yeast to humans, yet the roles that they play there and how they interact with actomyosin filaments remain unclear. It has been evident since the work of Schroeder, and more recently Carvalho, that the CR disassembles as it closes, since its closure results in a decrease in its circumference but does not increase its thickness or width.

From many studies since these pioneering works, we have learned much about the CR, its constituent parts and their biochemical activities. Yet we still do not understand how those components are organized and coordinated with one another to promote CR assembly and closure, particularly in animal cells. Indeed, some of the most enduring and fundamental questions in the field that remain unanswered include: How does the CR generate tension? How does the CR maintain tension while closing and disassembling at the same time? How is the CR anchored to the plasma membrane? How are the different filament systems of the CR (F-actin, myosin II, septins) coordinated with one another? This article seeks to address these questions. The following sections will briefly summarize the current state of knowledge of the key players involved in CR assembly and function, before describing novel models for how the actomyosin and septin sub-networks of the CR collaborate to generate tension during CR assembly and regulate it to drive CR closure.

Rho: The Master Activator of Cytokinesis

The small molecular weight GTPase Rho has emerged as the master activator of cytokinesis, and specifically, CR assembly. From the onset of cytokinesis, RhoA (Rho1 in Drosophila) undergoes dynamic cycles of activation/inactivation at the equatorial plasma membrane with activation through GDP to GTP exchange catalyzed by a specific guanine nucleotide exchange factor (GEF), ECT2 Pebble in Drosophila and inactivation promoted by GTP hydrolysis catalyzed by GTPase activating proteins (GAPs). ECT2/Pebble forms a complex with the centralspindlin complex, comprising kinesin-6 (MKLP1/KIF23 in mammals, Pavarotti in Drosophila, ZEN4 in *C. elegans*) and RacGAP (MgcRacGAP in mammals, Tumbleweed/RacGAP50C in Drosophila, CYK4 in *C. elegans*), which is required both to activate the GEF activity (via the RacGAP component) and localize it to the equator (via the kinesin-6 component).

Although centralspindlin-ECT2/Pebble complexes localize to the central spindle at the cell interior, ECT2/Pebble is specifically active as a Rho GEF only at the plasma membrane. There, active Rho-GTP in turn binds and activates specific effector proteins (described below), while RhoGAPs stimulate GTP hydrolysis to rapidly inactivate Rho. Although ECT2/Pebble clearly controls the major Rho-dependent events during cytokinesis, the RhoGAPs responsible for inactivation of specific Rho-effector complexes are less clear. The RacGAP component of the centralspindlin complex required for ECT2/Pebble activation has long been a candidate and its involvement in Rho inactivation is supported by the analysis of GAP-defective MgcRacGAP in Xenopus embryos.

However, RacGAP exhibits preferential GAP activity toward Rac and Cdc42 rather than Rho *in vitro*. Genetic experiments in *C. elegans* embryos have led to conflicting models in which the CYK4 GAP domain either targets Rac, or acts non-canonically to activate Rho. Another candidate GAP for Rho inactivation at the CR is p190RhoGAP-A/ARHGAP35. M-phase GAP (MP-GAP:ARHGAP11A in mammals, RGA-3/4 in *C. elegans*) also acts to globally suppress Rho and restrict cortical contractility to the equator, although no ortholog exists in Drosophila. Finally, an additional level of regulation of the Rho GTPase cycle comes from guanine nucleotide dissociation inhibitors (GDIs), which can directly extract active Rho from the plasma membrane.

While our understanding of the dynamic control of Rho activity is far from complete, it is clear that active Rho-GTP binds and activates multiple effectors that are essential for cytokinesis. These include Diaphanous-related formins, which polymerize unbranched actin filaments.

Rho-GTP also activates Rho-kinase, which in turn activates myosin II, through both stimulatory phosphorylation of the myosin regulatory light chain (MRLC) and inhibitory phosphorylation of the myosin phosphatase. Together, these Rho-dependent events provide the textbook description for actomyosin-based CR assembly.

However, Rho controls a more expansive network than just formins and Rho-kinase. Rho-GTP also binds and recruits to the CR Anillin and Citron kinase (called Sticky in Drosophila. Anillin is a conserved scaffold protein that has emerged as a master organizer of the CR. Citron kinase/Sticky does not appear to play important roles at the CR but becomes essential for formation of the subsequent midbody ring (MR). The MR is a stable cortical ring structure that forms after CR closure at the center of the intercellular bridge, where it encircles the densely packed zone of interdigitating microtubule plus-ends of the midbody. Although the mechanisms of MR formation are poorly defined, MRs contain numerous CR-derived proteins including Anillin, Citron kinase/Sticky, myosin, centralspindlin, as well as CEP55 in mammalian cells. The MR persists after the midbody microtubules have depolymerized and it recruits ESCRT proteins to mediate abscission.

Finally, in considering the different Rho-dependent sub-networks, our observations also provide insight into the bigger picture view of how cytokinetic ring structures mature during successive stages of cytokinetic progression. The actomyosin sub-network drives CR assembly and closure, while the anillo-septin sub-network promotes CR closure and disassembly. Finally, an Anillin-Citron kinase sub-network promotes MR formation (Fig. 5).

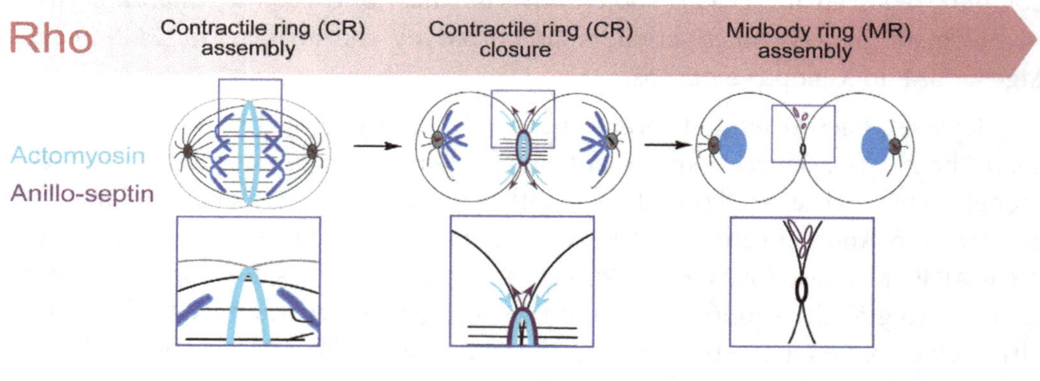

Fig. 5. The Rho-dependent network drives cytokinetic progression from CR assembly, through closure/disassembly and to midbody ring assembly.

Thus, maturation of the cell cortex during cytokinesis reflects a shifting importance of different sub-networks controlled by the master activator, Rho, and coordinated by the master organizer, Anillin. Mapping how these different sub-networks are integrated with one another throughout cytokinetic progression remains an important challenge.

CHAPTER

RED CELL ANTIGENS AND ANTIBODY-MEDIATED HYPERSENSITIVITY 9

RED BLOOD CELLS IN ANIMALS

The function of RBCs is to carry oxygen to the tissues at pressures sufficient to permit its rapid diffusion. This is accomplished through the following mechanisms: a carrier molecule, hemoglobin (Hgb); a vehicle (RBC) capable of bringing the intact Hgb to the cellular level; and a metabolism geared to protect both the RBC and the Hgb from damage. Interference with synthesis or release of Hgb, production or survival of RBCs, or metabolism causes disease.

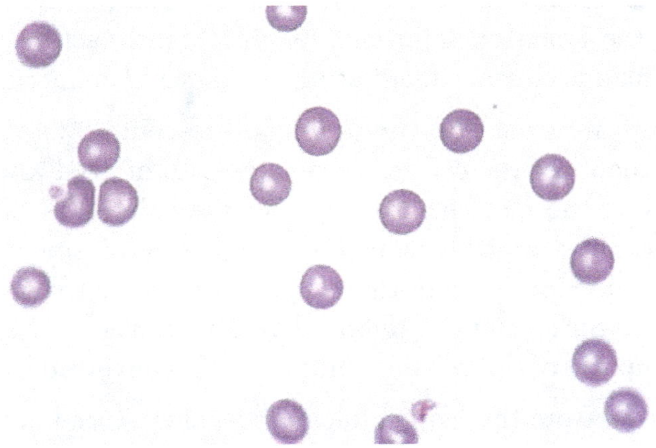

Fig. 1. Red Blood Cells

The function of RBCs is to carry oxygen to the tissues at pressures sufficient to permit its rapid diffusion. This is accomplished through the following mechanisms: a carrier molecule, hemoglobin (Hgb); a vehicle (RBC) capable of bringing the intact Hgb to the cellular level; and a metabolism geared to protect both the RBC and the Hgb from damage. Interference with synthesis or release of Hgb, production or survival of RBCs, or metabolism causes disease.

Red Blood Cells

Hgb is a complex molecule, formed of four heme units attached to four globins (two α and two β globins). Iron is added in the last step by the ferrochelatase enzyme. Interference with the normal production of heme or globin leads to anemia. Causes include copper or iron deficiency and lead poisoning. Hemoglobinopathies such as thalassemias and sickle cell anemia, important genetic diseases of people, have not been seen in other animals. In these diseases, the production of globins (α or β or both) does not balance heme production, and the Hgb is not functional. The only known hemoglobinopathy of animals is porphyria. Although described in several species, it is most important as a cause of photosensitivity in cattle.

Red cell mass, and thus oxygen-carrying capacity, remains constant over time in healthy animals. Mature RBCs have a finite life span; their production and destruction must be carefully balanced, or disease ensues.

Erythropoiesis is regulated by erythropoietin, which increases in the presence of hypoxia and regulates RBC production. In most species, the kidney is both the sensor organ and the major site of erythropoietin production, so chronic renal failure is associated with anemia. Erythropoietin acts on the marrow in concert with other humoral mediators to increase the number of stem cells entering RBC production, to shorten maturation time and to cause early release of reticulocytes. Other factors that affect erythropoiesis are the supply of nutrients (e.g., iron, folate, or vitamin B_{12}) and cell-cell interactions between erythroid precursors, lymphoid cells, and other components of the hematopoietic microenvironment. Factors that may suppress erythropoiesis include chronic debilitating diseases and endocrine disorders.

Two mechanisms exist for removal of senescent RBCs; both conserve the principal constituents of the cell for reuse. Removal of aged RBCs normally occurs by phagocytosis by the fixed macrophages of the spleen. As the RBC ages it may change antigenically, acquiring senescent antigens and losing its flexibility due to impaired ATP production. Both of these changes increase the risk that the cell will become trapped in the spleen and removed by macrophages. After phagocytosis and subsequent disruption of the cell membrane, Hgb is converted to heme and globin.

Iron is released from the heme moiety and either stored in the macrophage as ferritin or hemosiderin or released into the circulation for transport back to the marrow. The remaining heme is converted to bilirubin, which is released by the macrophages into the systemic circulation, where it complexes with albumin for transport to the hepatocytes; there, it is conjugated and excreted into the bile. In extravascular hemolytic anemias, RBCs have a shortened life span, and the same mechanisms occur at an increased rate.

Approximately 1% of normal aging RBCs are hemolyzed in the circulation, and free Hgb is released. This is quickly converted to Hgb dimers that bind to haptoglobin and are transported to the liver, where they are metabolized in the same manner as products from RBCs removed by phagocytosis. In intravascular hemolytic anemia, more RBCs are destroyed in the circulation (hemoglobinemia) than can be bound to haptoglobin. The excess Hgb and, therefore, iron are excreted in the urine (hemoglobinuria).

The principal metabolic pathway of RBC is glycolysis, and the main energy source in most species is glucose. Glucose enters the RBC by an insulin-independent mechanism, and most is metabolized to produce ATP and reduced nicotinamide adenine dinucleotide (NADH). The energy of ATP is used to maintain RBC membrane pumps so as to preserve shape and flexibility. The reducing potential of the NADH is utilized via the methemoglobin reductase pathway to maintain the iron in Hgb in its reduced form (Fe^{2+}).

The glucose not used in glycolysis is metabolized via a second pathway, the hexose monophosphate (HMP) shunt. No energy is produced via the HMP shunt; its principal effect is to maintain reducing potential in the form of reduced nicotinamide adenine dinucleotide phosphate (NADPH). In conjunction with the glutathione reductase/peroxidase system, NADPH maintains the sulfhydryl groups of globin in their reduced state.

Some disorders are the direct result of abnormal RBC metabolism and interference with glycolysis. Inherited deficiency of pyruvate kinase, a key glycolytic enzyme, causes ATP deficiency, which leads to reduced RBC life span and hemolytic anemia. Excessive oxidant stress may overload the protective HMP shunt or methemoglobin reductase pathways, causing Heinz body hemolysis or methemoglobin formation, respectively. Hemolytic anemia caused by a drug, such as acetaminophen in cats, is an example of this mechanism.

A decreased RBC mass (anemia) may be caused by blood loss, hemolysis, or decreased production. In acute blood loss anemia, RBCs are lost, but mortality is usually related to loss of circulating volume rather than to loss of RBC. Iron is the limiting factor in chronic blood loss. Hemolysis may be caused by toxins, infectious agents, congenital abnormalities, or antibodies directed against RBC membrane antigens. Decreased RBC production may result from primary marrow diseases (eg, aplastic anemia, hematopoietic malignancy, or myelofibrosis) or from other causes such as renal failure, drugs, toxins, or antibodies directed against RBC precursors. Malignancy of RBCs or their precursors may be acute (eg, erythroleukemia) or chronic (e.g., polycythemia vera). Animals with erythroleukemia are anemic despite having a marrow filled with rubriblasts, whereas those with polycythemia vera have erythrocytosis.

HYPERSENSITIVITY DISEASES IN ANIMALS

Excessive activity of the adaptive immune system can lead to inappropriate immune responses collectively called hypersensitivities. In general, inappropriate innate immune responses do this by triggering inflammation that leads to collateral damage to nearby tissues or organs, or by producing vastly excessive amounts of inflammatory cytokines. Excessive adaptive immune responses, in contrast, can cause damage by multiple mechanisms.

One simple classification divides these hypersensitivity reactions into four distinct types. Each involves very different mechanisms. Type I hypersensitivity is mediated by IgE antibodies and mast cells; Type II by IgG and/or IgM antibodies and complement; Type III by immune complexes, complement and neutrophils; and Type IV by T lymphocytes.

Type I Hypersensitivity

Type I, or immediate hypersensitivity, encompasses IgE-mediated responses to foreign antigens. These reactions may be minor and local or may be severe and generalized. In its most extreme form, type 1 hypersensitivity or allergy is expressed as a lethal shock syndrome called **anaphylaxis**.

Anaphylaxis is an acute systemic manifestation of the interaction of an antigen (allergen) binding to IgE on mast cells and basophils. The antigen binding triggers the mast cell to release a complex mixture of **inflammatory mediators**, including:

- histamine
- leukotrienes
- eosinophil chemotactic factors
- platelet activating factor
- kinins
- serotonin
- proteases
- cytokines

Some of these molecules directly affect both the vascular system, causing vasodilation and increased vascular permeability, and the smooth muscles, causing contraction. Other mediators attract eosinophils to the reaction site.

The severity of anaphylaxis depends on the type of antigen, the amount of IgE produced, the amount of antigen received, and the route of exposure. If the animal has been previously sensitized by exposure to an allergen (antigen) and produces high levels of IgE antibodies, then injection of the sensitizing antigens directly into the bloodstream can result in anaphylactic shock and related allergic reactions such as hives, urticaria, and facial-conjunctival edema.

If the sensitizing allergen enters through the mucous membranes or the skin, allergic reactions tend to be more localized. Antigens that can trigger anaphylactic and allergic reactions are numerous and include the venom of stinging and biting insects, some vaccines, drugs, foods, and blood products.

Systemic Anaphylaxis (Generalized Anaphylactic Reactions)

Anaphylactic shock occurs in sensitized animals within seconds to minutes after exposure to the allergen. In most domestic species, the lungs are the primary target organs, and the portal-mesenteric vasculature is a secondary target; this is reversed in dogs. Mast cell degranulation releases histamine and other mediators that cause constriction of bronchial airways or pulmonary veins, pooling of blood and edema in the pulmonary vascular bed, and severe respiratory distress. Mast cell degranulation in the portosystemic vasculature causes venous dilation and pooling of blood in the intestine and liver.

Clinical signs may be localized or generalized and include:

- restlessness and excitement
- pruritus around the head or site of exposure
- facial edema
- salivation
- lacrimation
- vomiting
- abdominal pain
- diarrhea
- dyspnea
- cyanosis
- shock
- incoordination
- collapse
- convulsions
- death

In dogs, the major organ affected by anaphylactic shock is the liver, and signs are associated with constriction of hepatic veins, resulting in portal hypertension and visceral pooling of blood. GI signs rather than respiratory signs are more apt to be seen in dogs. Immediate treatment, in addition to treating respiratory distress, consists of the systemic administration of epinephrine. Additional treatments include intravenous fluids to control shock and corticosteroids if needed. Ancillary support of blood pressure and respiration may also be necessary.

Urticarial reactions (hives) of the skin and subcutis and acute edema of the lips, conjunctiva, and skin of the face (facial-conjunctival angioedema) are less severe forms of Type I hypersensitivity. Hives are the least severe reaction and may not be associated with other clinical abnormalities. Facial-conjunctival edema is more severe and can be associated with mild to moderately severe systemic anaphylaxis. Urticarial reactions and facial-conjunctival edema occur in most species and usually resolve spontaneously within 24 hours. Not all urticarial reactions are mediated by Type I hypersensitivity.

Localized Allergic Reactions

Allergic rhinitis, manifest by serous nasal discharge and sneezing, is less common in domestic animals than in people. Often, it is seasonal, correlating with pollen exposure. Nonseasonal rhinitis may be associated with exposure to ubiquitous allergens, such as molds, animal danders, bedding, and feeds. Recurrent airway obstruction in horses is probably a response to chronic exposure to molds present in hay and poorly ventilated stables. Recent research on "equine asthma" has defined a type of the condition in which there is predominantly a neutrophilic response in the airway. Summer snuffles is a seasonal allergic rhinitis occurring in Guernsey or Jersey cattle placed on certain types of flowering pastures in late summer and early autumn.

Allergic rhinitis can be diagnosed tentatively by the following:

- identification of eosinophils in the nasal exudate
- demonstration of a favorable response to antihistamines
- disappearance of signs when the offending allergen is removed, or
- occasionally, its seasonal nature

Skin testing is not an accurate means to identify the causes of nasal allergies in animals.

Chronic allergic bronchitis has been diagnosed in dogs. A dry, harsh, hacking cough that is easily precipitated by exertion or by pressure on the trachea is a characteristic clinical sign. The disease may be seasonal. It is not usually associated with other signs of illness. The bronchial exudate is rich in eosinophils and free of bacteria. Chest radiographs are normal, and there may or may not be a low-grade peripheral eosinophilia. The condition is treated with bronchodilators and expectorants (aminophylline and potassium iodide or guaifenesin). Glucocorticoids will alleviate clinical signs, especially when their use can be limited to certain seasons or to low-dose, alternate-day therapy. Avoidance of the offending allergen(s) usually is not possible.

Allergic bronchiolitis is most common in cats. It is manifest by a low-grade cough, wheezing, some dyspnea, and increased peribronchiolar density on radiographs, and it may be mistaken for other conditions such as allergic asthma or lungworm disease. Early in the course of the disease, clinical signs can be reduced by antihistamine therapy, but if the disease increases in severity, moderate to high dosages of corticosteroids may be necessary. The offending allergen usually is not identified.

Pulmonary infiltration with eosinophilia occurs **most frequently in dogs** but has been recognized in all species. It is associated with diffuse inflammatory infiltrates in the lungs and a pronounced peripheral eosinophilia; frequently, serum globulins are increased. Unlike allergic bronchitis, affected animals are often dyspneic or tire easily with exercise. The bronchial exudate contains numerous eosinophils. The specific offending allergen is rarely identified. Glucocorticoids are the treatment of choice. A similar syndrome is also associated with resident or migratory parasitic infections of the lungs in young animals.

Allergic asthma occurs most frequently **in cats**, in which the signs are similar to those in people. It occurs more frequently in summer and in some cats can be triggered by going outdoors. Indoor cats can also get asthma, often from reaction to dust mite allergens. Individual attacks can be transient and mild or can be protracted and severe (status asthmaticus). Mild attacks may manifest as wheezing and coughing; in severe attacks, there may be expiratory dyspnea, hyperinflation of the lungs, aerophagia, cyanosis, and frantic attempts to obtain air. Eosinophils are found in bronchial wash fluids of asthmatic cats.

Intestinal allergies (food allergies) are principally seen in dogs and cats, particularly kittens. **Allergic gastritis** is manifest by vomiting, which occurs 1 to >12 times weekly within 1–2 hours of eating. The vomitus may be tinged with bile. In cats, vomiting may be the sole sign; dogs may also have intermittent loose feces. Cats and dogs with allergic gastritis are usually healthy except for vomiting.

Allergic enteritis is associated with a mild inflammation of the small intestine but with little or no eosinophilia. Feces usually are normal in volume and frequency but vary from semiformed to watery. They may be extremely odorous, especially in cats. Affected animals may be excessively thin despite good appetite. Skin lesions and poor coat are commonly associated with food allergies in cats but less commonly in dogs. The allergy often develops following episodes of viral, bacterial, or protozoal enteritis, a phenomenon known as allergic breakthrough.

Eosinophilic enteritis, the most severe form of allergic intestinal disease, manifests by moderate to severe inflammation of the intestines and a pronounced eosinophilia. Diarrhea, weight loss, and poor coat condition are usually evident. The prevalence of allergic colitis is greater in cats than in dogs, although in general it is not common. In dogs, it is often associated with frequent defecation and soft, mucus-laden and sometimes bloody feces; in cats, it most frequently manifests by more normal feces coated or spotted with fresh blood.

Atopic dermatitis is a complex, pruritic, chronic skin disorder that occurs in many species but has been studied mostly in dogs. Some animals with atopic dermatitis may have a genetic predisposition that leads to excessive production of reaginic (IgE) antibodies. It has been estimated that ~10% of all dogs suffer from atopy, with a breed predisposition in terriers, Dalmatians, and retrievers. There is increasing evidence that dogs with atopic dermatitis have a skin barrier defect and that most allergens enter through the skin. Atopic dogs often chew at their feet and axillae. Excessive sweating is especially noticeable in hairless areas. The severity of the skin lesions are greatly increased by licking, scratching, flea infestation, and secondary bacterial or yeast infection. Atopic skin lesions in cats are either miliary (small scabs) and widespread or are larger and more localized. Localized lesions are often pruritic.

In cats, food allergens probably are a more common cause of skin lesions than are inhaled allergens. Sweet itch is a seasonal allergic dermatitis of horses associated with certain insect bites, especially night-feeding *Culicoides*. Intensely pruritic lesions appear along the dorsum from the ears to tail head and perianal area. Similar allergic skin reactions to insect bites can be seen around the ears and face of cats and dogs. (For diagnosis and treatment, see Atopic Dermatitis.)

Type II Reactions

Type II hypersensitivity reactions occur when an antibody binds to antigens located on the surface of cells. This bound antibody can then activate the classical complement pathway, resulting in cell lysis, or phagocytosis. Many different antigens may trigger this cell destruction, but an infection in a genetically predisposed animal appears to be a major triggering pathway. Cross-reactive antibodies can develop during infections. These cross-reactive antibodies directed toward an infectious agent may also bind to normal tissue antigens and trigger antibody-mediated cytotoxicity. Pathogens such as *Babesia* or *Haemobartonella*, which parasitize cells, trigger an immune response that destroys those cells as part of the protective mechanism. As another example, drug metabolites can bind to erythrocytes and create a new epitope that stimulates an antibody response, thereby causing destruction of the cells by antibody and complement.

The most common manifestations of Type II hypersensitivity involve blood cells. These include hemolytic anemia if RBCs are involved, leukopenia involving WBCs, or thrombocytopenia involving platelets. Under some circumstances, a cytotoxic attack on vascular epithelial cells will cause a vasculitis with local vascular leakage.

Bovine Neonatal Pancytopenia

In 2007, a dramatic hemorrhagic disease affecting calves appeared in Europe; upon investigation it was found to result from the use of a bovine viral diarrhea vaccine. The vaccine virus was grown in bovine kidney cells. As a result, it stimulated antibody formation in some recipient cows directed against the cell's MHC molecules. These antibodies were concentrated in their colostrum. When their calves suckled, the ingested antibodies destroyed the calf's bone marrow stem cells and resulted in a massive and lethal pancytopenia. The offending vaccine has been withdrawn.

Type III Reactions

Antigen-antibody complexes (immune complexes) deposited in small blood vessels fix complement in situ and cause acute inflammation. Activation of complement by immune complexes results in production of complement byproducts that are chemotactic for neutrophils. The neutrophils are unable to ingest the complexes that are stuck in the blood vessel walls and they release their granule contents in the tissue. These granules contain toxic enzymes that cause severe tissue damage. The most frequently affected sites of immune complex deposition are the joints, skin, kidneys, lungs, and brain.

The prerequisite for the development of immune-complex disease is the persistent presence of soluble antigen and antibody. These form insoluble immune complexes that become trapped on the basement membrane of small blood vessels. The deposited immune complexes then activate the classical complement pathway. Complement fragments attract neutrophils and are also directly vasoactive, triggering a vasculitis. These antigens may persist for a number of reasons, including chronic infections and certain cancers, especially lymphoreticular neoplasms. Chronic antigen exposure may also occur with inhaled antigens, and, in such cases, immune complexes can form in the alveolar walls. Lastly, some animals respond to self-antigens, which then act as a source of chronic antigen exposure. In many cases, the origin of the antigen within these immune complexes cannot be determined.

The location of the immune complexes is largely determined by the route by which antigen enters the body. Inhaled antigens give rise to a pneumonitis, antigens that enter through the skin cause local skin lesions, and antigens that access the bloodstream form immune complexes that are deposited in renal glomeruli or joints. **Clinical signs** are therefore variable but may include:

- fever
- cutaneous signs (such as erythema multiforme)

- polyarthritis (shifting-leg lameness or painful, swollen joints)

Other signs include ataxia, behavior change, proteinuria, isosthenuria, polydipsia, polyuria, or nonspecific signs such as vomiting, diarrhea, or abdominal pain. Diagnosis is based on the elimination of more common causes of clinical signs. Supporting evidence to confirm the diagnosis includes establishing a temporal relationship if a drug or infectious agent is suspected as the cause, identifying chronic infections or malignancies, and performing histopathology and immunohistochemistry on biopsies to identify immune-mediated vasculitides or nephritis.

Therapy should include supportive treatment, removal of the causative agent, or treatment of the underlying disorder, such as appropriate antibiotic therapy for bacterial infections, surgical drainage of abscesses or infected tissue, therapy for heartworm disease, and the withdrawal of the offending drugs. Immunosuppressive therapy may be needed to prevent the continued deposition of immune-complexes.

Membranoproliferative Glomerulonephritis

Membranoproliferative glomerulonephritis is caused by immune complexes that form within the bloodstream and are filtered out in the glomeruli. In effect, the insoluble complexes collect on the glomerular basement membrane. Depending on their size, they may be deposited on the subendothelial or subepithelial surface of the membrane. Secondary glomerulonephritis occurs as a side effect of chronic infectious, neoplastic, or immunologic disorders. Animals with idiopathic glomerulonephritis (>50% of cases) usually have signs of renal disease, whereas secondary glomerulonephritis is often a relatively minor part of a more serious disease.

Hypersensitivity Pneumonitis

When inhaled antigens meet circulating antibodies in the walls of the lung alveoli, immune complexes form in the alveolar walls and trigger acute inflammation. Hypersensitivity pneumonitis is most common in large animals exposed over a long time to antigenic dusts. The most potent antigens of this type are those contained in the spores of thermophilic actinomycetes from moldy hay. Inhalation of these spores causes farmer's lung disease in humans and a similar condition in cattle. Hypersensitivity pneumonitis is characterized by the onset of respiratory distress 4–6 hours after exposure to moldy hay. The most effective treatment is removal of the source of the antigen; otherwise, corticosteroid therapy may help.

Vasculitis

Vasculitis mediated by immune complexes occurs in animals, especially dogs and horses. Lesions are most prevalent in the dermis of the distal limbs and mucous membranes of the mouth, particularly the palate and tongue (dogs) and lips (horses).

Involvement of the nose, ears, eyelids, cornea, and anus is less common. Early lesions develop as reddened areas that rapidly form shallow erosions. A scab quickly forms over dermal erosions. Edema of the limbs is common in horses and a less frequent but equally striking sign in dogs. Vasculitis is a feature of systemic lupus in some animals but most often is idiopathic. Drug-induced vasculitis has been well recognized in dogs. The vasculitis is detected on histopathologic and immunohistopathologic examination of superficial and deep biopsies taken from the margins of lesions.

Vasculitis is treated by withdrawal of offending drugs and, if necessary, by immunosuppressive drug therapy. Glucocorticoids used alone or in combination with other agents such as azathioprine or cyclophosphamide are usually used to treat non-drug-induced cases.

Periarteritis Nodosa

(Polyarteritis Nodosa, Necrotizing Polyarteritis)

Periarteritis nodosa is a rare disease of domestic animals caused by deposition of immune complexes and inflammation in walls of small and medium-sized arteries. Among farm animals, it is **most common in pigs**, usually associated with erysipelas and streptococcal infections, and is attributed to a type III reaction to these bacteria or to their vaccines. It has been reported in cats, although it may be mistaken for the noneffusive form of feline infectious peritonitis.

Canine Rheumatoid Arthritis

Canine rheumatoid arthritis results from excessive, uncontrolled inflammation around joints. It manifests initially as a shifting lameness with soft-tissue swelling around involved joints. Within weeks or months, the disease localizes in individual joints, and characteristic radiographic changes develop. The earliest radiographic changes consist of soft-tissue swelling and a loss of trabecular bone density in the area of the joint. Lucent cyst-like areas frequently are seen in the subchondral bone. The most prominent lesion is a progressive erosion of cartilage and subchondral bone in the area of synovial attachments, resulting in loss of articular cartilage and collapse of the joint space. Angular deformities often occur, and luxation of the joint is a frequent sequel. Deformities are most frequent in the carpal, tarsal, and phalangeal joints and less frequent in the elbow and stifle.

The primary lesion in canine rheumatoid arthritis is nonsuppurative, proliferative synovitis. This is followed by joint erosion and eventually leads to fibrous ankylosis.

An erosive arthritis has also been recognized in cats. It tends to occur in older, male cats and frequently is associated with infection with feline syncytia-forming virus. The development of this disease in cats is much more insidious than in dogs.

Canine rheumatoid arthritis responds poorly to systemic glucocorticoids alone. Immunosuppressive agents with anti-inflammatory activity such as cyclophosphamide and azathioprine are used with glucocorticoids to treat this disorder; NSAIDs such as aspirin, carprofen, etodolac, or meloxicam may bring relief.

Plasmacytic-Lymphocytic Synovitis

Plasmacytic-lymphocytic synovitis is possibly a variant of rheumatoid arthritis. It occurs in medium-sized and large dogs. Although multiple joints often are involved, the disease has a predisposition for the stifle. The most common clinical signs are hindlimb lameness and anterior drawer motion of the stifles. Lymphocytes, plasma cells, and neutrophils are present in the synovial fluid, although in some cases the fluid is essentially normal. Examination of the joint shows synovial proliferation and stretching or rupture of the cruciate ligaments.

Idiopathic Polyarthritis

Arthritis of unknown etiology is **most common in large dogs**, particularly German Shepherds, Doberman Pinschers, retrievers, spaniels, and pointers. In toy breeds, it is most frequent in Toy Poodles, Yorkshire Terriers, and Chihuahuas, or mixes of these breeds. There is no evidence of a primary chronic infectious disease process or of systemic lupus erythematosus. Arthritis is often the sole manifestation.

Diagnosis is based on the history of cyclic antibiotic-unresponsive fever, malaise, and anorexia, with stiffness or lameness. Bony changes are not seen on radiographs until the disease is well established. Even then, radiographic changes are mild and can mimic degenerative joint disease. Synovial fluid contains leukocytes but is sterile.

The disease may be controlled with daily high-dose glucocorticoids followed by low-dose, alternate-day therapy. Treatment usually can be discontinued after 3–5 months. Dogs that do not respond well to such therapy (>50%) may be treated with more potent immunosuppressive drugs such as azathioprine or cyclophosphamide in addition to glucocorticoids. Gold salts help augment glucocorticoid therapy in some animals.

Other Type III Reactions

Purpura hemorrhagica of horses is a severe nonthrombocytopenic purpura that often follows a *Streptococcus equi* infection; it occurs when immune complexes of antibody and streptococcal antigen are deposited in vascular basement membranes.

Anterior uveitis ("blue-eye") is an immune complex–mediated reaction that frequently occurs in the recovery stage of infectious canine hepatitis. It results from the reaction of serum antibodies with uveal endothelial cells infected with canine adenovirus 1. Similarly, severe equine recurrent uveitis is associated with immunologic reactions to Leptospira or Onchocerca spp. This periodic ophthalmia results from autoimmune attack. Antibodies against some serovars of Leptospira can cross-react with retinal antigens and so trigger severe ophthalmia. Uveitis caused by Toxoplasma and feline infectious peritonitis virus infections of cats may also have an immunologic basis.

Type IV Reactions

Cell-mediated immune reactions occur when antigen triggers type 1, cell-mediated responses. Multiple cytokines are produced, as well as activated macrophages and cytotoxic T cells. The infiltration of mononuclear cells and the release of inflammatory molecules from these cells results in the pathologic processes of cell-mediated immune reactions. The antigens usually responsible for the development of Type IV reactions include intracellular bacteria or parasites, some viruses, reactive chemicals, and (in certain situations) cellular autoantigens. The lesions commonly occur in the skin (allergic contact dermatitis) when the antigen comes into contact with the skin. Examples of antigens that cause type IV responses are metals such as nickel and chemicals that may be on lawns or carpets (these can cause contact dermatitis on the ventral abdomen of dogs that lie on their ventrum on such surfaces). The diagnosis is based on eliminating other causes of disease and on histology. The goals of treatment are to identify and eliminate the source of antigen responsible for the reaction and to provide anti-inflammatory or immunosuppressive therapy as required.

Granulomatous Reactions

T cell–mediated granulomatous reactions may also occur around persistent infectious foci. These reactions to microorganisms such as mycobacteria, *Coccidioides* spp, *Blastomyces* spp, and *Histoplasma* spp, and possibly feline infectious peritonitis virus, may be a result of chronic cell-mediated immune reactions and localized macrophage activation. Although cell-mediated immunity effectively controls these types of infections in most animals, for poorly understood reasons, these same mechanisms are only partially effective in others. These granulomatous reactions are characterized by the development of a fibrous stroma and an infiltration of macrophages, giant cells, and lymphocytes around the persistent antigen.

Lymphocytic Choriomeningitis

Lymphocytic choriomeningitis, a viral infection of mice, results from the destruction of virus-infected cells by T cells, leading to CNS damage and a choriomeningitis.

Old-dog Encephalitis

Old-dog encephalitis may also result from cell-mediated immune mechanisms directed against cells persistently infected with canine distemper virus. The initiating canine distemper virus infection is usually clinically inapparent and may precede the development of encephalitis by many years.

Allergic Contact Hypersensitivity

Allergic contact hypersensitivity results from chemicals reacting with and modifying normal dermal proteins. The modified proteins trigger a cell-mediated immune response, which causes inflammation and damages the skin (eg, poison oak and poison ivy reactions in people). This reaction has been described in dogs, cattle, and horses and usually occurs as a result of contact with sensitizing chemicals incorporated in plastic food dishes, plastic collars, and drugs placed on the skin.

Organ-Specific Autoimmunity

Along with primary and secondary immunodeficiencies, the third type of immunologically mediated disease involves the development of autoimmunity. This is an immune response directed against normal cellular components. These diseases are readily divided into organ-specific diseases affecting a single body organ or into diseases directed against widespread antigens and as a result affect multiple organ systems.

Autoimmune Thyroiditis

Autoimmune thyroiditis in dogs is characterized by destruction of the thyroid gland by an autoimmune process that has both humoral (Type II) and cell-mediated (Type IV) components. It is particularly prevalent in Doberman Pinschers, Beagles, Golden Retrievers, and Akitas. Hypothyroidism may be the sole manifestation of the disease or may be a clinical or subclinical component of a broader autoimmune disorder such as systemic lupus erythematosus or panendocrinopathy.

Autoimmune Adrenalitis

Autoimmune adrenalitis has been reported in dogs. The adrenal glands are slowly destroyed by a plasmacytic-lymphocytic infiltrate. When sufficient glandular tissue is destroyed, the dogs develop Addison disease (adrenocortical insufficiency. The condition is sometimes associated with autoimmune thyroiditis.

Immune-mediated Hemolytic Anemia (IMHA) and Thrombocytopenia

The production of autoantibodies against erythrocyte or platelet antigens leads to anemia and thrombocytopenia, **the most common Type II reactions.** Antibody and complement attach to RBCs either directly or indirectly via an absorbed antigen and then mediate RBC destruction, resulting in a severe, life-threatening anemia. Concurrent thrombocytopenia is found in 60% of cases. IMHA can be associated with systemic lupus erythematosus or with lymphoreticular malignancies. Drugs or infections may trigger episodes of hemolytic anemia or thrombocytopenia in many species. More often than not, the initiating cause is unknown.

Immune-mediated hemolytic anemia occurs in several clinical forms: peracute, acute or subacute, chronic, cold agglutinin disease, and red cell aplasia. Most cases are treatable, but relapses are common.

Peracute IMHA is seen mainly in middle-aged, larger breeds of dogs. Affected dogs are acutely depressed and have a rapid decrease in PCV within 24–48 hours, with bilirubinemia, variable icterus, and sometimes hemoglobinuria. Initially, the anemia is nonresponsive, but it may respond within 3–5 days. Thrombocytopenia may also be present. Antiglobulin tests are often negative, and spherocytes may or may not be present, but tube or slide agglutination of RBCs is marked. The autoagglutination is not dispersed by saline dilution, hence the term hemolytic anemia with in-saline agglutinins. The serum usually contains autoantibodies that cause agglutination of most donor RBCs.

The prognosis of peracute IMHA is poor even with prompt and vigorous therapy. The most effective therapy involves immediate use of high dosages of glucocorticoids plus cyclophosphamide, together with a compatible blood transfusion. If incompatible blood must be used, the animal should first be heparinized and maintained on heparin for 10 days. Even without transfusion, heparinization may be beneficial for the first 2 weeks or more. Bovine hemoglobin blood substitute and human immunoglobulins can be used as supportive therapy until immunosuppressive treatment reduces the destruction of RBCs.

Acute IMHA is the most common form of the disease, with a breed **predilection in Cocker Spaniels.** Initial signs are pallor, fatigue, and less commonly, icterus. Hepatosplenomegaly is a prominent sign. The WBC count may be increased due to bone marrow hyperplasia. Autoagglutination of RBCs is uncommon, and the antiglobulin test is generally positive. These animals usually respond well to glucocorticoid therapy. If a favorable response is not seen within 7–10 days, cytotoxic drugs (cyclophosphamide or azathioprine) should be added to the regimen.

Chronic IMHA differs from the acute form in that the PCV falls to a constant level and remains there for weeks or months. The bone marrow is either normal or hyperresponsive, and the antiglobulin test is often negative. Chronic IMHA is relatively more common in cats than in dogs. Usually, the anemia is responsive early in the course of disease but responds minimally or not at all by the time it becomes severe. Initial treatment is with glucocorticoids; if there is no response within 2 weeks, cytotoxic drugs may be added to the regimen.

Cold agglutinin disease is an IMHA of dogs and horses. Its cause is usually unknown but it may be secondary to infection, other autoimmune diseases, or neoplasia. The IgM autoantibodies can be agglutinating or nonagglutinating. Complete agglutination does not occur at body temperature but only when the blood is chilled; thus, it is more frequent in colder climates and seasons. Initial signs may be of a hemolytic disease; in the agglutinating type, vascular blockage may lead to necrosis of the nose, tips of the ears and tail, digits, scrotum, and prepuce. Diagnosis is based on a reversible autoagglutination that occurs only at 4°C. The direct antiglobulin reaction is usually negative for IgG, frequently positive for C3, and usually positive for IgM if the reaction is performed in the cold. Mortality is high. In the absence of an obvious initiating cause such as infection or neoplasia, the disease is best controlled with high doses of glucocorticoids in combination with cyclophosphamide.

Red cell aplasia is most common in dogs. It occurs in two forms, one in postweanling to adolescent puppies and the other in adults. Unlike in IMHA, the bone marrow shows a selective depression of erythroid elements; granulocytes and platelets are unaffected. Therefore, the peripheral anemia is unresponsive. The immune attack is directed against erythroid stem cells, and the antiglobulin test is usually negative. Treatment is usually as for chronic IMHA, but recovery may be very slow.

Immune-mediated thrombocytopenia is common in dogs. It occurs more often in females than males. The most frequent clinical signs are hemorrhages of the skin and mucous membranes. Melena, epistaxis, and hematuria may be accompanying features and can cause profound anemia. Hemolytic anemia and thrombocytopenia sometimes occur together. Immune-mediated thrombocytopenia usually is diagnosed on the basis of low peripheral platelet counts despite a pronounced megakaryocytosis in the marrow. Occasionally, megakaryocytes may be selectively absent from the marrow. Tests for antiplatelet antibodies are difficult to conduct, so diagnosis is usually made on clinical presentation and response to therapy.

Animals with immune-mediated thrombocytopenia that show only petechial and ecchymotic hemorrhages, with no significant blood loss and megakaryocytes in the marrow, may be treated initially with glucocorticoids. The clinical signs should abate and the platelet count begin to rise after 5–7 days. If the platelet count has not increased significantly by 7–10 days, cyclophosphamide, azathioprine, or vincristine can be added to the glucocorticoid regimen.

In animals with megakaryocytes in the marrow and severe blood loss, a more rapid response to therapy is desirable. Such animals are treated with a single injection of vincristine combined with daily glucocorticoids; a favorable response usually occurs after 3–5 days. If the blood loss is life-threatening, platelet-rich whole blood should be administered. If the platelet count has risen by day 7, remission is maintained on glucocorticoids alone. If there is no response after 7 days, a second dose of vincristine is given. If the platelet count is still low after 2 weeks, vincristine is discontinued and either cyclophosphamide or azathioprine is added.

Animals with thrombocytopenia and no megakaryocytes respond much more slowly to glucocorticoids, or to glucocorticoids and vincristine. Preferred treatment for these animals is with prednisolone and cyclophosphamide, and a response should not be expected earlier than 1–2 weeks after beginning therapy. Treatment may be discontinued in most animals with immune-mediated thrombocytopenia

1–3 months after the platelet count returns to normal. Some animals have a persistent thrombocytopenia despite drug therapy, or they can be maintained in remission only with chronic, high-dose treatment. The alternatives are to allow the animal to live with the thrombocytopenia if signs are minimal or to use longterm combination drug therapy with glucocorticoids and either vincristine, azathioprine, or cyclophosphamide. Splenectomy is seldom curative by itself but may allow use of lower and safer dosages of immunosuppressive drugs.

Autoimmune Skin Diseases

In autoimmune skin diseases, affected animals make autoantibodies against the intracellular cement proteins in the epidermis. This promotes local proteolysis, leading to separation of the epidermal cells (acantholysis) and development of vesicles within the skin.

Pemphigus foliaceus is the most common of these diseases, occurring more often in dogs than in cats and horses. It is characterized by the development of erosions, ulcerations, and thick encrustations of the skin and mucocutaneous junctions. The absence of lesions in the mouth, and the widespread thick, crusty nature of the skin lesions, tend to differentiate pemphigus foliaceus from the much rarer pemphigus vulgaris. Autoantibodies in the skin react with intracellular cement (desmoglein), resulting in its degradation and separation of the cornified and uncornified cell layers. Immunosuppression is required to treat the disease. High doses of glucocorticoids are used initially, but low-dose, alternate-day therapy is used once the disease is under control. More potent immunosuppressive drugs such as cyclophosphamide or azathioprine may be used with glucocorticoids in cases unresponsive to steroids alone. Animals that respond poorly to initial therapy, or that require high dosages of drugs to control lesions, have a poor longterm prognosis.

Pemphigus vulgaris is a less common autoimmune skin disease than pemphigus foliaceus. It is characterized by vesicle formation along the mucocutaneous junctions of the mouth, anus, prepuce, and vulva, and in the oral cavity. Other areas of the skin are only mildly involved. Because the epidermis of animals is relatively thin (compared with human skin), these blisters rupture rapidly and form erosions; consequently, characteristic bullae are seldom seen. The vesicles develop as a result of suprabasilar acantholysis. Secondary bacterial infection often complicates the lesions, and if untreated, the disease is often fatal. It is treated with high doses of glucocorticoids alone or in combination with other drugs such as cyclophosphamide, azathioprine, or gold salts. Pemphigus vulgaris is difficult to maintain in remission, and the longterm prognosis of affected animals is fair to poor.

Bullous pemphigoid is a rare canine skin disease recognized most often in Collies and Doberman Pinschers. Lesions are often widespread but tend to be concentrated in the groin. The involved skin resembles a severe scald. Bullae also develop; they are subepidermal and may be full of eosinophils. Autoantibodies to the basal lamina can be detected in immunohistopathologic sections. The treatment of choice is prednisolone and azathioprine used in combination; remission is frequent, but continual drug therapy at relatively high dosages may be required to keep the disease under control. The longterm prognosis is poor.

Myasthenia Gravis

Myasthenia gravis is an autoimmune disease in which autoantibodies directed against the acetylcholine receptors of muscle cells cause receptor degradation or blockage and thus block neuromuscular transmission. The disease is characterized by extreme generalized muscle weakness, accentuated by mild exercise. Megaesophagus due to paralysis of esophageal muscles is a frequent primary or accompanying complaint in dogs. Thymomas are often associated with myasthenia gravis in people but are uncommon in domestic species. Administration of a short-acting anticholinesterase (edrophonium chloride) produces a dramatic increase in muscle strength. Treatment is with a long-acting anticholinesterase. Chronic immunosuppressive drug therapy for this disease is logical. Autoantibodies to the acetylcholine receptors can be detected in the serum of affected animals by an indirect immunohistopathologic assay using normal muscle as a substrate.

Immune-mediated Meningitis

Immune-mediated meningitis occurs in adolescent or young adult **Beagles, Boxers, German Shorthaired Pointers, and Akitas** but is rare in other pure and mixed breeds. The **clinical signs** consist of:

- cyclic episodes of fever
- severe neck pain and rigidity
- reluctance to move
- depression

Each attack lasts 5–10 days, with intervening periods of complete or partial normality lasting about a week. During attacks, protein and neutrophils in the CSF are increased. The primary lesion is a meningeal arteritis, but occasionally other organs are affected as well. The disease is often self-limiting, so that over several months attacks become milder and less frequent. Glucocorticoids reduce the severity of attacks. In some animals, the disease becomes chronic and only partially amenable to therapy.

A more severe form of this meningitis has been reported in young Bernese Mountain Dogs. The disease in this breed is somewhat cyclical, but the resolution in intervening periods is shorter than in other species. CSF abnormalities resemble those seen in other breeds. The condition requires longterm, high-dose glucocorticoid therapy.

A syndrome of meningitis, often associated with polyarthritis, is seen in young Akitas. The dogs show severe episodes of fever, depression, cervical pain and rigidity, and generalized stiffness. Affected dogs grow slowly and often appear unthrifty. The condition responds poorly to glucocorticoid and immuno-suppressive therapy. Most affected dogs are euthanized as young adults. A milder and more drug-responsive form of the disease has been reported in older Akitas and may be associated with pemphigus foliaceus, uveitis, and plasmacytic-lymphocytic thyroiditis.

Keratitis Sicca

Keratitis sicca is a "dry eye" syndrome that occurs in dogs. It can occur in either a primary form or secondary to chronic use of sulfonamides. It results from immune-mediated destruction of the lacrimal glands and is similar to Sjögren syndrome of people. Affected dogs may respond favorably to cyclosporine eye drops.

MULTIORGAN AUTOIMMUNITY

Systemic Lupus Erythematosus (SLE)

This complex autoimmune disease occurs in dogs, is rare in cats, and has been reported in large animals. It has two consistent immunologic features: immune complex disease and a tendency to produce multiple autoantibodies. Clinically, it reflects a combination of Type II and III mechanisms. Antibodies to nucleic acids (called antinuclear antibodies, ANA) are the diagnostic hallmark of SLE, but in many individuals, antibodies to RBCs, platelets, lymphocytes, clotting factors, , and thyroglobulin are also present. The presence of ANA can be diagnostic of the disease. Either the immune complex or the autoantibody component of the disease tends to predominate in a given animal.

Immune complex deposition around small blood vessels may lead to:

- synovitis
- dermal reactions
- oral erosions and ulcers
- myositis
- neuritis
- meningitis
- arteritis
- myelopathy

- glomerulonephritis
- pleuritis

Glomerulonephritis is one of the major, life-threatening complications of SLE in cats. Autoimmune hemolytic anemia or thrombocytopenia, or both, are the most common presentations of SLE in animals.

SLE is characterized by the presence of ANA, and tests for these or the associated lupus cells may help in diagnosis. However, some healthy animals may have ANA, and not all animals with SLE have detectable ANA in their blood. Diagnosis of SLE must therefore be based on the entire clinical syndrome—not just on the presence or absence of ANA.

SLE usually can be treated with glucocorticoids. Initially, they are used in high daily doses, and when remission occurs, alternate-day, low-dose therapy is used. Drug treatment should be continued for 2–3 months after all clinical signs have resolved. Cyclophosphamide or azathioprine, or both, are used in combination with glucocorticoids in animals with SLE that is difficult to control with glucocorticoids alone.

CHAPTER

REGULATION OF ADAPTIVE IMMUNITY 10

The adaptive immune system is a sophisticated defense system. It can recognize and respond to foreign invaders and can learn from the experience so that the body responds faster and more effectively when exposed to the invader a second time. There is, however, a risk associated with this—the risk of collateral damage. One of the reasons why the adaptive immune system is so complex is that much effort must be put into ensuring that it will only attack foreign or abnormal tissues and will ignore normal healthy tissues. As might be anticipated, many different mechanisms minimize the chances of developing autoimmunity. In addition, immune responses are regulated to ensure that they are appropriate with respect to both quality and quantity (Fig. 1).

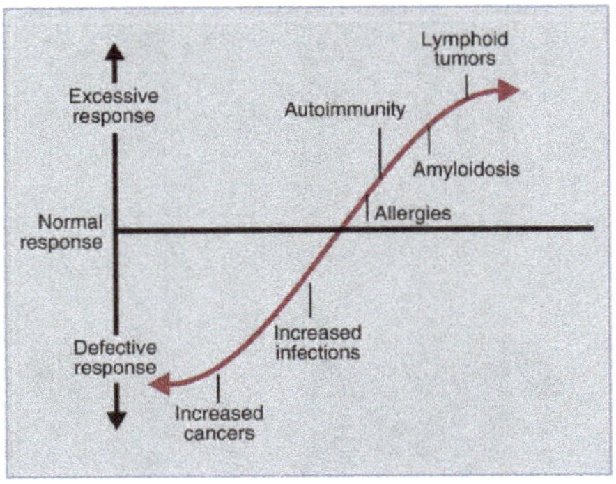

Fig. 1. Some of the bad things that can happen if the immune system is not carefully regulated.

Since both T and B cells generate antigen-binding receptors at random, it is clear that the initial production of self-reactive cells cannot be prevented. An animal cannot control the amino acid sequences and hence the binding specificity of these receptors. As a result, when first generated, as many as 50% of the T cell antigen receptors (TCRs) and B cell antigen receptors (BCRs) may bind self-antigens. If autoimmunity is to be avoided, lymphocytes with these inappropriate receptors must either be destroyed or turned off.

Tolerance

Tolerance is the name given to the situation in which the immune system will not respond to a specific antigen. Tolerance is primarily directed against self-antigens from normal tissues. In 1948 two Australian immunologists, Burnet and Fenner, recognized this need for self-tolerance and suggested that immature lymphocytes would become tolerant to an antigen if they first met it early in fatal life.

Support for this suggestion came from observations on chimeric calves. In 1945 Owen noted that when cows are carrying twin calves, blood vessels in the two placentas commonly fuse. As a result, the blood of the twins intermingles freely, and bone marrow stem cells from one animal colonize the other. Each calf is born with a mixture of blood cells, some of its own and some originating from its twin. In dizygotic (non-identical) twins, this is called a chimera. These "foreign" blood cells persist indefinitely because each chimeric calf is fully tolerant to the presence of its twin's cells (Fig. 2). Burnet and Fenner suggested that this could only happen because each calf was exposed to the foreign cells early in fetal life during a period when lymphocytes become tolerant upon encountering antigens. Cells from an unrelated calf would be rejected normally if administered after birth.

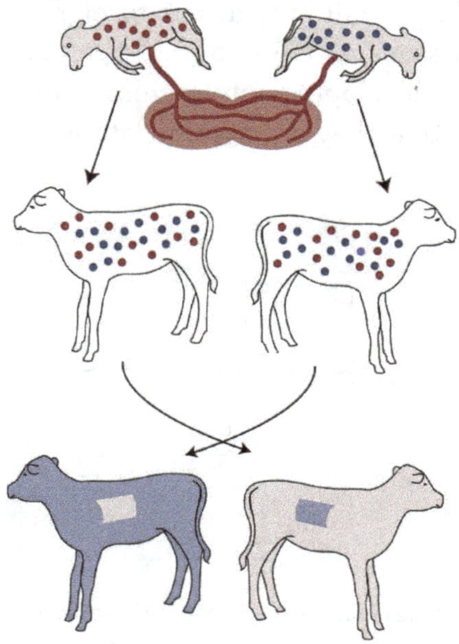

Fig. 2 Fusion of the placentas of dizygotic twin calves results in the development of calf chimeras. Hematopoietic stem cells from each animal colonize the bone marrow of the other. Each chimera is tolerant to its twin's cells and will accept a skin graft from its twin despite the genetic differences.

Subsequent studies have shown that self-tolerance is of two types, central and peripheral. In central tolerance, immature self-reactive lymphocytes within the thymus, bursa, or bone marrow either die or alter their receptor specificity. In peripheral tolerance, mature lymphocytes that encounter self-antigens either die, are turned off, or are suppressed by Treg cells. By reconstituting lethally irradiated mice with T or B cells derived from normal or tolerant donors, tolerance can be shown to occur in both cell populations. However, their susceptibility to peripheral tolerance differs. T cells can be made tolerant rapidly and easily within 24 hours and remain in that state for more than 100 days. In contrast, B cells develop tolerance in about 10 days and return to normal within 50 days.

T CELL TOLERANCE

Central T Cell Tolerance

Negative Selection

Tolerance will result if there are no functional T cells with receptors that can bind self-antigens (Fig. 3).

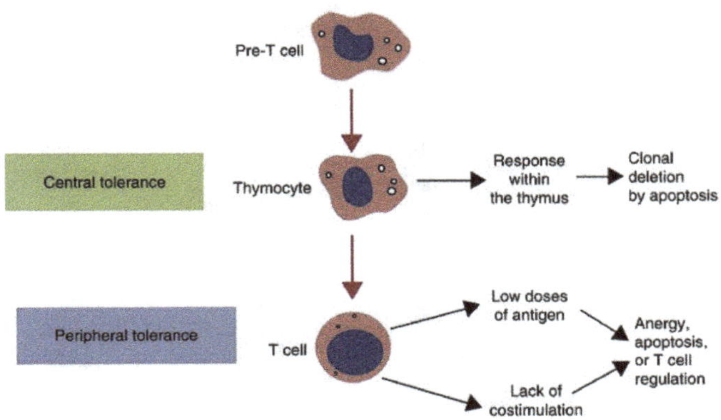

Fig. 3 The principal ways by which T cells are made tolerant.

Although the body generates an enormous diversity of TCRs, far fewer receptors are actually used by mature T cells than might be anticipated. Several processes serve to limit receptor diversity. First, the mechanisms used to generate diverse TCRs inevitably result in the production of nonfunctional receptors. For example, two thirds of possible gene arrangements will be out of frame. Cells with these nonfunctional TCRs undergo apoptosis. As T cells mature within the thymus, positive selection ensures that the cells that recognize self-MHC molecules survive. At this point, however, the cells whose receptors bind too strongly to self-antigens die by apoptosis (Fig. 4). The timing and extent of this apoptosis depend on the affinity of the TCR for a self-antigen. T cells that bind self-antigens strongly die earlier and more completely than weakly binding cells. Thus the T cells that eventually leave the thymus have been purged of dangerous, self-reactive cells.

The negative selection process is assisted by the presence of many different self-antigens in the thymus. Normally each tissue possesses its own tissue-specific antigens. Thus "skin antigens" are usually restricted to the skin, whereas "liver antigens" are restricted to the liver, and so forth. However, the epithelial cells in the thymic medulla show uniquely "promiscuous" gene expression. Thymic epithelial cells use a transcription regulator, called the autoimmune regulator (AIRE), that promotes the expression of many different proteins once thought to be restricted to other tissues. Examples include insulin, thyroglobulin, and myelin basic protein. In this way, the thymic epithelial cells ensure that self-reactive T cells encounter many normal tissue antigens and are therefore eliminated. In addition, some normal tissue antigens may be taken up by macrophages and carried to the thymus. Self-reactive T cells that respond to these antigens are also eliminated. However, this raises another question: What about self-antigens that are not expressed in, or do not enter, the thymus? For example, antigens in the eye, testis, or brain are not processed in this way, and as a result central tolerance to these antigens does not develop.

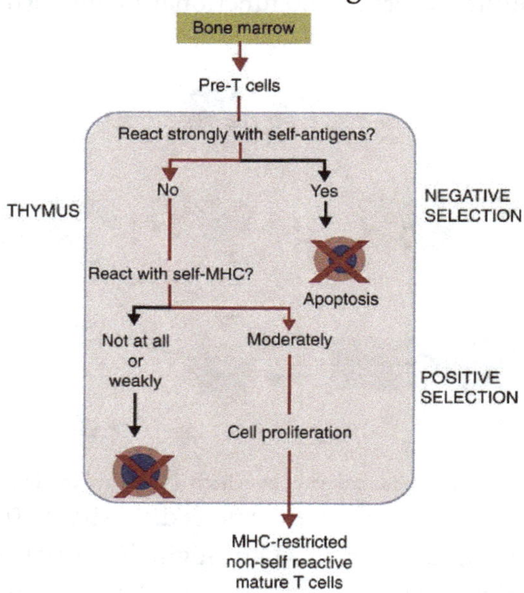

Fig. 4. How the thymus induces central T cell tolerance by negative selection. Surviving T cells are unreactive to autoantigens yet can still respond to foreign antigenic peptides in association with MHC molecules as a result of positive selection.

Positive and negative selection acting together ensure that cells that can bind self-MHC molecules are positively selected and those that bind the MHC molecules with very low or very high affinity are subsequently deleted. As a result, the moderate-affinity clones survive and can recognize foreign antigens. An additional factor that probably determines thymocyte survival is the dose of antigen presented to the cells. If the amount of a specific antigen is high (as one might anticipate for a self-antigen), multiple TCRs will be occupied on each thymocyte and trigger apoptosis. In contrast, if the amount of an antigen is low, this will occupy only a few TCRs, and the weak signal may cause positive selection and thymocyte proliferation.

Receptor Editing

When the antigen receptors of a developing T cell bind to self-antigens, another strategy employed to prevent autoimmunity is receptor editing. Although cell maturation stops when it leaves the thymus, the *RAG* genes remain active and as a result, V(D)J recombination continues. Consequently, the *TCR* genes continue to diversify, and changed receptors are expressed on the cell surface. This process is called receptor editing. If a cell successfully edits its receptors, its maturation can proceed. Failure to do so will result in its apoptosis. This is a potentially hazardous process since it permits the development of self-reactive T cells that have not undergone careful selection within the thymus.

Peripheral T Cell Tolerance

Clonal Anergy

Low-affinity self-reactive T cells may survive the selection process and leave the thymus and must then be suppressed by peripheral tolerance mechanisms. One form of peripheral tolerance is clonal anergy, the prolonged, antigen-specific suppression of T cell function. Clonal anergy can be triggered by the signals received by the T cell. T cells normally require multiple signals from several sources in order to respond to antigen. If these signals are insufficient or inappropriate, T cell responses to antigen will be suppressed.

Indeed, occupation of the TCR in the absence of co-stimulation causes tolerance. For example, protein solutions normally contain some aggregated molecules. These aggregated molecules are readily taken up and processed by dendritic cells and thus are highly immunogenic. If a solution of such a protein, such as bovine ã-globulin, is ultracentrifuged so that all the aggregates are removed, then the aggregate-free solution will induce anergy. This is due to the lack of co-stimulation from antigen-presenting cells (APCs) (Fig. 5).

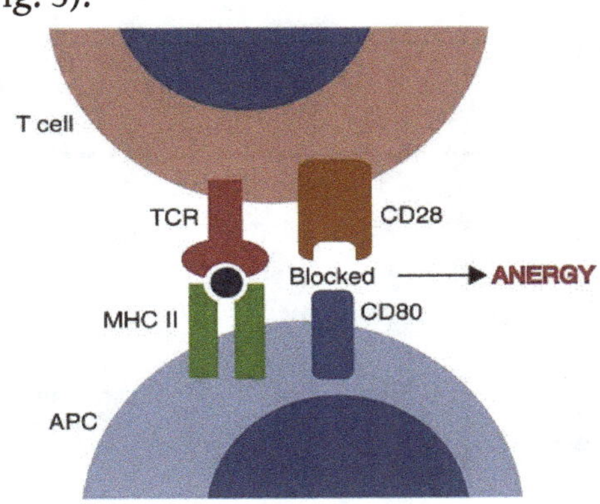

Fig. 5 Peripheral tolerance through clonal anergy will develop if a TCR is stimulated by antigen in the absence of simultaneous co-stimulation through the CD28/CD80 or CD28/CD86 pathway.

Binding to the TCR by an antigen alone activates the tyrosine kinases and phospholipase C of the T cell and raises its intracellular Ca^{2+}. This results in enhanced production of IêB that inhibits NF-êB and effectively prevents the cell from making cytokines, especially IL-2. Tolerant Th1 cells produce about 1% to 3% of normal IL-2 levels and much less IFN-ã and TNF-á. Once induced, their anergy can last for several weeks. Induction of the transcription factor FoxP3 also silences anti-inflammatory cytokine genes and leads to the production of Treg cells.

Triggering of T cell responses normally requires prolonged interactions with antigen-presenting cells. Tolerance induction, on the other hand, is characterized by relatively short interactive episodes. Thus a key difference between T cell activation and anergy may simply be the duration of their encounter with APCs.

Very high doses of an antigen can induce a form of clonal anergy called immune paralysis (Fig. 6). The high doses of the antigen probably bypass APCs, reach the Th cell receptors directly, and in the absence of co-stimulation trigger anergy.

B Cell Tolerance

Unlike the TCR repertoire, B cell antibody diversity is generated in two phases. The first phase involves VDJ rearrangement or gene conversion in the primary lymphoid organs; the second phase involves random somatic mutation in secondary lymphoid organs. B cells therefore have several opportunities to generate receptors that can bind self-antigens. It has been estimated that 55% to 75% of early immature B cells have self-reactive receptors, so suppression of these self-reactive B cells must begin at an early stage in an animal's development.

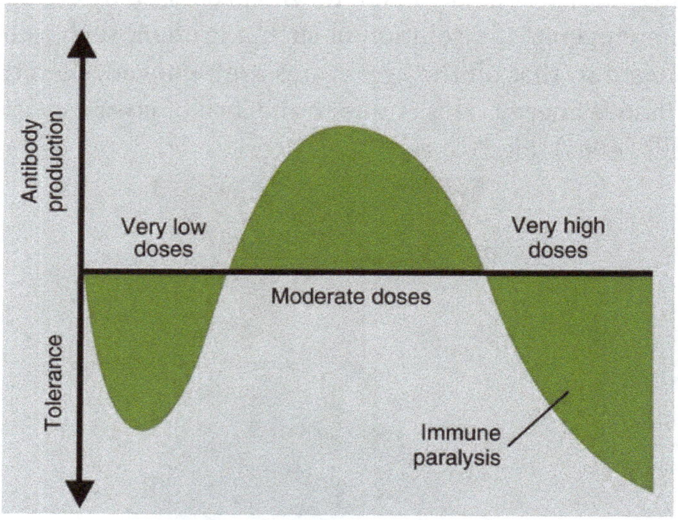

FIG. 6 The ability of different doses of antigen to induce peripheral tolerance. Both very low and very high doses can induce tolerance. Moderate doses, in contrast, induce an immune response.

Immature B cells within the bone marrow can be made tolerant once they have arranged their V-region genes and are committed to express complete immunoglobulin M (IgM) molecules. When these immature cells encounter and bind antigen, the BCR transmits a signal that arrests cell development, blocks synapse formation, and triggers apoptosis. An immature B cell population can be rendered tolerant by one millionth of the dose of an antigen required to make mature B cells tolerant. Immature B cells may also undergo receptor editing as described previously. If receptor editing fails to generate a non-self-reactive B cell, it will die.

Peripheral B Cell Tolerance

Peripheral B cell tolerance is induced by multiple mechanisms, including apoptosis, clonal anergy, clonal exhaustion, and blockage of BCRs.

Because BCRs undergo random somatic mutation within germinal centers, self-reactive B cells can still develop in secondary lymphoid organs. These cells will not, however, make autoantibodies if APCs and helper T cells are absent or if Treg cells are active (Figure 20-8). This is not, however, a foolproof method of preventing self-reactivity. In the absence of T cell help, B cells may be activated by pathogen-associated molecular patterns (PAMPs) such as bacterial lipopolysaccharide (LPS), flagellins, or unmethylated CpG DNA acting through their toll-like receptors (TLRs). B cells may also be activated by either cross-reacting epitopes or a foreign carrier molecule stimulating nontolerant helper T cells (Fig. 7).

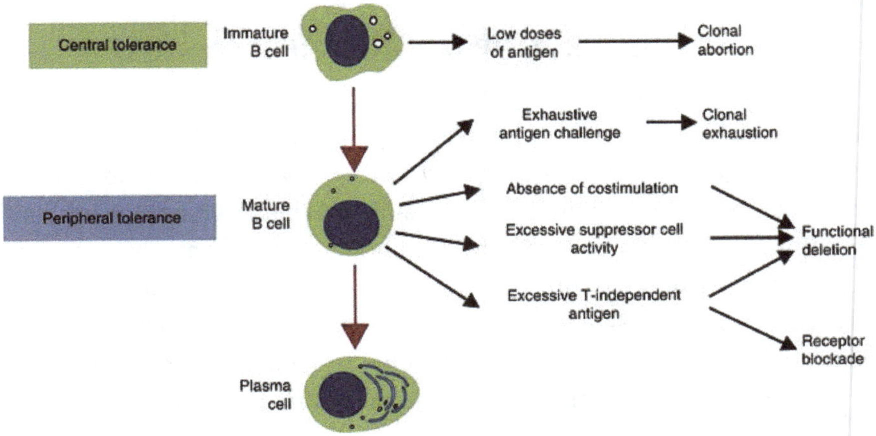

FIg. 7. Central and peripheral tolerance mechanisms in B cells.

As with T cells, B cell anergy occurs when the B cells encounter antigens in the absence of co-stimulation. B cells are difficult to maintain in a tolerant state, however, and will reactivate rapidly unless steps are taken to maintain tolerance. Self-reactive B cells must also bind to a critical threshold of self-antigen to be made tolerant. This results in selective silencing of high-affinity B cells. Presumably the failure of low-affinity anti-self B cells to become tolerant poses little threat of autoimmune disease because the low-affinity antibodies will not cause tissue destruction.

B cells subjected to repeated exhaustive antigenic stimulation may differentiate into short-lived plasma cells. If all B cells develop into such plasma cells, no memory B cells will remain to respond to antigen, and tolerance will result. Some polymeric antigens such as pneumococcal polysaccharide can bind irreversibly to BCRs, freezing the B cell membrane and blocking any further responses by these cells. The B cells recover once the antigen is removed.

Orally administered proteins may also induce tolerance. The mechanisms depend on the amount of an antigen fed. High doses induce clonal deletion and anergy, whereas lower doses induce the development of Treg cells.

Duration of Tolerance

The duration of tolerance depends on the persistence of an antigen and on the ability of the bone marrow to generate fresh T or B cells. When an antigen is completely eliminated, tolerance fades. If, however, an antigen is persistent, such as occurs in calf chimeras or with an animal's own self-antigens, tolerance persists. In the continued presence of an antigen, newly formed antigen-sensitive cells will undergo apoptosis as soon as their receptors bind self-antigen. Treatment that promotes bone marrow activity, such as low-dose X-irradiation, hastens the fading of tolerance, whereas immunosuppressive drug treatment has the opposite effect.

CONTROL OF IMMUNE RESPONSES

Tolerance is not the only mechanism of immune regulation employed by the body. The magnitude of immune responses must also be regulated. An inadequate immune response may lead to immunodeficiency and increased susceptibility to infection. An excessive immune response may result in the development of allergies or autoimmunity. Failure to control the lymphocyte proliferation that occurs during immune responses may permit development of lymphoid cell tumors. Failure to control the immune response to the fetus may lead to abortion. The immune responses must therefore be carefully regulated to ensure that they are appropriate in both quality and quantity. As might be anticipated, many different control mechanisms exist.

Antigen Regulation of Immune Responses

Adaptive immune responses are antigen driven. They commence only on exposure to an antigen, and once its concentration drops below a critical threshold, they stop. If an antigen persists, the stimulus persists and the immune response is prolonged. Prolonged responses occur after immunization with slowly degraded antigens such as the bacterial polysaccharides, or with antigens incorporated in oil or insoluble adjuvants. Antigens that do not reach organized lymphoid tissues, irrespective of their origin, fail to induce either immunity or tolerance. Thus self-antigens restricted to sites such as the brain, or infectious agents such as papillomaviruses that never enter lymphoid organs, are usually ignored by the immune system.

Antibody responses are also regulated by antigen. Rigid polymeric antigens such as those on a bacterial surface or antigens linked to TCR activators such as LPS can induce B-cell responses in the absence of T cell help. On the other hand, no polymeric, flexible antigens such as soluble proteins induce B cell responses only in the presence of CD^{4+} T cells. Antigen concentration also affects this because the lower the antigen concentration, the greater is the need for T cell help.

Antigen Processing and Immune Regulation

The nature of the immune response may vary in different parts of the body as a result of processing by different dendritic cell populations. Langerhans cells seem especially suited for promoting T cell responses, whereas follicular dendritic cells prime B cells. DC1 cells are optimized to present antigens to Th1 cells, whereas DC2 cells present antigens to Th2 cells. Adjuvants also influence the type of immune response through their effects on APCs. Thus, lipids conjugated to protein antigens commonly induce cell-mediated responses rather than antibody production and localize in T cell rather than B cell areas of lymphoid tissues.

CHAPTER

ALLERGY 11

Animal allergies are common, particularly in people who have other allergies or asthma. People may have an allergy to any animal, especially those with fur or feathers. However, most animal allergies result from a person coming into contact with cats and dogs.

According to the Asthma and Allergy Foundation of America, up to 30% of people with allergies in the United States may experience an allergic reaction to cats and dogs.

People are about twice as likely to have a cat allergy than a dog allergy.

In this article, we will examine animal allergies and their causes. We will also look at the symptoms of animal allergies and potential treatments.

Pet allergy is an allergic reaction to proteins found in an animal's skin cells, saliva or urine. Signs of pet allergy include those common to hay fever, such as sneezing and runny nose. Some people may also experience signs of asthma, such as wheezing and difficulty breathing.

Most often, pet allergy is triggered by exposure to the dead flakes of skin (dander) a pet sheds. Any animal with fur can be a source of pet allergy, but pet allergies are most commonly associated with cats and dogs.

If you have a pet allergy, the best strategy is to avoid or reduce exposure to the animal as much as possible. Medications or other treatments may be necessary to relieve symptoms and manage asthma.

Although concern is ongoing about the risks of zoonotic disease transmission from animal exposure, allergic diseases caused by animal allergens may be a greater public health and clinical problem because of the prevalence of disease and potential for mortality. Diagnosing and managing animal allergy can be challenging in part because many people are reluctant to give up their pets.

Pets and other animals can develop allergic conditions that may be triggered by the allergens that cause problems in people. In addition, because of the similarity of animal and human disease, animals serve as research models for human beings. Therefore increased communication among public health, human health, and veterinary clinicians may lead to improved management and prevention of allergic conditions.

VETERINARY CLINICIANS

- Communication with human health clinicians can help explore alternatives to removing a pet from the household of an allergic person.
- Allergic conditions in an animal may suggest an indoor air contaminant with human health relevance. Veterinarians treating an animal with an allergic condition can inquire about human beings with problems related to allergies or airborne contaminant exposures and whether causative agents have been identified. Contact with the treating health care provider may help coordinate household allergen management.

ANIMAL ALLERGY IN HUMAN BEINGS

Human beings can become sensitized to a wide range of animal allergens (Table 1). As much as 10% of the general population and 50% of persons with atopy (allergic predisposition) may be sensitized to dogs and cats. Other animals causing significant allergy in human beings include rodents, horses, insects, and birds.

Table 1 Sources of Animal Allergens Associated with Human Allergy

Animal Species	Source of Allergen
Rats and mice	Urine, hair, saliva
Guinea pigs	Urine, dander, saliva, hair
Rabbits	Urine, saliva, hair
Cats	Dander, saliva
Dogs	Dander
Birds	Feathers, serum
Horses	Serum, dander
Cattle	Hair, dander
Reptiles	Scales3
Nonhuman primates	Hair
Cockroaches	Feces, saliva, debris from dead animals4
Mites	Feces

Much symptomatic animal allergy is associated with pet ownership, but allergy can also be a significant occupational problem for individuals working with animals, including laboratory animal workers[3] and veterinarians. Occupational allergens include rodent urine, cat dander, and horse dander. Because animal allergens may persist in the environment long after elimination of a pet and can be carried distances in dust, cat and dog allergens may be present in homes where no pets are present and in schools.

ALLERGY TO CATS AND DOGS

A common misconception is that human beings are allergic to cat and dog hair and that short-haired breeds of cats and dogs are less allergenic than long-haired breeds. In fact, human allergy to cat and dogs is related to specific protein allergens, such as Fel d 1 and Can f 1, respectively, rather than hair *per se.* For this reason, despite advertising claims to the contrary, there are currently no "nonallergenic" breeds of cats and dogs. However, some species appear to provoke allergies in certain individuals and efforts are under way to develop breeds with lower allergenic potential. Cats produce a number of proteins that can act as human allergens. The one considered the most important, Fel d 1, is produced by sebaceous and salivary glands, basal squamous epithelial skin cells, and anal glands of cats.[6] It can be carried on particles less than 5 microns in diameter that can remain airborne for long periods of time. A naturally selected line of cats with deficient Fel d 1 is being developed. Dog breed, gender, and seborrhea appear to influence the levels of Can f 1 allergen detected on fur. Cat and dog allergens may persist for extended periods in a house even after a pet has left, and both Fel d 1 and Can f 1 have been detected in homes without pets.

Risk Factors for Pet Allergy

Despite the prevalence of pet allergy, it is not clear whether having a pet in the house increases the overall risk of allergy. Host factors play an important role, especially the presence of atopy, defined as "the genetic propensity to develop immunoglobulin E [IgE] antibodies in response to exposure to allergen." Studies have shown that children born into families that already own dogs (where there is no history of atopy) have a lower risk of allergic disease by 2 years of age compared with families that did not have a dog. The genetic basis of allergic predisposition is a subject of active scientific investigation. The timing of allergen exposure also appears to play a role. Although it has been reported that early exposure to cats can increase the risk of early sensitization and development of an immune response to cat allergens, other studies have shown a protective effect for pet ownership early in life, and still others have demonstrated inconsistent results regarding the development of early clinical allergic disease (particularly asthma). Farm exposure in early life is also associated with an allergy-protective effect in human beings.

COMMON ANIMALS AND ALLERGENS

People with animal allergies usually react to harmless proteins that are present in an animal's:

- dander
- saliva
- urine
- feces

Dander is tiny flakes of dead skin cells in an animal's fur, hair, or feathers that may induce allergy. Like cats and dogs, smaller mammals, such as rats, guinea pigs, hamsters, rabbits, and birds, also shed dander.

Allergens are substances that cause an allergic reaction. Pet hair itself is not an allergen. However, it may collect dander, saliva, and urine and carry other allergens, such as pollen or dust.

Animals without fur, such as reptiles, amphibians, and fish, do not shed dander and have less chance of triggering an allergic reaction.

The number of people with animal allergies is increasing, and so is ownership of pets.

According to the American Academy of Allergy, Asthma & Immunology, nearly 62% of households in the United States have pets, and over 161 million of these pets are cats or dogs.

Causes

When an allergen, such as animal skin flakes, pollen, or mold, causes inflammation inside the nose, allergic rhinitis occurs.

Allergic rhinitis happens when the immune system mistakenly identifies a harmless allergen, such as a specific animal protein, as a threat.

When people with allergies to animal proteins inhale them or have them touch their skin, the immune system may trigger a reaction.

The immune system responds to an allergen by releasing histamine. Histamine is a chemical in the body that causes the nose, throat, and skin symptoms that people associate with an allergic reaction.

Antihistamines, such as Benadryl and Zyrtec, are medications that may help alleviate allergy symptoms.

Some people with animal allergies may experience allergic contact dermatitis. This type of dermatitis occurs when an allergen contacts the skin and causes an allergic reaction.

Proteins from animals may become airborne on microscopic particles. Dander may remain airborne for long periods or collect on furniture or clothing.

Animal saliva may stick to furniture, clothing, and carpets and become airborne once dry.

Symptoms

Animal allergies produce an inflammatory response in the nasal passages, lungs, or skin.

Nasal passage and lung symptoms of an animal allergy may include:

- itchy nose, eyes, roof of the mouth, or throat
- runny nose
- stuffy nose
- sneezing
- red or watery eyes
- blue-tinted skin under the eyes
- difficulty breathing
- wheezing when exhaling
- interrupted sleep due to shortness of breath

Skin symptoms of an animal allergy may include:

- raised red patches, or hives
- itchy skin
- eczema
- a burning sensation
- swelling or tenderness

For some people, symptoms are minor and appear after several days of coming into contact with a pet. For others, coughing and shortness of breath may occur within 15–30 minutes of inhaling an allergen.

Sometimes, pet allergies may worsen asthma symptoms or trigger a severe asthma episode.

ITCHING AND ALLERGY IN DOGS

Coping with an itchy pet can be an extremely frustrating experience for a pet owner and can truly test the limits of the human-animal bond. Persistent scratching and chewing by a dog can also result in open wounds to the skin and pain to your pet.

The following information is intended to help provide pet owners with a basic understanding of the most common underlying causes of itching and allergies in small animals. Here's a summary of the most common underlying causes of itching and allergies in small animals.

What are the most common causes of chronic itching?

Itching in dogs can involve not only scratching but also chewing, licking, and rubbing. The two most common causes of itching are external parasites and allergies. Examples of itchy external parasites on dogs are fleas and small bugs called sarcoptic mange mites.

What are the major types of allergies in dogs?

Allergies are a common cause of skin and ear conditions in dogs. People with allergies usually have "hay fever" (watery eyes, runny nose and sneezing) or asthma. However, dogs with allergies rarely have respiratory signs from their allergies and instead usually have red and itchy skin, hair loss, or recurring skin or ear infections.

What are the major types of allergies in dogs?

Flea allergy

Flea allergic dermatitis is the most common skin disease in dogs. For the flea allergic patient, 100% flea control is essential for remaining symptom-free.

"But doctor, I never see fleas on my pet." You may not see them, but that doesn't mean they aren't there! Flea allergy is caused by the flea's saliva, and it only takes a few bites to cause a problem. Also, an itchy dog often scratches so much that adult fleas are hard to find because they are removed from the body.

"If fleas are the problem, why is my pet still itchy in the winter?" In warm climates or in our homes, fleas may survive in low numbers year-round. Because flea allergy is so common, many veterinarians recommend instituting complete flea control before proceeding with tests for itching. For most allergic dogs, year-round flea treatment is an important part of reducing itch.

Food allergy

Some pets develop hypersensitivities to foods. Various food proteins, carbohydrates, or even preservatives or dyes can all be potential food allergens. There is currently no accurate blood or skin test to determine if your dog has a food allergy. The only method of diagnosing a food allergy is by placing your dog on a carefully selected prescription or homemade hypoallergenic diet for several weeks, which is called a food trial. The diet only contains ingredients your dog has never eaten before. If the allergy signs resolve, a food challenge is performed by feeding the former diet and watching for a return of the itching. If this occurs, a diagnosis of food allergy is confirmed.

Atopic dermatitis

Atopic dermatitis is a type of allergy. Skin or ear inflammation occurs in response to a variety of normally harmless substances, such as plant pollens, house dust mites, and other environmental allergens. Allergy tests of the skin or blood help us compile a list of allergens for a "vaccine" (allergen specific immunotherapy) to decrease the pet's sensitivity.

Secondary infections

Allergies are often the underlying cause of recurring skin and/or ear infections. Bacterial and yeast infections, though secondary to the allergy, can increase your pet's level of itching. Long-term treatment with antibiotics and anti-yeast medications is commonly required, along with medicated bathing programs.

THE HYGIENE HYPOTHESIS

The Hygiene Hypothesis and the Bacterial World

Even before high-throughput sequencing techniques were established that allow a deeper view into the microbial world on our body surfaces, Noverr and Hufnagle proclaimed the "Microbiota Hypothesis" by which they claimed the microbiota to be indispensable for developing and maintaining a tolerogenic immune status. A similar idea concept was proposed earlier by Holt, Sly and Björkstén. The rediscovery of the microbiota and its powerful metabolic and immunologic interplay with the mucosal surfaces of the host underlined and complemented the principals of this basic idea. Microbiome research has made significant achievements over the past 15 years; here we can emphasize only a few aspects that might be relevant in the context of the Hygiene Hypothesis and the development of allergies.

Phylogenetic Impacts

An intriguing concept to better understand the complex symbiotic interplay at organ surfaces was suggested by McFall-Ngai in 2007. In her evolutionary perspective she shed light on findings made in invertebrates which not only lack an endoskeleton but also an adaptive immune system. Thus, invertebrates have to exclusively rely on their innate immune system, which to our current understanding, lacks an immunological memory. Analyses of the intestinal microbiota in such animals have shown—in contrast to vertebrates—a rather low diversity in the community of their microbial residents. Only a handful of strains could be identified as stable colonizers on the gastrointestinal surfaces while most bacteria travel through as transient visitors.

Some invertebrates, like insects, separate bacterial colonies from epithelial host cells by a peritrophic matrix composed of chitin and other compounds. During the course of evolution, the microbial colonization of epithelia started to get more complex and in turn the host was challenged to develop new strategies to manage these diversifying communities. To permanently recognize a specific bacterium as beneficial or harmful, an adaptive immune response that provides an immunological memory over generations of immune cells was needed. Mutual adaption of both partners, the bacterial community, as well as the complex network of adaptive immune cells, led to a sophisticated metabolic and immunologic interplay with a highly digestive and defensive performance. This symbiosis is based on early education of the host's immune cells by a diverse microbial community to successfully discriminate dangerous pathogens from beneficial symbionts and own healthy cells. Finally McFall-Ngai stated, that complex systems might be prone to failure and allergies and autoimmune disorders might be a consequence of this .

Ontogenetic Impacts

A number of recently published reports substantiated the impact of the early life microbiota on immune maturation and the development of allergic disorders in early infancy. The developmental starting point of the infant gut microbiota is still unknown, but undoubtedly, the process of delivery seems to be a key point in the development of the neonatal microbiota. Meconium, the neonate's first intestinal discharge, was shown to contain various bacterial strains indicating that the perinatal gut is colonized by bacteria. In a landmark study, Dominguez-Bello et al. reported that the neonatal microbiota differs between vaginally born infants and neonates delivered by Caesarian (C)-section. The authors found a high abundance of *Bacteroides, Bifidobacterium*, and *Lactobacillus spec.* in meconium samples obtained from vaginally delivered newborns, while *Staphylococcus, Streptococcus, Corynebacterium*, and *Propionibacterium* spp. were found predominantly in meconium samples of C-section born neonates.

Colonization of the neonate's colon by *Lactobacilli* and *Bifidobacteria* transferred from the maternal vaginal compartment during vaginal passage might provide advantages for the newborn due to the metabolic properties of these bacteria that foster the adaptation to milk-based feeding. These bacteria are capable of metabolizing breast milk-derived lactose and human milk oligosaccharides (HMOS) and were shown to provide immune-modulating short chain fatty acids (SCFAs) and conjugated trans-linoleic acids (tCLAs), which are shown to reduce pro-inflammatory eicosanoid production by regulating the transcription of cyclooxygenase 2 (COX2-) and to induce anti-inflammatory M-2macrophage differentiation.

However, how sustainable and decisive are these mode of delivery-associated differences beyond the neonatal age? Researchers recently showed that function and composition of the microbiota significantly diversifies in all body sites within the first 6 weeks of life, resembling the corresponding maternal body site microbiota at this time point. Infant's mode of delivery or other prenatal factors seems to have no impact on this development. Data from the Copenhagen Prospective Studies on Asthma in Childhood$_{2010}$ (COPSAC$_{2010}$) cohort underlined the importance of the maturation of the microbiota on the further development of the gut microbiome and the risk of asthma later in life. In that study, researchers compared the gut microbiome of vaginally and C-section delivered infants from birth to 1 year of life in the context of asthma development at school age. Marked differences between C-section and vaginally delivered infants were observed by 1 week and by 1 month of life, but only minor differences between these groups were found by 1 year of age. An increased risk for school-age asthma was only observed in a subgroup of C-section-born infants that maintained the C-section-associated composition for at least 1 year. The authors conclude that vaginal delivery and/or subsequent maturation of the infant microbiota might support a more robust and stable microbiota in the offspring that is more adaptive to the challenges later in life. Further exposure to the maternal microbiota, as well as nutritional impacts (e.g., cessation of breastfeeding) within the first month of life, might foster the maturation of the gut microbiome in early infancy.

Nutritional Impacts

How is the microbiota linked to the rising atopic epidemic observed in the recent decades? A recently published study conducted in indigenous tribes living in the Brazilian Amazonas-Orinoco Basin may help to answer this question. In this study the gut microbiome of the semi-nomadic gatherer/hunter people of the Yanomami who maintained a primitive close-to-nature life-style was compared to subjects representing populations that are characterized by a westernized or non-ancestral life-style in rural and urban settings. The Yanomami microbiota was significantly more diverse than those of the westernized counterparts. Moreover, an additional study comparing Venezuelan with Brazilian Yanomami indicated a high level of adaptability to specific environmental conditions of the microbiota in these peoples. While a high taxonomic diversity was found in both sub-tribes, the composition of microbiota was significantly different. These findings point to environmental and life-style factors that influence the composition of the microbiota the absence of which may thus foster the loss of taxonomic and metabolic diversity in westernized societies.

Diet is one of the most prominent environmental factors that differ between modern and ancient life-styles. While dietary habits in indigenous people such as the Yanomami strongly depend on the sometimes limited food supply due to seasonal cycling, people living in developed societies have access to high in calories food ready at any time and in abundance. Moreover, diet in indigenous cultures is often based on high-fiber products derived from plants that are easy to culture such as plantain, manioc or sweet potatoes, all rich in inulin. High-fiber diet and, in particular inulin, is known as an effective enhancer of beneficial bacteria such as *Bifidobacteria* in the colon that stabilize gut homeostasis.

Translating these findings into a clinical approach, McLoughlin et al. applied soluble inulin to asthmatics in a short-term placebo-controlled-trial and could report an array of beneficial effects in patients orally treated with inulin. In comparison to the placebo group, inulin-treated patients displayed a significantly reduced number of eosinophils in the sputum and, overall, reported a significantly improved asthma control. Inhibition of histone deacetylase 9 (HDAC9) in sputum cells upon a combined application of inulin and a multi-strain probiotic mixture of *Lactobacillus acidophilus, Lactobacillus rhamnosus* GG and *Bifidobacterium animalis* subspecies *lactis* indicated that epigenetic pathways are involved in the mechanisms by which lactic acid bacteria modulate host responses in combination with the prebiotic gavage.

A number of recently recognized metabolites released by beneficial symbiotic bacteria convey immunomodulatory effects, mainly in the gut but also on other mucosal surfaces.

In particular, SCFAs derived from dietary fibers and released in the lumen of the colon contribute to immune modulation and inhibition of pro-inflammatory cytokines when absorbed by gut epithelial cells. By binding to chemoattractant G protein 43 receptor, SCFAs are capable of regulating inflammatory responses as shown for intestinal inflammation. Tryptophan, an amino acid produced by an array of beneficial microorganisms, is degraded to indole derivatives which may bind to the aryl hydrocarbon receptor (AHR) and by this regulate the activity of immune cells at the epithelial barrier. That involves AHR-dependent differentiation of regulatory T cells associated with anti-inflammatory IL-10 expression. Further, Th2-cells are inhibited on the transcription factor level in favor of a Th1 response.

A number of beneficial bacteria contribute to the orchestration of T cell subsets at the gut epithelial barrier. *Bacteroides sp.* and *Clostridium* clusters IV and XIVa colonizing the gut epithelium are known to stimulate intestinal epithelial cells to release thymic stromal lymphopoietin (TSLP), transforming growth factor (TGF)-ß and interleukin (IL)25- which in combination may induce tolerogenic effects in dendritic cells (DCs), e.g., by secretion of TGF-β and retinoic acid. Both factors initiate differentiation of naïve T cells to regulatory T cells upon activation of the nuclear transcription factor forkhead box P (FoxP3).

These regulatory mechanisms are challenged by "pathobionts" or other damage factors. In presence of these stressors, overexpansion of Th1, Th2 and Th17 effector cell subsets might result in an inflammatory response in the infected organ or, by migration of these cells, at distant sites. Namely, *Clostridium difficile*, which is associated with wheezing and atopic sensitization, was shown to initially disturb the intestinal balance when acquired early in childhood.

Traveling from the gastrointestinal to the respiratory tract the microbiota established in the lung might also play a role in the development of allergic disorders, namely of allergic asthma. Though the gut is known to play a major role in establishing and regulating immune defense mechanisms, the "gut-lung axis" alone might not completely explain the rise of allergic asthma. As many studies focused on the lung microbiome, it has become clear that there is a strong relationship between frequently inhaled environmental microbes, microbial colonization of the respiratory tract, and the prevalence of allergic asthma.

For example, results from the "Multidisciplinary Study to Identify the Genetic and Environmental Causes of Asthma in the European Community (GABRIEL) Advanced Studies (GABRIELA)" study suggested a transfer of built-environment-associated bacteria into the respiratory tract. Indoor dust samples from farm houses and nasal swabs from farm children displayed a higher bacterial diversity than those samples collected in rural non-farm children.

New evidence was added recently by studies conducted in the Finnish part of the PASTURE-study. Kirjavainen et al. reported that the ecological diversity of the so-called "indoor microbiota" is inversely linked to the prevalence of allergic asthma. Substantiating former farm studies, this report further validated the hypothesis that microbial diversity and composition in the natural environment is linked to a reduced risk of early-onset allergic asthma and that traditional farming is a proxy for this effect.

But what are the cellular and molecular mechanisms associated with high microbial diversity? Interestingly, the farm studies consistently showed an inverse association between a highly diverse environmental microbiota and allergic asthma, but this did not account to other allergic manifestations such as hay fever or atopic sensitization. On the other hand, endotoxin exposure protects against atopy but fosters the risk of non-allergic asthma and early onset of wheeze when inhaled in higher concentrations.

These findings derived from the farm studies still challenge the Hygiene Hypothesis and might point out that microbial colonization and exposure to microbial compounds have to be considered separately. Integration of beneficial environmental bacteria into the microbial community of the respiratory tract leads to a tolerogenic mucosal symbiosis that establishes a local T-cell balanced anti-inflammatory milieu at the epithelium, probably enhanced by a well-balanced gut microbiota. Endotoxins are potent activators of innate TLR-signaling and can attenuate B cell driven sensitization and formation of IgE-antibodies.

Already in 2003, Vercelli postulated a switch from Th2-driven allergic responses at low endotoxin exposure to a pronounced Th1 response in the lung under high levels of environmental endotoxin. This might explain the elevated prevalence of non-allergic asthma in environments overloaded with endotoxin.

TREATMENT AND MANAGEMENT

Managing an animal allergy involves avoiding the allergy-causing animal whenever possible. Minimizing exposure to the animal may help reduce allergic reactions and their severity.

To help control symptoms, a doctor may recommend medications, such as:

- **Antihistamines:** These may reduce the amount of histamine causing an allergic reaction and alleviate itching, runny nose, and sneezing.
- **Corticosteroids:** These steroid nasal sprays may reduce inflammation and ease sneezing and a runny or stuffy nose.
- **Decongestants:** These lessen swelling in the nasal passages, which makes breathing through the nose easier.
- **Leukotriene modifiers:** A doctor may prescribe these when antihistamines and corticosteroids are not a suitable option. They block the actions of certain chemicals the body releases, and they reduce inflammation and nasal congestion.
- **Immunotherapy:** This involves exposure to incremental increases of an allergen, which may reduce sensitivity to the substance over time.

Remedies

It can be challenging to eliminate exposure to animal allergens, particularly if the animal is a pet or the person works with animals. People may also encounter animal allergens that other people carry around on their clothing.

The following suggestions may help reduce exposure to animal allergens:

- **Create a pet-free zone:** Making chosen areas of the house pet-free can help lessen allergens in those areas.
- **Remove furnishings that attract dander:** Pet dander collects on carpets, curtains, and horizontal blinds. If possible, replace carpet with tile, vinyl flooring, or wood that cleans easily.
- **Clean the carpet frequently:** Choosing carpets with a low pile and regularly steam cleaning them may help reduce pet dander in the room.
- **Wash pets frequently:** Washing a pet every week may decrease airborne allergens.
- **Ask for help:** Ask someone without a pet allergy to clean the pet's bedding, cage, or litter tray. The helper could also brush the pet outside to remove some dander.

- **Change clothing:** After spending long periods with a pet, change clothing to reduce allergen exposure.
- **Try high-efficiency filters:** High-efficiency particulate air purifiers may decrease the amount of airborne allergens.

Some people with animal allergies may be more sensitive to some breeds of cats or dogs than others.

People may consider breeds that shed less to be hypoallergenic. However, dogs and cats that are nonallergic do not exist.

When introducing a new pet to the home, a trial period can help determine whether a person has an allergy to the animal.

Allergy testing

A doctor may refer a person to an allergy specialist, known as an allergist, for allergy testing. Allergy testing determines the precise trigger of a person's symptoms.

Types of allergy tests include:

Skin test

During a skin test, an allergist places a tiny amount of allergen on the skin. Then they prick or scratch the skin to see whether any swelling appears. Test results are typically available within 15 minutes.

Intradermal test

If results from a skin test are unclear, an allergist may use an intradermal test. During this type of test, an allergist will use a syringe to inject the allergen under the skin.

Blood test

Sometimes an allergist may not perform a skin test due to a person having a skin condition. In this case, a doctor may order a blood test to screen for specific allergy-causing antibodies to various animal allergens.

A blood test may also indicate how sensitive a person is to a specific allergen.

Summary

Animal allergies are a common occurrence, especially among people with other allergies or asthma.

An animal allergy occurs when people come into contact with proteins in pet dander, saliva, or urine. The immune system mistakenly flags the protein as a threat and produces histamine, which causes allergy symptoms.

The most effective way to prevent animal allergy symptoms is to avoid the animal. However, there are steps people can take to reduce exposure to allergens from their pets.

Treatment options are available to help relieve inflammation and control allergy symptoms.

CHAPTER 12

IMMUNODEFICIENCY

Immunodeficiency diseases manifest clinically as a predisposition to infections. They are usually recognized when an animal makes multiple visits to a veterinarian for infections that would normally be relatively easy to control. Two major groups of immunodeficiency disease occur. One group is inherited as a result of mutations or other genetic disease. These primary or congenital immunodeficiency diseases usually develop in very young animals (<6 months of age). The second group of immunodeficiency diseases are secondary to some other stimulus such as a viral infection or tumor.

These secondary or acquired diseases tend to occur in adult animals. One other general rule in diagnosing immunodeficiencies is that defects in the innate and antibody-mediated immune systems tend to result in uncontrollable bacterial infections, whereas defects in the cell-mediated immune system tend to result in overwhelming viral and fungal infections.

DEFECTS IN INNATE IMMUNITY

Phagocytosis is a central feature of innate immunity and inflammation. Phagocytic cells are found either in the tissues (histiocytes, synovial macrophages, Kupffer cells, etc) or in the bloodstream (neutrophils and monocytes). Phagocytes have receptors for immunoglobulins and complement on their surfaces that assist in the engulfment (opsonization) of foreign material coated with specific antibody (opsonins) or complement, or both.

Phagocytosis involves chemotaxis of the phagocyte toward foreign, noxious, or damaged tissues; adherence of microorganisms to the plasma membrane of the phagocyte; ingestion of the organisms into a phagosome; and subsequent activation of the respiratory burst and lysosomal enzymes in the phagosome, leading to microbial death and destruction.

DEFECTS IN PHAGOCYTOSIS

Defects in phagocytic activity can be due to acquired or congenital defects in any of the above processes or simply to a deficiency of phagocytic cells themselves. They often manifest as an increased susceptibility to bacterial infections of the skin, respiratory system, and GI tract. These infections respond poorly to antibiotics. Secondary phagocytic deficiencies include disorders that lead to profound and chronic loss of leukocytes. Some of the conditions in which secondary infections can be lethal include:

- feline leukemia virus infection
- feline panleukopenia virus infection
- feline immunodeficiency virus infection
- tropical canine pancytopenia
- idiopathic granulocytopenias
- drug-induced granulocytopenias (anticancer drugs, estrogens, anticonvulsants, sulfonamides, etc)
- myeloproliferative disorders

A cyclic decrease of all cellular elements, most notably neutrophils, occurs in the peripheral blood and lowers the resistance to infection of certain lines of gray Collies and Collie crosses.

Congenital abnormalities that lead to impaired phagocytosis are well documented in people. Deficiencies of opsonins, chemotactic abilities, and myelo-peroxidase, have been recognized in humans but not in other animals. Chediak-Higashi syndrome results from a defect in phagosomal function and has been recorded in cats, mink, cattle, and orcas. For example, mink with the Aleutian coat color mutation are susceptible to chronic parvovirus infection and so develop Aleutian disease. Other strains of mink are susceptible to infection with this virus but do not develop clinical disease. This is due to Chediak-Higashi syndrome.

Chronic granulomatous disease has been recognized as an X-linked defect in some Irish Setters (canine granulocytopathy syndrome). Some lines of Weimaraners develop bacterial septicemias (usually manifested by bone and joint infections) as puppies. The underlying causes of these defects are unknown; some of the affected dogs have lower than normal levels of IgM and IgG, and their leukocytes have a bactericidal defect.

LEUKOCYTE ADHESION DEFICIENCY

Leukocyte adhesion deficiency is an autosomal recessive primary immunodeficiency. It has been described in people, Irish Setters, and Holstein calves. The deficiency results from the absence of an integrin, an adhesive glycoprotein expressed on leukocytes. Clinically, it is characterized by recurrent severe bacterial infections, impaired pus formation, and delayed wound healing. Infected animals usually have severe fever, anorexia, and weight loss. Response to antibiotic therapy is usually poor. Extreme, persistent leukocytosis may occur (>100,000 WBC/mL) and consists predominantly of mature neutrophils. The integrin deficiency prevents blood leukocytes from binding to vascular endothelial cells. As a result, they cannot leave blood vessels or enter the tissues, so they cannot contribute to the defense of tissues against infections.

COMPLEMENT DEFICIENCIES

A congenital deficiency of C3 has been described in Brittany Spaniels. These dogs developed recurrent bacterial infections, especially skin diseases and pneumonias. Although complement is necessary for opsonization and neutrophil chemotaxis, bacterial infections do not always develop in people or laboratory animals with complement deficiencies because the existence of multiple pathways provides a way to activate the system even if one pathway is blocked. Diagnosis is based on a blood test showing reduced C3 levels. A congenital deficiency in the C1 inhibitor has been recognized in humans and occurs rarely in dogs and pigs. This can lead to uncontrolled complement activation and inflammation. Affected animals have recurrent bouts of facial edema.

There is no specific treatment for complement deficiencies. Vaccination and antibiotics are used to prevent and treat infection. As with all inherited diseases, subsequent breeding programs must be carefully assessed to prevent the reappearance of the disease in future generations.

DEFICIENCIES IN ADAPTIVE IMMUNITY

Immunoglobulin Deficiencies

Immunoglobulin deficiencies may also be acquired or congenital. Acquired deficiencies occur in neonates that do not receive adequate maternal antibodies (failure of passive transfer) or in older animals due to conditions that decrease active immunoglobulin synthesis. Failure of passive transfer occurs in species that use colostrum as the major source of maternal antibodies. It is commonly associated with recurrent infections in calves, lambs, piglets and foals. Failure of passive transfer can occur when a young animal fails to nurse properly during the first several days of life or when the dam's colostrum contains low levels of specific antibodies.

Defects in the absorption of immunoglobulin from ingested milk may also occur. Immunoglobulin levels <400 mg/dL in a post-nursing serum sample indicate a failure of passive transfer in foals. Premature weaning of calves is a problem in dairy herds and is a leading cause of failure of passive transfer in dairy calves. Newborn animals that do not receive sufficient maternal antibodies often succumb to fatal bacterial or viral infections of the GI and respiratory tracts.

Hypogammaglobulinemia of clinical significance can be associated with any disorder that interferes with antibody synthesis. Tumors, such as myelomas or lymphosarcomas that secrete large amounts of monoclonal antibody, can be associated with profound antibody deficiencies. This is because the tumor cells outcompete normal immunoglobulin-producing cells, or because regulatory pathways inhibit immunoglobulin production.

Animals with myelomas that produce monoclonal antibodies may have secondary infections. Some viruses, such as canine distemper and canine or feline parvovirus, may damage the immune system so severely that antibody production is virtually stopped. Secondary invasion by organisms such as *Pneumocystis* spp may then occur.

Congenital hypogammaglobulinemia has been recognized either alone or in combination with defects in cell-mediated immunity (combined immunodeficiency, see below). Deficiencies in IgG subclasses have been seen in some breeds of cattle; IgM deficiency has been described in horses; and IgA deficiencies have been described in Beagles, German Shepherds, and Chinese Shar-Peis. Cattle with IgG subclass deficiency are usually asymptomatic. Older foals with IgM deficiencies develop respiratory infections. Dogs with IgA deficiency, like their human counterparts, are prone to chronic skin infections, chronic respiratory infections, and possibly allergies.

IgA deficiency of Beagles appears to be due to a defect in its secretion because IgA-positive cells are present in normal numbers. Some German Shepherds have lower IgA levels than other breeds and a higher prevalence of intestinal infections. IgA deficiency in Shar-Peis is highly variable; some have negligible serum and secretory levels, and some have normal serum levels and low or negligible secretory levels. Like German Shepherds, affected Shar-Peis may have allergic disease. Patients with these immunodeficiency syndromes may have a higher than usual prevalence of diseases such as autoimmune hemolytic anemia, thrombocytopenia, and systemic lupus erythematosus. Longterm treatment with broad-spectrum antibiotics is required and is often unsatisfactory.

Transient hypogammaglobulinemia has been recognized most frequently in foals and puppies. It may be more common in Spitz-type puppies than in other breeds. It results from a delayed onset of immunoglobulin production in a newborn. Puppies with this condition develop recurrent respiratory infections at 6–1 months of age but usually recover by 8 months.

Affected foals frequently develop clinical signs of hypogammaglobulinemia (usually respiratory infections) at ~6 months of age when their maternal antibody reaches a very low level. After another 3–5 months, they begin to produce immunoglobulin. Appropriate antibiotic treatment and supportive therapy is often sufficient.

Deficiencies in Cell-mediated Immunity

Deficiencies in cell-mediated immune responses are associated with **thymic aplasia**, an absent or very small thymus. This has been seen in some inbred lines of dogs, cats, and cattle, as well as mice. This condition in laboratory mice has been used to create inbred strains of athymic mice (commonly known as nude mice because they lack hair) that are widely used in immunologic research.

Combined Immunodeficiency Diseases

If both humoral and cell-mediated immune responses are deficient, they are classified as combined immunodeficiencies (CIDs). These result from inherited defects in the earliest lymphocyte progenitors. An autosomal recessive CID has been identified in Arabian foals and Basset Hounds. It results from a defect in DNA repair enzymes and prevents the production of functional antigen receptors. Sporadic cases of CID have also been seen in Toy Poodle, Rottweiler, and mixed-breed puppies. Affected dogs are frequently asymptomatic during the first several months of life but become progressively more susceptible to microbial infections as maternal antibody wanes. Puppies with CID are clinically normal until 6–12 weeks of age.

The most common cause of death from CID is canine distemper as a consequence of routine immunization with modified live virus distemper vaccines. Arabian foals with CID frequently succumb to adenovirus pneumonia or other infections when ~2 months old. The foals are persistently lymphopenic. Precolostral serum samples have no detectable IgM antibody. Immunoglobulin levels are normal at first but then progressively decline when compared with levels in healthy foals. At necropsy, the thymus may be difficult to identify and structurally abnormal. Lymphocytes are depleted in the lymph nodes, Peyer's patches, and spleen. A PCR test can confirm CID in foals and the presence of the mutated gene in heterozygote animals. As a result of such testing, the prevalence of equine CID has declined significantly.

Selective Immunodeficiencies

Many immunodeficiency diseases have yet to be fully analyzed, so their precise mechanisms remain unknown. For example, Rottweiler puppies have a breed predilection for severe and often fatal canine parvovirus infections. Their resistance to other infections is essentially normal, and the basis of this selective immunodeficiency is unknown.

Persian cats have a predilection toward severe, and sometimes protracted, dermatophyte infections. In some Persian cats, the fungal infections invade the dermis and cause granulomatous disease (mycetomas).

Focal and systemic aspergillosis, as well as mycoses due to related fungi, affect certain types of dogs. Long-nosed breeds, in particular German Shepherds and shepherd-crosses, are prone to develop focal aspergillosis in the nasal passages. Systemic aspergillosis is seen almost exclusively in German Shepherds. It is characterized by fungal pyelonephritis, osteomyelitis, and discospondylitis. The organism can be isolated readily from blood and urine.

Diagnosis

Recurrent persistent infections in young animals suggest some form of immunodeficiency. A complete differential leukocyte count will reveal whether the cells are present in appropriate numbers. Turbidity tests are relatively easy to perform and are used to diagnose failure of passive transfer of immunity. They may also provide useful diagnostic information. Specific immunoglobulin deficiencies can be detected by means of a quantitative immunoassay such as radial immunodiffusion.

Primary immunodeficiencies as genetic diseases are generally not treatable but, if diagnosed, steps should be taken to ensure that parent animals that carry defective traits are no longer used for breeding.

VIRAL INFECTIONS CAUSING IMMUNODEFICIENCY

Canine Distemper Virus Infection

Canine distemper virus (CDV) causes canine distemper, a common disease of dogs worldwide that is associated with a high degree of morbidity and mortality. The virus also infects several other species, including foxes, raccoons, skunks, ferrets, and free-ranging and captive felids. Disease in dogs is most prevalent in regions where vaccination of young dogs against the disease is either not performed or is poorly timed, and epidemics continue to occur in shelter environments in developed countries.

Canine distemper virus is a Morbillivirus related to measles virus and has been used to study the pathogenesis of measles virus infection. Morbilliviruses are enveloped RNA viruses that survive poorly in the environment. Based on genetic variation within the viral hemagglutinin (H) gene, a multitude of different strains of CDV exist that vary in their geographic distribution, cell tropism, and virulence. Although CDV infects a variety of different cell types, including epithelial, mesenchymal, neuroendocrine, and hematopoietic cells, the marked tropism of CDV for immune cells is critical in respect to its ability to cause immunosuppression. Viral components involved in CDV-induced immuno-deficiency include the viral hemagglutinin; the V protein (a nonstructural phosphoprotein); and the nucleocapsid (N) protein.

Dogs are generally exposed to CDV through contact with infected oronasal secretions. The virus initially infects monocytes within lymphoid tissue in the upper respiratory tract and tonsils and is subsequently disseminated via the lymphatics and blood to the entire reticuloendothelial system. Direct viral destruction of a significant proportion of the lymphocyte population, and especially CD4+ T cells, occurs within the blood, tonsils, thymus, spleen, lymph nodes, bone marrow, mucosa-associated lymphoid tissue, and the hepatic Kupffer cells.

This viral destruction is associated with an initial lymphopenia and transient fever that occurs a few days after infection. Subsequently, there is a second stage of cell-associated viremia, after which CDV infects cells of the lower respiratory; gastrointestinal tract; central nervous system; urinary tract; and red and white blood cells, including additional lymphoid cells.

Elimination of CDV by the host depends on humoral and CMI. Because the virus is lymphocytolytic, the outcome of infection depends on the rate at which the host is able to remove the virus before the virus has sufficient time to cause severe immune system injury. Dogs mounting a partial immune response may undergo recovery from acute illness but fail to eliminate the virus completely, leading to a spectrum of more chronic disease manifestations that often involve the uvea, lymphoid organs, footpads, and especially the CNS. Opportunistic infections may also have the chance to develop in these dogs.

Dogs with canine distemper may develop profound lymphopenia and leucopenia. Lymphopenia results from generalized depletion of T and B cells in a variety of tissues (Fig. 1). CD4+ T cells are preferentially depleted during the acute phase, which is followed by CD8+ cell depletion. Necrosis of hematopoietic cells within the bone marrow may result in leucopenia.

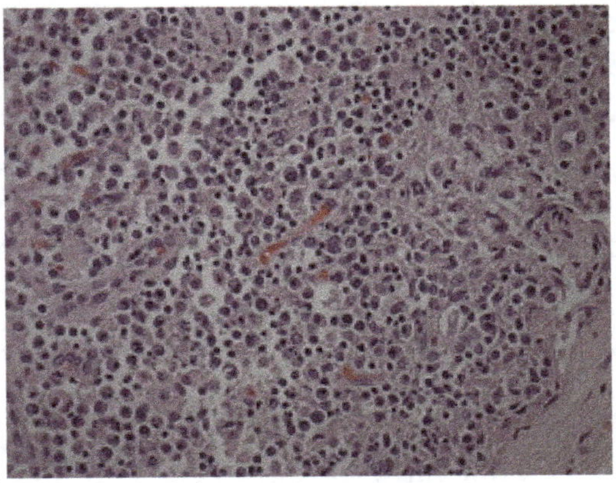

Fig. 1. Severe cortical lymphoid necrosis in a mandibular lymph node from a 5-month-old female spayed German Shepherd cross that was euthanized as a result of canine distemper virus infection.

Infection of ferrets has been used as a model of CDV-induced immunosuppression.

CDV infection of ferrets leads to dramatic reduction in cell-mediated immune function with markedly depressed lymphocyte proliferative activity, and to some extent delayed type hypersensitivity responses. The virus enters lymphocytes following binding of the viral H gene to the primary receptor for the virus, signaling lymphocyte activation molecule (CD150, SLAM). The expression of SLAM appears to be upregulated in response to CDV infection. SLAM is also expressed on antigen-presenting cells, such as dendritic cells and activated monocytes, and infection of these cells, which may predominate in the chronic phase of infection, has been hypothesized to be associated with impaired antigen presentation.

Infection of dendritic cells within the thymus may lead to impaired maturation and selection of T cells, with subsequent release of immature CD-5 T cells, including cells that may have the potential for autoreactivity. Lymphocyte apoptosis also occurs independent of viral infection in canine distemper, although the mechanisms have not yet been elucidated. The presence of the viral V protein is essential to permit rapid replication of CDV in T cells and critical in CDV-mediated immunosuppression. This protein almost completely antagonizes alpha interferon, TNF-alpha, Il-6, gamma-interferon, and Il-2 in the acute phase of infection.

Suppression of the cytokine response is associated with severe immunosuppression and a fatal outcome in ferrets. Finally, the N protein of Morbilliviruses may interfere with the immune response through the binding of the CD32 (Fc-gamma) receptor on B cells, resulting in impaired differentiation of B cells into plasma cells. Binding of this receptor on dendritic cells is associated with impairment of antigen presentation by dendritic cells and resulting disruption of T cell function.

The most common secondary infections in canine distemper are secondary bacterial infections that contribute to bronchopneumonia. *Bordetella bronchiseptica* is also a common co-pathogen in dogs with distemper. Dogs may be diagnosed with bordetellosis in the early stages of distemper, the underlying CDV infection being overlooked. Other opportunistic infections that have been identified in dogs with distemper include toxoplasmosis, salmonellosis, nocardiosis, and generalized demodicosis. In one study from Brazil, canine distemper was the most common underlying immunosuppressive disease predisposing to nocardiosis in dogs.

Infection with *Pneumocystis carinii* was associated with CDV infection in a mink, and concurrent neosporosis and canine distemper was reported in a raccoon.

Canine Parvovirus 2 and Feline Panleukopenia Virus Infection

Although parvoviruses do not cause chronic, persistent infections in dogs and cats, parvoviral replication creates the perfect storm for development of acute and severe opportunistic bacterial infections. The combination of leukopenia, disruption of the gastrointestinal barrier, and the immature immune system of the young animals that are most susceptible to these viruses is associated with the common development of sepsis, which is frequently the cause of death.

Canine parvovirus 2 (CPV-2) and feline panleukopenia virus (FPV) are small, nonenveloped DNA viruses. Since its emergence in 1978, CPV has subsequently mutated to CPV-2a; CPV-2b; and in the last decade, CPV-2c, which was first documented in Italy and has subsequently spread to dogs on every continent, with the exception of Australia. The CPV-2c strain appears to be particularly virulent and there has been some debate regarding the ability of current vaccines to protect against it and the ability of commercially available SNAP ELISA tests to detect the virus.

CPV and FPV have tropism for rapidly dividing cells. As such, they exert an effect on the host that resembles the outcome of treatment with a chemotherapeutic drug. The virus binds and enters cells using the transferrin receptor. Cells preferentially involved are the crypt cells of the gastrointestinal tract, bone marrow, and lymphoid tissue. Leukopenia results from sequestration of neutrophils within damaged gastrointestinal tissue and is compounded by destruction of white cell precursors within the bone marrow. Damage to the gastrointestinal barrier can result in translocation of enteric bacteria. In the face of the massive immunosuppression that ensues as a result of virus-induced neutropenia and lymphopenia, the host fails to contain bacterial replication and bacteremia and sepsis ensue. Treatment of secondary infections with broad-spectrum parenteral antimicrobial drugs is critical to permit recovery of dogs and cats from parvoviral infection. Bacterial causes of sepsis reported in infected animals include *Escherichia coli*, *Salmonella* spp, and *Clostridium difficile*. *Giardia* infection also exacerbates illness.

Immunosuppression may also contribute to replication of other co-infecting enteric viruses, such as enteric coronavirus, which in turn exacerbate the damage to the gastrointestinal mucosa. Similarly, CPV-induced immunosuppression potentiates the development of postvaccinal canine distemper encephalitis.

The importance of secondary infections in the pathogenesis of parvovirus infections is highlighted by the fact that experimental infection of germfree cats is not associated with development of clinical illness, despite the associated reduction in white cell count.

FELINE RETROVIRAL INFECTIONS

Feline leukemia virus and feline immunodeficiency virus are common causes of viral-induced immunodeficiency in cats, although the underlying mechanisms by which they exert immunodeficiency are still incompletely understood. Subtypes of FeLV and FIV are defined based on variations in the *env* gene sequence, which also influences their pathogenicity.

FELINE LEUKEMIA VIRUS INFECTION

There are four different subtypes of the gamma retrovirus FeLV: FeLV-A, FeLV-B, FeLV-C, and FeLV-T. Each subtype uses a different receptor to enter cells. All cats infected with FeLV-B, FeLV-C, and FeLV-T are co-infected with FeLV-A, with FeLV-A being the only type that is transmitted between animals. The other subtypes arise through recombination or point mutation within FeLV-A during the course of infection and influence the clinical expression of disease. FeLV-T, a T-cell tropic variant, is unique amongst gamma retroviruses in that it requires two host proteins to enter and infect cells. As a result of its T-cell tropism, FeLV-T infection may be particularly associated with immunodeficiency in cats.

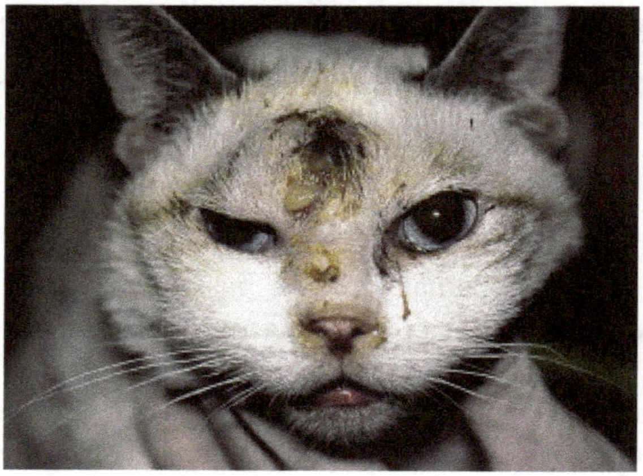

Fig. 2. Siamese cat with FeLV infection and concurrent severe cryptococcal rhinosinusitis that was refractory to therapy with antifungal drugs.

Transmission of FeLV-A primarily occurs through prolonged, close contact with salivary secretions, although other routes of transmission, including through biting, can also occur. After an initial phase of viremia, FeLV replicates within rapidly dividing lymphoid, myeloid, and epithelial cells, such as those lining the intestinal crypts.

As with distemper, when cellular destruction exceeds the ability of the host's immune system to suppress viral replication, persistent viremia and progressive FeLV-related disease results.

Clinical outcomes of FeLV infection include tumor development, especially lymphoma or leukemia; non-regenerative anemia; marrow failure, which in turn can result from myelophthisis, myelodysplasia, or myelofibrosis; neurologic manifestations, such as anisocoria; reproductive failure; gastrointestinal disease; and immunodeficiency. The development of opportunistic infections may result from marrow failure or cell-mediated immunodeficiency. The immunosuppressive properties of FeLV have been linked at least in part to the transmembrane viral envelope peptide, p15E.

This viral protein inhibits T- and B-cell function, inhibits cytotoxic lymphocyte responses, alters monocyte morphology and distribution, and has been associated with impaired cytokine production and responsiveness. Kittens persistently infected with FeLV have impaired T-cell, and to a lesser extent, B-cell function. Infected cats may develop lymphopenia, thymic atrophy, and depletion of lymphocytes within lymph node paracortical zones. CD4+ T-cell malfunction may contribute to a decreased humoral and cellular immune response in affected cats. The response to vaccination may also be impaired. Neutrophil function is also impaired in cats that are FeLV-infected.

Opportunistic infections documented in cats that are FeLV-infected include bacterial infections of the upper and lower urinary tract, hemoplasmosis, respiratory tract infections, feline infectious peritonitis (FIP), and chronic stomatitis, although there is little evidence in the literature to support an increased prevalence of these infections in cats with FeLV as opposed to cats not infected with FeLV. Some infections, such as cryptococcosis, appear to occur with the same frequency in cats that are FeLV positive as in cats that are FeLV negative, but may be more severe and refractory to therapy (Fig. 2).

FELINE IMMUNODEFICIENCY VIRUS INFECTION

FIV is a lentivirus that is primarily transmitted between cats by biting. FIV invades cells via the primary receptor CD134, which is expressed on feline CD4+ T lymphocytes; B lymphocytes; activated macrophages; and the secondary receptor CXCR4, a chemokine receptor.

The mechanisms of immunosuppression in FIV infection are complex, and despite more than 20 years of research on the subject, not completely understood. Paradoxically, immune suppression and immune hyperactivation have been documented in infected cats. A comprehensive review of the subject is beyond the scope of this article but has been recently published elsewhere.

Central to FIV-induced immunosuppression is a progressive reduction in CD4+ T-cell numbers. The number of CD4+ T cells in peripheral blood declines shortly after infection, owing to initial viral replication within target activated CD4+ T cells and macrophages. After this acute phase of infection, numbers of CD4+ T cells rebound and viremia is suppressed. Neutropenia can also occur during this phase and it has been suggested that this may result from neutrophil apoptosis. CD4+/CD25+ T regulator cells have recently been shown to be infected and activated during acute infection. When activated, these cells inhibit proliferation and induce apoptosis of other activated CD4+ or CD8+ T cells, which may also contribute to persistence of FIV and further immunosuppression.

Evidence also points to altered dendritic cell function during acute FIV infection. The impairment of T-cell function in acute FIV infection has been suggested to result from cytokine dysregulation, immunologic anergy, and increased apoptosis. In turn, this is associated with an inability to mount a primary immune response to opportunistic pathogens.

A prolonged asymptomatic period follows, sometimes lasting years or even the lifetime of the cat, which is associated with a gradual decline in CD4+ T-cell numbers; a reduction in the CD4+/CD8+ ratio; generalized lymphoid depletion; and in some cats, hyperglobulinemia, which results from B-cell hyperactivation. In addition to a decline in cell numbers, although activated, paradoxically, T cells develop a reduced ability to respond to antigenic stimulation. Altered lymphocyte expression of cell surface molecules, including CD4, cytokine receptors and major histocompatibility complex (MHC) II antigens, and continued alteration of dendritic cell function, also contribute to immunosuppression. Dysregulation of cytokine production occurs. Cats chronically infected with FIV fail to produce Il-2, Il-6, and Il-12 in response to *T gondii* infection, instead producing elevated levels of the antiinflammatory cytokine Il10-.

Ultimately these changes lead to opportunistic infections, most commonly bacterial infections of the mouth; chronic bacterial skin infections; persistent viral upper respiratory tract infections; mycobacterial infections; hemoplasmosis; toxoplasmosis; and parasitic infections, such as demodicosis and severe flea burdens.

FELINE CORONAVIRUS INFECTION

FIP virus infection is associated with a profound, virus-induced depletion of CD4+ and CD8+ cells and hypergammaglobulinemia, suggesting virus-induced dysregulation of the immune response. The mechanism of T cell depletion is not clear, because the virus does not infect lymphocytes, only monocytes and macrophages. Infection of antigen-presenting cells, specifically dendritic cells, by the virus has been hypothesized to cause T-cell apoptosis. Despite the profound T-cell deficiency that accompanies FIP, opportunistic infections are rarely reported, perhaps partly as a result of the rapidly fatal clinical course of disease.

BACTERIAL INFECTIONS CAUSING IMMUNODEFICIENCY

Perhaps the best examples of bacterial infections causing immunodeficiency are those of the tick-borne pathogens Ehrlichia canis and Anaplasma phagocytophilum, which are described later in this article. Bartonella spp. and hemotropic mycoplasmas (hemoplasmas) may also be capable of inducing chronic immunodeficiencies. Human infection with Bartonella bacilliformis infection may be immunosuppressive and many patients have succumbed with secondary bacterial infections, especially salmonellosis. Impaired leukocyte function, cyclic CD8+ lymphopenia, and diminished expression of adhesion molecules and MHC Class II molecules by CD8+ and B lymphocytes, respectively, were documented in one study of Bartonella vinsonii subspecies berkhoffii-infected dogs.

Hemoplasma-induced immunosuppression is not a new phenomenon and has been recognized as a problem in experiments involving chronically infected laboratory rodents and in sheep chronically infected with *Mycoplasma ovis*. The clinical importance of immunosuppression induced by *Bartonella* spp and hemoplasmas in cats and dogs requires further investigation.

EHRLICHIA CANIS INFECTION

Ehrlichia canis is a gram negative intracellular bacteria that causes canine monocytic ehrlichiosis (CME), arguably the most important infectious disease of dogs exposed to ticks worldwide. The organism is transmitted by the brown dog tick, *Rhipicephalus sanguineus*. The organism infects monocytes, in which it forms morulae. In the United States, disease is diagnosed most frequently in dogs living in the southeastern and southwestern states, but because of chronic, subclinical infection, dogs can be transported to non-endemic regions and subsequently develop disease. Different strains of *E canis* exist but the degree by which these vary in virulence is poorly characterized.

The course of CME has been divided into acute, subclinical, and chronic phases, although in naturally infected dogs, these phases are often not readily distinguishable. Clinical signs of acute disease include depression, inappetence, fever, and weight loss. Ocular and nasal discharges, edema, hemorrhages, and neurologic signs may also occur. The organism replicates in reticuloendothelial cells with generalized lymphadenopathy and splenomegaly, and transient cytopenias, especially thrombocytopenia, may occur.

After the acute phase, which may last up to 6 weeks, a subclinical phase may develop that lasts months to years. During this phase, the organism appears to evade host immune responses through antigenic variation. Ultimately, a small percentage of these infected dogs develop chronic CME. Chronic CME is characterized by signs that include lethargy, inappetence, fever, weight loss, bleeding tendencies, pallor, lymphadenopathy, splenomegaly, dyspnea, anterior uveitis, polyuria/polydipsia, muscle wasting, polyarthritis, and edema.

Dogs with severe chronic ehrlichiosis may develop marrow failure, with aplastic pancytopenia. Severe disease may also be associated with a protein-losing nephropathy and development of neurologic signs. Some dogs have bone marrow plasmacytosis and peripheral granular lymphocytosis. Hyperglobulinemia is a frequent finding on the serum chemistry profile and usually results from a polyclonal gammopathy, although monoclonal gammopathies have also been reported. High antibody titers to *E canis*, occasionally exceeding 1:1,000,000, are also common.

The chronic phase may also be associated with development of secondary opportunistic infections. The precise underlying mechanism of the immunodeficiency that develops and how it relates to successful persistence of *E canis* has not been elucidated. Not all dogs that develop chronic infections are pancytopenic, so leukopenia alone does not explain the predisposition for opportunistic infection. Furthermore, the types of infections reported, such as viral papillomatosis; generalized demodicosis; protozoal infections, such as neosporosis and opportunistic mycoses, suggest a defect develops in CMI (Fig. 3).

E canis infection has also been suggested to predispose dogs to development of canine leishmaniasis. Infection of a canine cell line with *E canis* resulted in suppression of MHC Class II expression. In one study, acute experimental infection with *E canis* was not associated with measurable suppression of CMI or humoral immune responses. Alterations in immune responses during chronic infection require further evaluation.

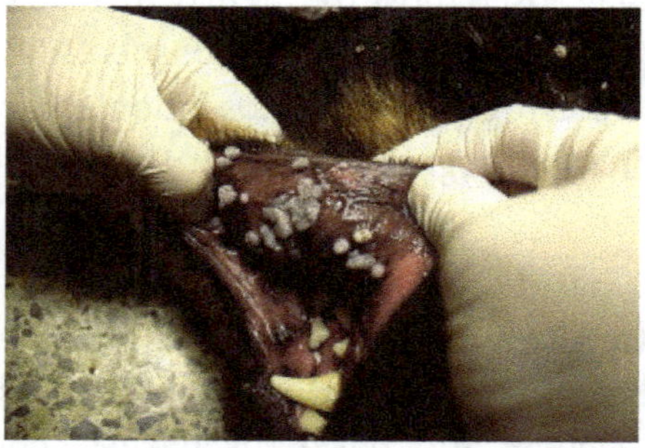

Fig. 3. Viral papillomatosis in a male neutered Rottweiler cross with chronic canine monocytic ehrlichiosis

Anaplasma Phagocytophilum Infection

Like E canis, Anaplasma phagocytophilum is an obligate, tick-transmitted intracellular bacteria that forms morulae within leukocytes. In contrast to E canis which infects monocytes, A phagocytophilum infects granulocytes, primarily the neutrophil, and causes granulocytic anaplasmosis, a disease of humans, dogs, horses, ruminants, and occasionally cats. The vector ticks are generally those belonging to the Ixodes persulcatus complex, primarily I scapularis and I pacificus in the United States, and I ricinus in Europe. Numerous small wild mammals, deer, and possibly birds, act as reservoir hosts for the organism. Several genetic variants have been identified and there is increasing evidence of strain variation in host specificity and pathogenicity.

Immunosuppression resulting from A phagocytophilum infection results primarily from impairment of neutrophil function by the bacteria. After inoculation into the host, A phagocytophilum attaches to sialylated ligands on the surface of neutrophils, after which it enters neutrophils via caveolae-mediated endocytosis, bypassing phagolysosomal pathways. A phagocytophilum then actively disables neutrophil bactericidal functions, in particular neutrophil superoxide production, thus promoting its own survival.

A phagocytophilum also reduces neutrophil mobility and phagocytosis, and reduces endothelial adherence and transmigration of neutrophils.

By inhibiting neutrophil apoptosis, the organism is able to survive in a well-differentiated cell that normally has a very short lifespan. The impairment of neutrophil function and leukopenia that develop as a result of A phagocytophilum infection is occasionally associated with development of opportunistic infections in some humans and animals with granulocytic anaplasmosis. The best example of this is tick pyemia, which is a debilitating lameness and paralysis that develops in infected lambs in Europe, most commonly as a result of disseminated Staphylococcus aureus or Pasteurella spp infection. Infection with A phagocytophilum may influence the outcome of infection with Borrelia burgdorferi, which can be co-transmitted by Ixodes ticks, possibly as a result of impaired neutrophil function.

IMMUNOSUPPRESSION CAUSED BY PROTOZOAL AND FUNGAL PATHOGENS

Leishmaniasis, caused by the protozoal parasite *Leishmania infantum*, is a chronic progressive disease transmitted by the sand fly. The mechanisms of immunosuppression induced by this organism are perhaps the best studied amongst protozoal parasites. The disease is most common in the Mediterranean basin and South America. The organism causes a systemic disease in dogs characterized by lymphadenopathy, crusting skin lesions, weight loss, anemia, ocular lesions, polyarthritis, and protein-losing nephropathy. The infection is often associated with other infections, especially ehrlichiosis and babesiosis, and occasionally with neoplastic disease, especially hematopoietic tumors.

Leishmania infantum invades mononuclear phagocytes, evading the phagolysosome, and survives within them through inhibition of the respiratory burst, inhibition of macrophage function and apoptosis, and impairment of antigen presentation through inhibition of MHC Class I and MHC Class II molecule expression. The protozoan also appears to impair macrophage and neutrophil chemotaxis, and interferes with Il12- transcription.

The *Leishmania* spp surface protein gp63 is a key protein that mediates entry and survival within macrophages. It also allows the organism to resist complement and was recently shown to bind to and suppress the activity of NK cells.

Several fungal pathogens are capable of causing immunosuppression, including *Aspergillus* spp, *Candida* spp, and *Cryptococcus* spp. *Cryptococcus neoformans* and *Cryptococcus gattii* are highly immunosuppressive fungal pathogens, although co-infections with other pathogens are rarely documented.

Cryptococcal organisms possess several potent virulence factors that are capable of suppressing or orchestrating the immune response in favor of fungal growth and persistence. The cryptococcal capsular polysaccharide, glucuronoxylomannan, has attracted the most attention in this regard.

It effectively inhibits phagocytosis and interferes with migration of leukocytes from the bloodstream into tissues by causing them to shed selectin. It can also deplete complement and directly inhibits T-cell responses.

There is a shift from a Th1 to a Th2 immune response, the Th1 response being normally required for organism clearance.

The cryptococcal urease enzyme was shown to promote accumulation of immature dendritic cells within the lung, and an associated shift in the immune response to a non-protective Th2-cytokine dominated response.

Summary

This review highlights the mechanisms of immunosuppression in just a small subset of the huge variety of infectious agents that are capable of inducing immunosuppression to promote their own survival within the host. The degree of immunosuppression and the mechanisms by which immunodeficiency develops are highly variable and complex. Pathogen surface molecules and cellular receptor tropisms play an important role in determining the initial immune cells infected. Because of the cascading mechanisms involved in normal immune cell recruitment, cytokine and antibody production, pathogens frequently disrupt the function of immune cells that do not undergo direct infection. Considerable research effort has been invested in understanding the mechanisms of pathogen-induced immunosuppression, with the hope that effective therapies may be developed that reverse the immunodeficiencies developed and in turn assist the host to clear persistent or life-threatening infectious diseases.

CHAPTER

CANCER AND VACCINES IMMUNOTHERAPY TREATMENT 13

IMMUNOTHERAPY HELPS THE BODY USE ITS OWN WEAPONS

According to Dr. John Yannelli, associate professor of immunology at the University of Kentucky, close to 10% of the 70 million dogs in the United States will develop cancer. The risk increases with age. More than 50% of dogs over age 10 will suffer from some type of cancer, and 25% of those will die from cancer.

For some canine cancers, immunotherapy is more than the latest buzzword. It's an effective treatment. Traditional cancer therapies either destroy cancers via radiation or surgery, or as with chemotherapy, attack the dog's cancer while also damaging their immune system. A big plus to immunotherapy is that it can be specific — targeting only abnormal cells and not affecting other normal cells.

What is immunotherapy?

Immunotherapy uses your dog's own immune system to fight and destroy cancer cells. A healthy immune system recognizes and destroys abnormal cells every day.

While the immune system is normally triggered by the rapid rate at which cancer cells replicate, it can be overtaken by cancer cells. They can multiply at too quickly for the immune system to react, or the cancer cells can sometimes hide from the immune system and escape immediate recognition. In these cases, the immune system may need to be stimulated to recognize the cancer cells and attack them.

A developing therapy

There are some caveats to using immunotherapy. Much of the information on immunotherapy for dogs has been extrapolated from human studies, and the canine immune system has not been studied as extensively as the human one. The "workhorse cells" of canine immune systems, lymphocytes, have not been fully characterized. This can make it harder to predict which dogs and which cancers are most likely to respond to immunotherapy.

One challenge with immunotherapy is predicting which patients will respond. There is a lot of research going on both to find ways to increase the number of patients that respond to immunotherapies and to identify biomarkers that will predict which patients will respond. Because there are very few immunotherapies available in veterinary medicine, there are not yet many hurdles to commercializing these products. Practitioners and owners need to be vigilant about requesting peer-reviewed efficacy and safety data on immunotherapy products that are commercially available.

Immunotherapy seems to work best with a smaller "cancer load," which means many cancers respond best after radiation, surgery or chemotherapy has helped shrink the cancer first. But that increases the cost of treatment and requires more owner compliance.

Limitations

In fairness to this evolving therapy, cancers in dogs are not as extensively identified as are human cancers from both appearance (phenotype) and genetic (genotype) perspectives. That makes it difficult to create unique immunotherapies that would be appropriate for an individual dog's tumors. Different dog breeds show varying susceptibility to cancers, and there are even variations in how cancers develop and respond to therapy in different breeds or lines within a breed. Much cancer research involves collaboration with human medical researchers. Dr. Kristy Richards '90, a groundbreaking cancer researcher and associate professor of biomedical sciences, studied canine lymphoma and how the treatments could benefit both people and dogs. One area she explored was chimeric antigen receptor (CAR) T cells.

T cells are one of the immune system's warriors that attack cancer cells and other pathogens. With CAR, an antibody becomes part of a T cell. Since it is on the surface, it can easily identify and bind with cancer cells. Of course, the T cell comes along with the antibody and can then kill the cancer cell. Richards described CAR as a "guided missile" heading for cancer cells.

Cancer vaccines

Cornell is participating in a national, multi-institutional CAR study evaluating an osteosarcoma vaccine for dogs. "The results are being analyzed elsewhere and results are not available yet," says Hume. But it's one of the comparative oncology projects that will hopefully benefit both people and dogs.

For research on canine cancers, most of the work is done with patients with naturally occurring cancers. For many owners, participating in a clinical trial helps financially while also contributing to cancer knowledge. The first cancer vaccine to have widespread use is Oncept from Merial. This vaccine was designed to prevent metastases of melanoma. In dogs, melanomas tend to occur in dark-pigmented dogs such as Scottish Terriers and are not directly related to sun exposure. If the melanoma appears in the mouth or nail beds, it tends to be very aggressive with rapid spread to local lymph nodes and to the lungs. This vaccine includes DNA from the human melanocyte protein tyrosinase.

Human tyrosinase is similar to the same enzyme in dogs and is part of pigment production. It is present in most melanomas. So when this vaccine is given, the dog mounts an immune response that cross-reacts to both the human and canine tyrosinase, and goes after any melanoma cells. A rare side effect is that the immune system indiscriminately goes after a dog's normal pigment cells, as well as the cancer cells leading to depigmentation or a graying of the coat.

Some concern has been expressed over the use of this vaccine, as the standard FDA clinical trials have not been completed.

In this case, the vaccine targets about 30 proteins found on cancer cells as a result of mutations. These proteins are not normally found on healthy dog cells, so the vaccine is designed to specifically target any abnormal cells that develop. The researchers hope to deter lymphoma, osteosarcoma, hemangiosarcoma and mast cell tumors (mastocytomas). These are fairly common and deadly canine cancers.

Autologous vaccines are being explored to help dogs with cancer. In an autologous vaccine, some of the dog's own tumor cells are extracted, deactivated and treated to stimulate an intense immune reaction. Multiple tumor antigens are present in the vaccine so theoretically the immune response should be very strong and very specific.

This immunotherapy requires your veterinarian to send a sample of the tumor to a laboratory that then creates the vaccine. Your dog eventually receives enough vaccine for a minimum of three weekly injections.

So far, the autologous vaccines have primarily been used against solid cancers such as anal sac adenocarcinomas and transitional cell carcinomas. Some dogs have seen regression of their tumors, others have had tumors stabilize and some have had no recurrence of a growth that was surgically removed. The Torigen Company has made personalized vaccines for more than 250 dogs and cats and will be publishing results soon.

CANCER IMMUNOTHERAPY

The field of cancer immunotherapy continues to evolve, and the past decade has witnessed several important breakthroughs in both the human and veterinary oncology fields. Monoclonal antibodies designed to block specific signaling pathways in tumor cells (e.g., trastuzumab [Herceptin]), to deplete malignant lymphoma cells (e.g., rituximab [Rituxan]), and to alter T-cell signaling (e.g., ipilimumab [Yervoy]) represent major advances in cancer immunotherapy. Although monoclonal antibodies are not yet available for targeted immunotherapy in veterinary medicine, a canine lymphoma–targeting antibody is expected soon. One notable recent advance in veterinary cancer immunotherapy is the development and approval of the first canine cancer vaccine (Oncept), which targets a melanoma antigen (tyrosinase) for immune recognition by T cells.

As the field of cancer immunotherapy advances, progress can be expected on several fronts. First, there is likely to be a continued focus on the development of new monoclonal antibodies targeting either tumor cells directly or key immune-regulatory molecules. Second, a number of new cancer vaccines currently are under development, most targeting tumor antigens that are shared by tumors of a certain histotype or in some cases by different tumor types. Third, there is also increasing emphasis on immune interventions designed to modify the immunosuppressive tumor microenvironment, including and especially tumor-associated macrophages.

Nonspecific Tumor Immunotherapy

Most cancer immunotherapeutics currently available in veterinary medicine are designed to activate multiple components of the innate immune system nonspecifically to generate antitumor immunity. Natural killer cells, macrophages, and dendritic cells are the primary effector cells responsible for generating antitumor activity following administration of nonspecific immune activators. Release of innate immune cytokines, especially interferon-á (IFN-á) and IFN-ã, also contributes significantly to antitumor activity by suppressing tumor cell growth and by inhibiting tumor angiogenesis. There is generally only a minor T-cell contribution to antitumor immunity following administration of nonspecific tumor immunotherapeutics.

Systemic Tumor Immunotherapy Using Toll-like Receptor and Nod-like Receptor Agonists

Most nonspecific cancer immunotherapeutics stimulate the innate immune system by activating Toll-like receptors (TLRs) or Nod (nucleotide-binding oligomerization domain)–like receptors (NLRs). The TLRs and their activating ligands with greatest relevance to cancer immunotherapy are TLR3 (activated by double-stranded RNA from viruses), TLR4 (activated by lipopolysaccharide), TLR7 and TLR8 (activated by viral nucleic acids and synthetic molecules such as imiquimod), and TLR9 (activated by bacterial DNA). NLRs are expressed primarily in the cytoplasm of immune and nonimmune cells and recognize bacterial cell wall peptides (Nod1 and Nod2) as well as viral nucleic acids (retinoic acid–inducible gene [Rig-I] and nucleotide-binding oligomerization domain, leucine-rich repeat, and pyrin domain containing [NLRP]), and in some cases eukaryotic DNA and uric acid and NACHT-, LRR-, and PYD-containing proteins (NALPs).

Liposome-encapsulated muramyl tripeptide phosphatidylethanolamine (L-MTP-PE) is a Nod2 agonist. L-MTP-PE has been evaluated previously as an immunotherapeutic for prevention of metastases from osteosarcoma and hemangiosarcoma. L-MTP-PE triggers activation of macrophages in the lungs and other tissues and generates production of tumor necrosis factor-á and other innate immune cytokines. Repeated intravenous administration of L-MTP-PE has been shown to prolong survival times significantly in dogs with osteosarcoma and hemangiosarcoma and is roughly equivalent to chemotherapy in overall effectiveness.

Systemic administration of cationic liposomes complexed to bacterial plasmid DNA (CLDC) triggers potent activation of innate immunity in dogs with cancer, presumably primarily by stimulating activation of TLR9. CLDC immunotherapy was shown to activate innate immunity in dogs with metastatic osteosarcoma and significantly improved overall survival times in treated dogs compared with untreated control animals. In addition, CLDC administration was associated with significant inhibition of tumor angiogenesis. Currently CLDC immunotherapy is being developed in Europe for the veterinary market.

Systemic administration of live attenuated bacteria (primarily engineered *Salmonella*) also has been evaluated as a novel cancer immunotherapy. The engineered *Salmonella* localizes to the hypoxic tumor environment following intravenous administration. This approach, in some cases, generated local control of tumor growth or tumor regression, presumably mediated by local activation of innate immunity.

Recombinant Cytokine Therapy

Natural killer cells and T cells can be activated by systemic administration of high doses of immune-stimulatory cytokines, primarily interleukin-2 (IL-2) and IFN-á. Immunotherapy with recombinant IL-2 is approved for treatment of melanoma and renal cell carcinoma in humans. Infusions of human IL-2 have been assessed in clinical trials in dogs with advanced cancer and have been reported to produce systemic immune activation (fever) and some antitumor activity. Although human recombinant IFN-á (Roferon, others) is administered systemically at high doses for treatment of melanoma and renal cell carcinoma in humans, the drug rarely is administered at high doses in companion animals for treatment of cancer. However, recombinant IFN-á has been used for treatment of certain oral malignancies in cats, including squamous cell carcinoma.

ELIAS CANCER IMMUNOTHERAPY

Elias Cancer Immunotherapy or ECI is a form of immunotherapy known as Autologous Adoptive Cell Therapy or Adoptive T-Cell Therapy. A dog's cancer-fighting.

T-cells are removed and activated in the laboratory and infused back into the dog so they can better kill cancer cells. ELIAS combines it with vaccination. They produce a vaccine using the dog's own tumor cells, so the immune system is first stimulated to recognize the unique proteins on the surface of the tumor cells.

How does it work?

Following the amputation of the affected limb and thorough screening to ensure the patient is a candidate for treatment, ECI is administered over 6-8 weeks and consists of two steps.

ELIAS Immunotherapy Treatment Steps

Step 1

The patient dog undergoes amputation surgery of the affected limb. A tumor sample is sent to ELIAS's lab, where a vaccine is created. This patient-specific vaccine is injected intradermally weekly for three weeks.

he goal of this step is to increase the number of primed T-cells that specifically target cancer neoantigens in the patient's body. (Neoantigens are new antigens or proteins formed by cancer-specific mutations and found on the surface of tumor cells).

Step 2

The white blood cells are removed from the patient in a procedure called apheresis. It takes 4-6 hours depending on the size of the dog and requires sedation.

The collected white blood cells are sent to ELIAS's lab.

In the lab, mononuclear white blood cells are stimulated using a T cell-specific super-antigen. The vaccine-primed precursor T-cells are differentiated and activated into effector T-cells that can attack cancer.

These activated T-cells are shipped back to the clinic where, roughly seven days after apheresis, the patient receives an infusion of the T-cells.

The dog also receives five subcutaneous IL-2 injections. IL2 is an immune-stimulating cytokine (molecules usually secreted by cells) and helps sustain in-vivo T-cell proliferation.

What do we know about the safety of the treatment?

ELIAS has been evaluating ECI for several years by working with different veterinary teaching hospitals and clinicians.

In a trial recently described in a scientific conference paper, a total of 14 dogs with osteosarcoma were enrolled and evaluated.

The dogs included lab retrievers, few golden retrievers, and Great Danes. The median age was 6.6 years old, and the median weight was 39 kg (85lb).

Ten out of fourteen dogs completed the entire treatment protocol.

For all dogs, the treatment proved to be very safe and the observed side effects were mild to moderate and transient.

What is the standard-of-care treatment for dogs with osteosarcoma and does this immunotherapy treatment extend survival times?

Standard-of-care treatment for many osteosarcoma patients consists of amputation surgery followed by chemotherapy. And ECI's median survival time was greater than historical survival times for dogs receiving surgery and chemotherapy treatment.

The median survival time for dogs getting surgery (without chemotherapy) is 134 days.

The median survival time for dogs receiving surgery+chemotherapy is 308 days.

ELIAS reported a median survival time of 415 days for dogs who had surgery and ECI treatment. (No chemotherapy)

This means that half the dogs who finished their treatment survived beyond 415 days.

The survival times and quality of life have been impressive for some dogs, according to ELIAS.

VACCINES AND IMMUNOTHERAPY

he immune system protects the body against "foreign invaders" such as bacteria and other microorganisms that can cause disease. Certain proteins and other molecules of these invaders are known as antigens, and the immune-system defenses of the body respond to antigens by producing antibodies (see Introduction to Infections).

Drugs can be used to affect the immune system in several ways. Specific immunotherapy is perhaps the most familiar type—it involves giving a specific antigen (such as a vaccine) to cause a specific, controlled immune system response. As a result, vaccines can provoke effective, and often very specific, longterm immunity. Nonspecific immunotherapy can cause the immune system to produce proteins and other compounds that strengthen immunity. It may also give the immune system an overall boost to help it resist infection. Nonspecific immunity includes adjuvants, which may be added to a vaccine to increase its effectiveness, and immunostimulants, which may be given to treat longterm disease in which the immune system may be suppressed.

Types of Vaccines

Several types of vaccines have been developed for use in animals. Traditionally, vaccines were grouped according to whether they contained living or killed organisms. Killed organisms are not as likely to provoke a strong immune response (providing immunity) as living ones. Because of this, vaccines that use killed organisms frequently also include additional compounds, called adjuvants, intended to increase the overall effectiveness of the vaccine. A **killed vaccine** may contain the entire killed organism or just the portion of the organism that provokes the immune response. A Type 1 recombinant vaccine is also classified as killed.

Although vaccines that include live organisms tend to be more effective, there are some challenges involved in developing them, because the live organisms can also cause disease if not modified in some way. **Attenuated vaccines** are vaccines containing live organisms that have been altered so that they are less likely to cause disease. They can reproduce, which will cause the animal to mount a strong immune response. However, even if vaccines are attenuated, they can sometimes revert to virulence, causing the disease they were intended to prevent. To further ensure safety, Type 2 recombinant vaccines, or **gene-deleted vaccines**, were developed to safeguard against attenuated vaccines reverting to a form that can cause disease. The specific genes that cause disease in the host are found and deleted. The resulting vaccine includes live organisms that can reproduce and generate a strong immune response in the host, but can never cause disease.

Live vectored vaccines, or Type 3 recombinant vaccines, are an alternate method of inducing strong immunity with no risk of reversion to virulence. Using technology, the genes that code for a protective protein are removed from the disease-causing organisms and placed into a "vector" organism that does not cause disease. This vector reproduces in the host, producing high levels of the protective protein. The host develops a strong immune response to this protein, which then protects it from exposure to the original disease-causing organism. These vaccines are essentially free of adverse effects and are very stable.

DNA vaccines make it possible to immunize an animal by just injecting it with the DNA coding for a protein from the disease-causing organism. In addition to preventing diseases, DNA vaccine technology can also be used to treat diseases, including certain cancers.

In most countries, the production of vaccines is strictly controlled and regulated by government authorities. All vaccines are checked for safety and potency.

Giving Vaccines

The simplest and most common method used to give a vaccine is with an injection in the muscle or under the skin. Intranasal vaccines are also available for specific diseases, but they can be difficult to give, especially to large animals. Vaccines can also be given in feed or drinking water, a method that is most often used in the poultry industry. Fish can be vaccinated by immersion in a solution of antigen, which is absorbed through their gills. Transdermal (absorbed through the skin) vaccines are also being developed.

Vaccination Schedules

Vaccines stimulate an immune response, which lasts a varying amount of time depending on the specific vaccine and disease-causing organism. This means that a specific method and schedule of subsequent vaccine administration is needed to maintain immunity. In young animals there are challenges to mounting an immune response that must be considered, including the age of the animal and overcoming the immunity passed to the newborn by the mother. In mature animals some vaccinations are usually given yearly, while vaccination every 2 to 3 years is sufficient to ensure immunity with others.

Pet owners should work with their veterinarian to determine the best vaccination schedule for their animal(s). Few vaccines are available for species of pets other than dogs, cats, and horses. Ferrets should be vaccinated against rabies and canine distemper. Psittacine birds (parrots and parakeets) should be vaccinated against avian polyomavirus.

Adverse Consequences

Modern, commercially produced, government-approved vaccines are generally very safe. The most common risks with vaccines include injection-site reactions (such as pain or swelling, which usually subside within a short time), allergic responses, incomplete inactivation, disease in animals with compromised immune systems, neurologic complications, and, rarely, contamination with other live agents. The stress of vaccination may be enough to activate an infection already present in the animal. Hypersensitivity reactions—which range from mild to anaphylactic shock—can also occur. All animals should be observed for a period of time following vaccination. Discuss with your veterinarian what signs you should watch for. In rare cases, certain vaccines have been linked to development of a type of skin cancer in cats at the site where the vaccine was given.

PASSIVE IMMUNITY

In addition to vaccination, there are other ways of creating or increasing immunity against disease. Passive immunity involves one animal producing antibodies by active immunization, and then transferring those antibodies to a susceptible animal to confer immediate protection. The natural (and very important) form of passive immunization is the transfer of maternal antibodies to offspring across the placenta and in the colostrum (the first milk that is full of essential antibodies). Antisera may be produced in dogs against distemper and in cats against panleukopenia (also known as feline parvovirus enteritis). The effects of passive immunity are only temporary, however, as they only last for as long as the transferred antibody lasts, generally a few weeks.

In the same way, antibodies can be harvested from a portion of the blood to create immune globulin, which can then be given to another animal to provide immunity. For example, tetanus immune globulin (tetanus antitoxin) is given to animals and humans to confer immediate protection against tetanus.

GLOSSARY

A

Anthelmintic: A product that kills helminths or worms

Antiseptic: A substance that can be applied to a surface to make it free from germs

Arrhythmia: A heart beat that does not have a normal rhythm

Ascities: An abnormal build up of fluid in the abdomen often causing it to look distended

Ataxia: An abnormal gait when walking or running

Aural: Relating to the ears

Auscultation: The act of listening with a stethoscope

B

Benign: A word used to describe tumours which do not spread

Bilateral: Meaning on both sides

Biopsy: Taking a small sample for further testing, usually refers to tumours or the skin

Bradycardia: A heart beat that is slower than normal

C

Cardiac: Relating to the heart

Cestodes: Another word for tapeworms

Chronic: Used to describe an illness that has been going on for a prolonged period of time

Colitis: Inflammation of the large intestine producing diarrhoea, often with blood

Congenital: A condition that has been present since birth

Cryptorchid: One or both testicles have not descended and are retained in the abdomen

Cystitis: Inflammation of the bladder resulting in discomfort when urinating

Cytology: The study of cells through a microscope

D

Debride: Removing dead tissue from a wound

Defecation: The act of passing faeces

Diuretics: Drugs used to prevent or reduce water retention in the body

Dyspnoea: Difficulty with breathing

Dystocia: Difficulties in giving birth or whelping

E

Ectoparasites: Parasites that live on the skin such as fleas, lice and ticks

Endocrine: Relating to hormones

Endoscopy: Using a small light source and sometimes camera to visualise the inside of the stomach, lungs, nasal cavity or colon.

Extra-cranial: Anything outside the skull

F

Faeces: Solid waste produced from the rectum

Fibrosis: Replacing normal body tissues with scar tissue

FLUTD: Feline Lower Urinary Tract Disease

Flystrike: When blowfly lay larvae on damaged skin which hatch into maggots and cause tissue damage, often extensive

G

Gastric: relating to the stomach eg. Gastritis is inflammation of the stomach

Gestation: The period of time for which an animal is pregnant

Gingivitis: Inflammation of the gums

H

Haematology: The study of bloods cells

Haematuria: Blood in the urine

Hernia: Abnormal movement of organs or fat through a hole such as the umbilicus

Hormone: A chemical messenger produced by one organ and having an effect on another

Hyper-: Too much or an excess of something eg. Hyperthyroidism is an excess of thyroid hormone

Hypo-: Not enough or a deficit in something eg. Hypoglycaemia is a low blood glucose level

Hypertension: High blood pressure

Hypotension: Low blood pressure

I

Iatrogenic: caused by the veterinarian

Icterus: Another word for jaundice or yellowing of the skin and mucous membranes

Immune Mediated: A disease process that is caused by the body's own immune system

Intestine: The intestines refers to the guts from the stomach to the rectum

Intra-cranial: Inside the skull

Intravenous: Into a vein, used to describe routes of administration of drugs

J

Jugular: The main vein in the body, returning to the heart

L

Lactation: Producing milk from the mammary glands

Laparotomy: Opening the abdominal cavity

Lateral: On the side eg. lateral recumbancy means lying on the side

Lethargy: Reduction in activity of an animal

M

Malignant: A word to describe a tumour that is likely to spread to other parts of the body

Mastitis: Inflammation and infection in the mammary glands

MucousMembranes: Moist membranes such as the gums and inside the nose

N

Nasal: Relating to the nose

Necrosis: Death of tissues eg. necrotic tissue is often found in wounds and abscesses

Neoplasia: Another word for tumours

NSAID: Non Steroidal Anti Inflammatory, a pain relief drug similar to Ibuprofen

O

Oncology: The study of tumours

Oral: Relating to the mouth

Orchitis: Inflammation of the scrotum

Otitis: Inflammation of the ear canal

Ovariohysterectomy: Removal of the ovaries and uterus as performed in routine neutering

P

Palpation: Another word for feeling eg. abdominal palpation is feeling the abdomen for abnormal masses.

Palliative: Care aimed at keeping an animal comfortable rather than treating a condition

Paralysis: Loss of use of a part of the body often the limbs

Parasite: An organism that lives off another animal eg. worms living in the intestines

Pathogen: An agent capable of causing disease such as a bacteria or virus

Perineal: Relating to the area around the anus

Peritoneal: Relating to the inside of the abdominal cavity

Pinna: The external flap of the ear

Platelets: Small blood cells responsible for blood clotting

Polydipsia: Excessive thirst

Polyphagia: Excessive hunger

Polyuria: Urinating larger volumes than normal

Probiotic: Bacteria that are beneficial to the health of the intestines

Purulent: Relating to pus eg. purulent discharge is pus like discharge

Pyometra: Infection in the uterus in un-neutered females

R

Radiograph: The proper term for an x-ray image

Regurgitation: Bringing up food as soon as it has been eaten

Renal: Relating to the kidneys

Respiration: The act of breathing

S

Sclera: The white part of the eye

Septic: Meaning something is infected

Splenic: Relating to the spleen

T

Tachycardia: A heart beat that is faster than normal

Thorax: Another word for the chest

Thrombus: A blood clot

Torsion: A twist, sometimes in an organ eg. a gastric torsion is a twisted stomach

Toxin: A poisonous substance capable of causing harm

Trachea: The wind pipe leading from the back of the mouth to the lungs

U

Unilateral: On one side

Ureter: The tube leading from the kidney to the bladder

Urethra: The tube leading from the bladder to the outside

Urination: The act of passing urine

Uveitis: Inflammation of the back and inside of the eye

V

Vascular: Relating to the blood vessels

Viscera: Another word for the organs

Z

Zoonoses: Diseases that can be passed from animals to humans

BIBLIOGRAPHY

Abualrous ET, Fritzsche S, Hein Z, Al-Balushi MS, Reinink P, Boyle LH, et al. F pocket flexibility influences the tapasin dependence of two differentially disease-associated MHC class I proteins. Eur J Immunol (2015) 45:1248–57. doi:10.1002/eji.201445307

Abualrous ET, Saini SK, Ramnarayan VR, Ilca FT, Zacharias M, Springer S. The carboxy terminus of the ligand peptide determines the stability of the MHC class I molecule H-2Kb: a combined molecular dynamics and experimental study. PLoS One (2015) 10:e0135421. doi:10.1371/journal.pone.0135421

Anders AK, Call MJ, Schulze MS, Fowler KD, Schubert DA, Seth NP, et al. HLA-DM captures partially empty HLA-DR molecules for catalyzed removal of peptide. Nat Immunol (2011) 12:54–61. doi:10.1038/ni.1967

Bade-Doding C, Theodossis A, Gras S, Kjer-Nielsen L, Eiz-Vesper B, Seltsam A, et al. The impact of human leukocyte antigen (HLA) micropolymorphism on ligand specificity within the HLA-B*41 allotypic family. Haematologica (2011) 96:110–8. doi:10.3324/haematol.2010.030924

Bailey A, Dalchau N, Carter R, Emmott S, Phillips A, Werner JM, et al. Selector function of MHC I molecules is determined by protein plasticity. Sci Rep (2015) 5:14928. doi:10.1038/srep14928

Bailey A, Van Hateren A, Elliott T, Werner JM. Two polymorphisms facilitate differences in plasticity between two chicken major histocompatibility complex class I proteins. PLoS One (2014) 9:e89657. doi:10.1371/journal.pone.0089657

Beerbaum M, Ballaschk M, Erdmann N, Schnick C, Diehl A, Uchanska-Ziegler B, et al. NMR spectroscopy reveals unexpected structural variation at the protein-protein interface in MHC class I molecules. J Biomol NMR (2013) 57:167–78. doi:10.1007/s10858-013-9777-z

Bello M, Correa-Basurto J. Molecular dynamics simulations to provide insights into epitopes coupled to the soluble and membrane-bound MHC-II complexes. PLoS One (2013) 8:e72575. doi:10.1371/journal.pone.0072575

Bjorkman PJ, Saper MA, Samraoui B, et al. The foreign antigen binding site and T cell recognition regions of class I histocompatibility antigens. Nature 1987; 329:512.

Bjorkman PJ. MHC restriction in three dimensions: a view of T cell receptor/ligand interactions. Cell 1997; 89:167.

Blanco-Gelaz MA, Suarez-Alvarez B, Diaz-Pena R, Lopez-Larrea C. HLA-B27 polymorphism at position 116 critically influences the association with TAP/tapasin, intracellular trafficking and conformational homodimers formation. Mol Immunol (2009) 46:1304–11. doi:10.1016/j.molimm.2008.11.023

Bouvier M, Wiley DC. Importance of peptide amino and carboxyl termini to the stability of MHC class I molecules. Science (1994) 265:398–402. doi:10.1126/science.8023162

Bouvier M, Wiley DC. Structural characterization of a soluble and partially folded class I major histocompatibility heavy chain/beta 2m heterodimer. Nat Struct Biol (1998) 5:377–84. doi:10.1038/nsb0598-377

Bowman GR, Pande VS, Noé F. An Introduction to Markov State Models and Their Application to Long Timescale Molecular Simulation. Heidelberg: Springer Science & Business Media (2014).

Brown JH, Jardetzky TS, Gorga JC, et al. Three-dimensional structure of the human class II histocompatibility antigen HLA-DR1. Nature 1993; 364:33.

Brown JH, Jardetzky TS, Gorga JC, Stern LJ, Urban RG, Strominger JL, et al. Three-dimensional structure of the human class II histocompatibility antigen HLA-DR1. Nature (1993) 364:33–9. doi:10.1038/364033a0

Buchete NV, Hummer G. Coarse master equations for peptide folding dynamics. J Phys Chem B (2008) 112:6057–69. doi:10.1021/jp0761665

Carven GJ, Chitta S, Hilgert I, Rushe MM, Baggio RF, Palmer M, et al. Monoclonal antibodies specific for the empty conformation of HLA-DR1 reveal aspects of the conformational change associated with peptide binding. J Biol Chem (2004) 279:16561–70. doi:10.1074/jbc.M314315200

Carven GJ, Stern LJ. Probing the ligand-induced conformational change in HLA-DR1 by selective chemical modification and mass spectrometric mapping. Biochemistry (2005) 44:13625–37. doi:10.1021/bi050972p

Chen M, Bouvier M. Analysis of interactions in a tapasin/class I complex provides a mechanism for peptide selection. EMBO J (2007) 26:1681–90. doi:10.1038/sj.emboj.7601624

Chen Y, Sidney J, Southwood S, Cox AL, Sakaguchi K, Henderson RA, et al. Naturally processed peptides longer than nine amino acid residues bind to the class I

MHC molecule HLA-A2.1 with high affinity and in different conformations. J Immunol (1994) 152:2874–81.

Chicz RM, Urban RG, Lane WS, Gorga JC, Stern LJ, Vignali DA, et al. Predominant naturally processed peptides bound to HLA-DR1 are derived from MHC-related molecules and are heterogeneous in size. Nature (1992) 358:764–8. doi:10.1038/358764a0

Chou CL, Sadegh-Nasseri S. HLA-DM recognizes the flexible conformation of major histocompatibility complex class II. J Exp Med (2000) 192:1697–706. doi:10.1084/jem.192.12.1697

Cuendet MA, Zoete V, Michielin O. How T cell receptors interact with peptide-MHCs: a multiple steered molecular dynamics study. Proteins (2011) 79:3007–24. doi:10.1002/prot.23104

Dalchau N, Phillips A, Goldstein LD, Howarth M, Cardelli L, Emmott S, et al. A peptide filtering relation quantifies MHC class I peptide optimization. PLoS Comput Biol (2011) 7:e1002144. doi:10.1371/journal.pcbi.1002144

Deng L, Cho S, Malchiodi EL, Kerzic MC, Dam J, Mariuzza RA. Molecular architecture of the major histocompatibility complex class I-binding site of Ly49 natural killer cell receptors. J Biol Chem (2008) 283:16840–9. doi:10.1074/jbc.M801526200

Doebele RC, Busch R, Scott HM, Pashine A, Mellins ED. Determination of the HLA-DM interaction site on HLA-DR molecules. Immunity (2000) 13:517–27. doi:10.1016/S1074-7613(00)00051-0

Dong G, Wearsch PA, Peaper DR, Cresswell P, Reinisch KM. Insights into MHC class I peptide loading from the structure of the tapasin-ERp57 thiol oxidoreductase heterodimer. Immunity (2009) 30:21–32. doi:10.1016/j.immuni.2008.10.018

Duquesnoy RJ, Trucco M. Genetic basis of cell surface polymorphisms encoded by the major histocompatibility complex in humans. Crit Rev Immunol 1988; 8:103.

Fabian H, Huser H, Narzi D, Misselwitz R, Loll B, Ziegler A, et al. HLA-B27 subtypes differentially associated with disease exhibit conformational differences in solution. J Mol Biol (2008) 376:798–810. doi:10.1016/j.jmb.2007.12.009

Fabian H, Loll B, Huser H, Naumann D, Uchanska-Ziegler B, Ziegler A. Influence of inflammation-related changes on conformational characteristics of HLA-B27 subtypes as detected by IR spectroscopy. FEBS J (2011) 278:1713–27. doi:10.1111/j.1742-4658.2011.08097.x

Fahnestock ML, Tamir I, Narhi L, Bjorkman PJ. Thermal stability comparison of purified empty and peptide-filled forms of a class I MHC molecule. Science (1992) 258:1658–62. doi:10.1126/science.1360705

Falk K, Rötzschke O, Rammensee HG. Cellular peptide composition governed by major histocompatibility complex class I molecules. Nature 1990; 348:248.

Falk K, Rotzschke O, Stevanovic S, Jung G, Rammensee HG. Allele-specific motifs revealed by sequencing of self-peptides eluted from MHC molecules. Nature (1991) 351:290–6. doi:10.1038/351290a0

Fallang LE, Bergseng E, Hotta K, Berg-Larsen A, Kim CY, Sollid LM. Differences in the risk of celiac disease associated with HLA-DQ2.5 or HLA-DQ2.2 are related to sustained gluten antigen presentation. Nat Immunol (2009) 10:1096–101. doi:10.1038/ni.1780

Ferrante A, Templeton M, Hoffman M, Castellini MJ. The thermodynamic mechanism of peptide-MHC class II complex formation is a determinant of susceptibility to HLA-DM. J Immunol (2015) 195:1251–61. doi:10.4049/jimmunol.1402367

Fisette O, Wingbermuhle S, Tampe R, Schafer LV. Molecular mechanism of peptide editing in the tapasin-MHC I complex. Sci Rep (2016) 6:19085. doi:10.1038/srep19085

Fleischmann G, Fisette O, Thomas C, Wieneke R, Tumulka F, Schneeweiss C, et al. Mechanistic basis for epitope proofreading in the peptide-loading complex. J Immunol (2015) 195:4503–13. doi:10.4049/jimmunol.1501515

Frayser M, Sato AK, Xu L, Stern LJ. Empty and peptide-loaded class II major histocompatibility complex proteins produced by expression in Escherichia coli and folding in vitro. Protein Expr Purif (1999) 15:105–14. doi:10.1006/prep.1998.0987

Gao B, Adhikari R, Howarth M, Nakamura K, Gold MC, Hill AB, et al. Assembly and antigen-presenting function of MHC class I molecules in cells lacking the ER chaperone calreticulin. Immunity (2002) 16:99–109. doi:10.1016/S1074-7613(01)00260-6

Gao GF, Tormo J, Gerth UC, Wyer JR, Mcmichael AJ, Stuart DI, et al. Crystal structure of the complex between human CD8alpha(alpha) and HLA-A2. Nature (1997) 387:630–4. doi:10.1038/42523

Garstka MA, Fritzsche S, Lenart I, Hein Z, Jankevicius G, Boyle LH, et al. Tapasin dependence of major histocompatibility complex class I molecules correlates with their conformational flexibility. FASEB J (2011) 25:3989–98. doi:10.1096/fj.11-190249

Glithero A, Tormo J, Doering K, Kojima M, Jones EY, Elliott T. The crystal structure of H-2D(b) complexed with a partial peptide epitope suggests a major histocompatibility complex class I assembly intermediate. J Biol Chem (2006) 281:12699–704. doi:10.1074/jbc.M511683200

Grandea AG III, Golovina TN, Hamilton SE, Sriram V, Spies T, Brutkiewicz RR, et al. Impaired assembly yet normal trafficking of MHC class I molecules in Tapasin mutant mice. Immunity (2000) 13:213–22. doi:10.1016/S1074-7613(00)00021-2

Grandea AG III, Van Kaer L. Tapasin: an ER chaperone that controls MHC class I assembly with peptide. Trends Immunol (2001) 22:194–9. doi:10.1016/S1471-4906(01)01861-0

Grotenbreg GM, Nicholson MJ, Fowler KD, Wilbuer K, Octavio L, Yang M, et al. Empty class II major histocompatibility complex created by peptide photolysis establishes the role of DM in peptide association. J Biol Chem (2007) 282:21425–36. doi:10.1074/jbc.M702844200

Gruen JR, Weissman SM. Evolving views of the major histocompatibility complex. Blood 1997; 90:4252.

Guce AI, Mortimer SE, Yoon T, Painter CA, Jiang W, Mellins ED, et al. HLA-DO acts as a substrate mimic to inhibit HLA-DM by a competitive mechanism. Nat Struct Mol Biol (2013) 20:90–8. doi:10.1038/nsmb.2460

Gunther S, Schlundt A, Sticht J, Roske Y, Heinemann U, Wiesmuller KH, et al. Bidirectional binding of invariant chain peptides to an MHC class II molecule. Proc Natl Acad Sci U S A (2010) 107:22219–24. doi:10.1073/pnas.1014708107

Guo HC, Jardetzky TS, Garrett TP, Lane WS, Strominger JL, Wiley DC. Different length peptides bind to HLA-Aw68 similarly at their ends but bulge out in the middle. Nature (1992) 360:364–6. doi:10.1038/360364a0

Gupta S, Hopner S, Rupp B, Gunther S, Dickhaut K, Agarwal N, et al. Anchor side chains of short peptide fragments trigger ligand-exchange of class II MHC molecules. PLoS One (2008) 3:e1814. doi:10.1371/journal.pone.0001814

Halloran PF, Wadgymar A, Autenried P. The regulation of expression of major histocompatibility complex products. Transplantation 1986; 41:413.

Hansen TH, Lybarger L, Yu L, Mitaksov V, Fremont DH. Recognition of open conformers of classical MHC by chaperones and monoclonal antibodies. Immunol Rev (2005) 207:100–11. doi:10.1111/j.0105-2896.2005.00315.x

Harris MR, Lybarger L, Myers NB, Hilbert C, Solheim JC, Hansen TH, et al. Interactions of HLA-B27 with the peptide loading complex as revealed by heavy chain mutations. Int Immunol (2001) 13:1275–82. doi:10.1093/intimm/13.10.1275

Hassan C, Chabrol E, Jahn L, Kester MG, De Ru AH, Drijfhout JW, et al. Naturally processed non-canonical HLA-A*02:01 presented peptides. J Biol Chem (2015) 290:2593–603. doi:10.1074/jbc.M114.607028

Hawse WF, Gloor BE, Ayres CM, Kho K, Nuter E, Baker BM. Peptide modulation of class I major histocompatibility complex protein molecular flexibility and the implications for immune recognition. J Biol Chem (2013) 288:24372–81. doi:10.1074/jbc.M113.490664

Hee CS, Beerbaum M, Loll B, Ballaschk M, Schmieder P, Uchanska-Ziegler B, et al. Dynamics of free versus complexed beta2-microglobulin and the evolution of interfaces in MHC class I molecules. Immunogenetics (2013) 65:157–72. doi:10.1007/s00251-012-0667-4

Hein Z, Uchtenhagen H, Abualrous ET, Saini SK, Janssen L, Van Hateren A, et al. Peptide-independent stabilization of MHC class I molecules breaches cellular quality control. J Cell Sci (2014) 127:2885–97. doi:10.1242/jcs.145334

Hopner S, Dickhaut K, Hofstatter M, Kramer H, Ruckerl D, Soderhall JA, et al. Small organic compounds enhance antigen loading of class II major histocompatibility complex proteins by targeting the polymorphic P1 pocket. J Biol Chem (2006) 281:38535–42. doi:10.1074/jbc.M606437200

Hulpke S, Baldauf C, Tampe R. Molecular architecture of the MHC I peptide-loading complex: one tapasin molecule is essential and sufficient for antigen processing. FASEB J (2012) 26:5071–80. doi:10.1096/fj.12-217489

Hunt DF, Henderson RA, Shabanowitz J, Sakaguchi K, Michel H, Sevilir N, et al. Characterization of peptides bound to the class I MHC molecule HLA-A2.1 by mass spectrometry. Science (1992) 255:1261–3. doi:10.1126/science.1546328

Kienast A, Preuss M, Winkler M, Dick TP. Redox regulation of peptide receptivity of major histocompatibility complex class I molecules by ERp57 and tapasin. Nat Immunol (2007) 8:864–72. doi:10.1038/ni1483

Kim A, Sadegh-Nasseri S. Determinants of immunodominance for CD4 T cells. Curr Opin Immunol (2015) 34:9–15. doi:10.1016/j.coi.2014.12.005

Knapp B, Fischer G, Van Hemelen D, Fae I, Maillere B, Ebner C, et al. Association of HLA-DR1 with the allergic response to the major mugwort pollen allergen: molecular background. BMC Immunol (2012) 13:43. doi:10.1186/1471-2172-13-43

Knapp B, Omasits U, Bohle B, Maillere B, Ebner C, Schreiner W, et al. 3-Layer-based analysis of peptide-MHC interaction: in silico prediction, peptide binding affinity and T cell activation in a relevant allergen-specific model. Mol Immunol (2009) 46:1839–44. doi:10.1016/j.molimm.2009.01.009

Knapp B, Omasits U, Schreiner W, Epstein MM. A comparative approach linking molecular dynamics of altered peptide ligands and MHC with in vivo immune responses. PLoS One (2010) 5:e11653. doi:10.1371/journal.pone.0011653

Krensky AM. The HLA system, antigen processing and presentation. Kidney Int Suppl 1997; 58:S2.

Kropshofer H, Arndt SO, Moldenhauer G, Hammerling GJ, Vogt AB. HLA-DM acts as a molecular chaperone and rescues empty HLA-DR molecules at lysosomal pH. Immunity (1997) 6:293–302. doi:10.1016/S1074-7613(00)80332-5

Kurimoto E, Kuroki K, Yamaguchi Y, Yagi-Utsumi M, Igaki T, Iguchi T, et al. Structural and functional mosaic nature of MHC class I molecules in their peptide-free form. Mol Immunol (2013) 55:393–9. doi:10.1016/j.molimm.2013.03.014

Lewis JW, Elliott T. Evidence for successive peptide binding and quality control stages during MHC class I assembly. Curr Biol (1998) 8:717–20. doi:10.1016/S0960-9822(98)70280-5

Lyngaa R, Pedersen NW, Schrama D, Thrue CA, Ibrani D, Met O, et al. T-cell responses to oncogenic Merkel cell polyomavirus proteins distinguish patients with Merkel cell carcinoma from healthy donors. Clin Cancer Res (2014) 20:1768–78. doi:10.1158/1078-0432.CCR-13-2697

Madden DR, Garboczi DN, Wiley DC. The antigenic identity of peptide-MHC complexes: a comparison of the conformations of five viral peptides presented by HLA-A2. Cell (1993) 75:693–708. doi:10.1016/0092-8674(93)90490-H

Madden DR. The three-dimensional structure of peptide-MHC complexes. Annu Rev Immunol (1995) 13:587–622. doi:10.1146/annurev.iy.13.040195.003103

Mage MG, Dolan MA, Wang R, Boyd LF, Revilleza MJ, Robinson H, et al. The peptide-receptive transition state of MHC class I molecules: insight from structure and molecular dynamics. J Immunol (2012) 189:1391–9. doi:10.4049/jimmunol.1200831

Matsumura M, Fremont DH, Peterson PA, Wilson IA. Emerging principles for the recognition of peptide antigens by MHC class I molecules. Science (1992) 257:927–34. doi:10.1126/science.1323878

McFarland BJ, Katz JF, Beeson C, Sant AJ. Energetic asymmetry among hydrogen bonds in MHC class II*peptide complexes. Proc Natl Acad Sci U S A (2001) 98:9231–6. doi:10.1073/pnas.151131498

Mohan JF, Petzold SJ, Unanue ER. Register shifting of an insulin peptide-MHC complex allows diabetogenic T cells to escape thymic deletion. J Exp Med (2011) 208:2375–83. doi:10.1084/jem.20111502

Mohan JF, Unanue ER. A novel pathway of presentation by class II-MHC molecules involving peptides or denatured proteins important in autoimmunity. Mol Immunol (2013) 55:166–8. doi:10.1016/j.molimm.2012.10.024

Narzi D, Becker CM, Fiorillo MT, Uchanska-Ziegler B, Ziegler A, Bockmann RA. Dynamical characterization of two differentially disease associated MHC class

I proteins in complex with viral and self-peptides. J Mol Biol (2012) 415:429–42. doi:10.1016/j.jmb.2011.11.021

Natarajan SK, Assadi M, Sadegh-Nasseri S. Stable peptide binding to MHC class II molecule is rapid and is determined by a receptive conformation shaped by prior association with low affinity peptides. J Immunol (1999) 162:4030–6.

Natarajan SK, Stern LJ, Sadegh-Nasseri S. Sodium dodecyl sulfate stability of HLA-DR1 complexes correlates with burial of hydrophobic residues in pocket 1. J Immunol (1999) 162:3463–70.

Noe F, Horenko I, Schutte C, Smith JC. Hierarchical analysis of conformational dynamics in biomolecules: transition networks of metastable states. J Chem Phys (2007) 126:155102. doi:10.1063/1.2714539

Nojima H, Kanou K, Kamiya K, Atsuda K, Umeyama H, Takeda-Shitaka M. Dynamic influence of the two membrane-proximal immunoglobulin-like domains upon the peptide-binding platform domain in class I and class II major histocompatibility complexes: normal mode analysis. Chem Pharm Bull (Tokyo) (2009) 57:1193–9. doi:10.1248/cpb.57.1193

Nojima H, Takeda-Shitaka M, Kurihara Y, Adachi M, Yoneda S, Kamiya K, et al. Dynamic characteristics of a peptide-binding groove of human HLA-A2 class I MHC molecules: normal mode analysis of the antigen peptide-class I MHC complex. Chem Pharm Bull (Tokyo) (2002) 50:1209–14. doi:10.1248/cpb.50.1209

Nojima H, Takeda-Shitaka M, Kurihara Y, Kamiya K, Umeyama H. Dynamic flexibility of a peptide-binding groove of human HLA-DR1 class II MHC molecules: normal mode analysis of the antigen peptide-class II MHC complex. Chem Pharm Bull (Tokyo) (2003) 51:923–8. doi:10.1248/cpb.51.923

Nurzia E, Narzi D, Cauli A, Mathieu A, Tedeschi V, Caristi S, et al. Interaction pattern of Arg 62 in the A-pocket of differentially disease-associated HLA-B27 subtypes suggests distinct TCR binding modes. PLoS One (2012) 7:e32865. doi:10.1371/journal.pone.0032865

Painter CA, Cruz A, Lopez GE, Stern LJ, Zavala-Ruiz Z. Model for the peptide-free conformation of class II MHC proteins. PLoS One (2008) 3:e2403. doi:10.1371/journal.pone.0002403

Painter CA, Negroni MP, Kellersberger KA, Zavala-Ruiz Z, Evans JE, Stern LJ. Conformational lability in the class II MHC 310 helix and adjacent extended strand dictate HLA-DM susceptibility and peptide exchange. Proc Natl Acad Sci U S A (2011) 108:19329–34. doi:10.1073/pnas.1108074108

Painter CA, Stern LJ. Conformational variation in structures of classical and non-classical MHCII proteins and functional implications. Immunol Rev (2012) 250:144–57. doi:10.1111/imr.12003

Park B, Lee S, Kim E, Ahn K. A single polymorphic residue within the peptide-binding cleft of MHC class I molecules determines spectrum of tapasin dependence. J Immunol (2003) 170:961–8. doi:10.4049/jimmunol.170.9.4869-a

Pashine A, Busch R, Belmares MP, Munning JN, Doebele RC, Buckingham M, et al. Interaction of HLA-DR with an acidic face of HLA-DM disrupts sequence-dependent interactions with peptides. Immunity (2003) 19:183–92. doi:10.1016/S1074-7613(03)00200-0

Paul S, Kolla RV, Sidney J, Weiskopf D, Fleri W, Kim Y, et al. Evaluating the immunogenicity of protein drugs by applying in vitro MHC binding data and the immune epitope database and analysis resource. Clin Dev Immunol (2013) 2013:467852. doi:10.1155/2013/467852

Pohlmann T, Bockmann RA, Grubmuller H, Uchanska-Ziegler B, Ziegler A, Alexiev U. Differential peptide dynamics is linked to major histocompatibility complex polymorphism. J Biol Chem (2004) 279:28197–201. doi:10.1074/jbc.C400128200

Pos W, Sethi DK, Call MJ, Schulze MS, Anders AK, Pyrdol J, et al. Crystal structure of the HLA-DM-HLA-DR1 complex defines mechanisms for rapid peptide selection. Cell (2012) 151:1557–68. doi:10.1016/j.cell.2012.11.025

Potolicchio I, Chitta S, Xu X, Fonseca D, Crisi G, Horejsi V, et al. Conformational variation of surface class II MHC proteins during myeloid dendritic cell differentiation accompanies structural changes in lysosomal MIIC. J Immunol (2005) 175:4935–47. doi:10.4049/jimmunol.175.8.4935

Praveen PV, Yaneva R, Kalbacher H, Springer S. Tapasin edits peptides on MHC class I molecules by accelerating peptide exchange. Eur J Immunol (2010) 40:214–24. doi:10.1002/eji.200939342

Prinz JH, Wu H, Sarich M, Keller B, Senne M, Held M, et al. Markov models of molecular kinetics: generation and validation. J Chem Phys (2011) 134:174105. doi:10.1063/1.3565032

Rabinowitz JD, Vrljic M, Kasson PM, Liang MN, Busch R, Boniface JJ, et al. Formation of a highly peptide-receptive state of class II MHC. Immunity (1998) 9:699–709. doi:10.1016/S1074-7613(00)80667-6

Raychaudhuri S, Sandor C, Stahl EA, Freudenberg J, Lee HS, Jia X, et al. Five amino acids in three HLA proteins explain most of the association between MHC and seropositive rheumatoid arthritis. Nat Genet (2012) 44:291–6. doi:10.1038/ng.1076

Reboul CF, Meyer GR, Porebski BT, Borg NA, Buckle AM. Epitope flexibility and dynamic footprint revealed by molecular dynamics of a pMHC-TCR complex. PLoS Comput Biol (2012) 8:e1002404. doi:10.1371/journal.pcbi.1002404

Reich Z, Altman JD, Boniface JJ, Lyons DS, Kozono H, Ogg G, et al. Stability of empty and peptide-loaded class II major histocompatibility complex molecules at neutral and endosomal pH: comparison to class I proteins. Proc Natl Acad Sci U S A (1997) 94:2495–500. doi:10.1073/pnas.94.6.2495

Roche PA, Cresswell P. Invariant chain association with HLA-DR molecules inhibits immunogenic peptide binding. Nature (1990) 345:615–8. doi:10.1038/345615a0

Rosen MK, Gardner KH, Willis RC, Parris WE, Pawson T, Kay LE. Selective methyl group protonation of perdeuterated proteins. J Mol Biol (1996) 263:627–36. doi:10.1006/jmbi.1996.0603

Rötzschke O, Falk K. Naturally-occurring peptide antigens derived from the MHC class-I-restricted processing pathway. Immunol Today 1991; 12:447.

Rupp B, Gunther S, Makhmoor T, Schlundt A, Dickhaut K, Gupta S, et al. Characterization of structural features controlling the receptiveness of empty class II MHC molecules. PLoS One (2011) 6:e18662. doi:10.1371/journal.pone.0018662

Sadegh-Nasseri S, Chen M, Narayan K, Bouvier M. The convergent roles of tapasin and HLA-DM in antigen presentation. Trends Immunol (2008) 29:141–7. doi:10.1016/j.it.2008.01.001

Saini SK, Abualrous ET, Tigan AS, Covella K, Wellbrock U, Springer S. Not all empty MHC class I molecules are molten globules: tryptophan fluorescence reveals a two-step mechanism of thermal denaturation. Mol Immunol (2013) 54:386–96. doi:10.1016/j.molimm.2013.01.004

Saini SK, Ostermeir K, Ramnarayan VR, Schuster H, Zacharias M, Springer S. Dipeptides promote folding and peptide binding of MHC class I molecules. Proc Natl Acad Sci U S A (2013) 110:15383–8. doi:10.1073/pnas.1308672110

Saini SK, Schuster H, Ramnarayan VR, Rammensee HG, Stevanovic S, Springer S. Dipeptides catalyze rapid peptide exchange on MHC class I molecules. Proc Natl Acad Sci U S A (2015) 112:202–7. doi:10.1073/pnas.1418690112

Santambrogio L, Sato AK, Fischer FR, Dorf ME, Stern LJ. Abundant empty class II MHC molecules on the surface of immature dendritic cells. Proc Natl Acad Sci U S A (1999) 96:15050–5. doi:10.1073/pnas.96.26.15050

Scherer MK, Trendelkamp-Schroer B, Paul F, Perez-Hernandez G, Hoffmann M, Plattner N, et al. PyEMMA 2: a software package for estimation, validation, and analysis of Markov models. J Chem Theory Comput (2015) 11:5525–42. doi:10.1021/acs.jctc.5b00743

Schlundt A, Gunther S, Sticht J, Wieczorek M, Roske Y, Heinemann U, et al. Peptide linkage to the alpha-subunit of MHCII creates a stably inverted antigen presentation complex. J Mol Biol (2012) 423:294–302. doi:10.1016/j.jmb.2012.07.008

Schmitt L, Boniface JJ, Davis MM, Mcconnell HM. Conformational isomers of a class II MHC-peptide complex in solution. J Mol Biol (1999) 286:207–18. doi:10.1006/jmbi.1998.2463

Schmitt L, Boniface JJ, Davis MM, Mcconnell HM. Kinetic isomers of a class II MHC-peptide complex. Biochemistry (1998) 37:17371–80. doi:10.1021/bi9815593

Schneeweiss C, Garstka M, Smith J, Hutt MT, Springer S. The mechanism of action of tapasin in the peptide exchange on MHC class I molecules determined from kinetics simulation studies. Mol Immunol (2009) 46:2054–63. doi:10.1016/j.molimm.2009.02.032

Schumacher TN, Heemels MT, Neefjes JJ, Kast WM, Melief CJ, Ploegh HL. Direct binding of peptide to empty MHC class I molecules on intact cells and in vitro. Cell (1990) 62:563–7. doi:10.1016/0092-8674(90)90020-F

Sekhar A, Kay LE. NMR paves the way for atomic level descriptions of sparsely populated, transiently formed biomolecular conformers. Proc Natl Acad Sci U S A (2013) 110:12867–74. doi:10.1073/pnas.1305688110

Sieker F, Springer S, Zacharias M. Comparative molecular dynamics analysis of tapasin-dependent and -independent MHC class I alleles. Protein Sci (2007) 16:299–308. doi:10.1110/ps.062568407

Sieker F, Straatsma TP, Springer S, Zacharias M. Differential tapasin dependence of MHC class I molecules correlates with conformational changes upon peptide dissociation: a molecular dynamics simulation study. Mol Immunol (2008) 45:3714–22. doi:10.1016/j.molimm.2008.06.009

Simone LC, Georgesen CJ, Simone PD, Wang X, Solheim JC. Productive association between MHC class I and tapasin requires the tapasin transmembrane/cytosolic region and the tapasin C-terminal Ig-like domain. Mol Immunol (2012) 49:628–39. doi:10.1016/j.molimm.2011.11.002

Smith KJ, Reid SW, Stuart DI, Mcmichael AJ, Jones EY, Bell JI. An altered position of the alpha 2 helix of MHC class I is revealed by the crystal structure of HLA-B*3501. Immunity (1996) 4:203–13. doi:10.1016/S1074-7613(00)80429-X

Sollid LM, Pos W, Wucherpfennig KW. Molecular mechanisms for contribution of MHC molecules to autoimmune diseases. Curr Opin Immunol (2014) 31:24–30. doi:10.1016/j.coi.2014.08.005

Springer S, Doring K, Skipper JC, Townsend AR, Cerundolo V. Fast association rates suggest a conformational change in the MHC class I molecule H-2Db upon peptide binding. Biochemistry (1998) 37:3001–12. doi:10.1021/bi9717441

Stadinski BD, Zhang L, Crawford F, Marrack P, Eisenbarth GS, Kappler JW. Diabetogenic T cells recognize insulin bound to IAg7 in an unexpected, weakly binding register. Proc Natl Acad Sci U S A (2010) 107:10978–83. doi:10.1073/pnas.1006545107

Stern LJ, Brown JH, Jardetzky TS, Gorga JC, Urban RG, Strominger JL, et al. Crystal structure of the human class II MHC protein HLA-DR1 complexed with an influenza virus peptide. Nature (1994) 368:215–21. doi:10.1038/368215a0

Suh WK, Derby MA, Cohen-Doyle MF, Schoenhals GJ, Fruh K, Berzofsky JA, et al. Interaction of murine MHC class I molecules with tapasin and TAP enhances peptide loading and involves the heavy chain alpha3 domain. J Immunol (1999) 162:1530–40.

Suthanthiran M, Strom TB. Renal transplantation. N Engl J Med 1994; 331:365.

Turnquist HR, Kohlgraf KG, Mcilhaney MM, Mosley RL, Hollingsworth MA, Solheim JC. Tapasin decreases immune responsiveness to a model tumor antigen. J Clin Immunol (2004) 24:462–70. doi:10.1023/B:JOCI.0000029118.51587.d9

Tynan FE, Borg NA, Miles JJ, Beddoe T, El-Hassen D, Silins SL, et al. High resolution structures of highly bulged viral epitopes bound to major histocompatibility complex class I. Implications for T-cell receptor engagement and T-cell immunodominance. J Biol Chem (2005) 280:23900–9. doi:10.1074/jbc.M503060200

Uchtenhagen H, Abualrous ET, Stahl E, Allerbring EB, Sluijter M, Zacharias M, et al. Proline substitution independently enhances H-2D(b) complex stabilization and TCR recognition of melanoma-associated peptides. Eur J Immunol (2013) 43:3051–60. doi:10.1002/eji.201343456

Urban RG, Chicz RM, Lane WS, Strominger JL, Rehm A, Kenter MJ, et al. A subset of HLA-B27 molecules contains peptides much longer than nonamers. Proc Natl Acad Sci U S A (1994) 91:1534–8. doi:10.1073/pnas.91.4.1534

Van Hateren A, Carter R, Bailey A, Kontouli N, Williams AP, Kaufman J, et al. A mechanistic basis for the co-evolution of chicken tapasin and major histocompatibility complex class I (MHC I) proteins. J Biol Chem (2013) 288:32797–808. doi:10.1074/jbc.M113.474031

Van Hateren A, James E, Bailey A, Phillips A, Dalchau N, Elliott T. The cell biology of major histocompatibility complex class I assembly: towards a molecular understanding. Tissue Antigens (2010) 76:259–75. doi:10.1111/j.1399-0039.2010.01550.x

Weber DA, Evavold BD, Jensen PE. Enhanced dissociation of HLA-DR-bound peptides in the presence of HLA-DM. Science (1996) 274:618–20. doi:10.1126/science.274.5287.618

Wieczorek M, Sticht J, Stolzenberg S, Gunther S, Wehmeyer C, El Habre Z, et al. MHC class II complexes sample intermediate states along the peptide exchange pathway. Nat Commun (2016) 7:13224. doi:10.1038/ncomms13224

Willcox BE, Thomas LM, Bjorkman PJ. Crystal structure of HLA-A2 bound to LIR-1, a host and viral major histocompatibility complex receptor. Nat Immunol (2003) 4:913–9. doi:10.1038/ni961

Wilson IA, Fremont DH. Structural analysis of MHC class I molecules with bound peptide antigens. Semin Immunol (1993) 5:75–80. doi:10.1006/smim.1993.1011

Wright CA, Kozik P, Zacharias M, Springer S. Tapasin and other chaperones: models of the MHC class I loading complex. Biol Chem (2004) 385:763–78. doi:10.1515/BC.2004.100

Yanaka S, Ueno T, Shi Y, Qi J, Gao GF, Tsumoto K, et al. Peptide-dependent conformational fluctuation determines the stability of the human leukocyte antigen class I complex. J Biol Chem (2014) 289:24680–90. doi:10.1074/jbc.M114.566174

Yaneva R, Springer S, Zacharias M. Flexibility of the MHC class II peptide binding cleft in the bound, partially filled, and empty states: a molecular dynamics simulation study. Biopolymers (2009) 91:14–27. doi:10.1002/bip.21078

Yin L, Trenh P, Guce A, Wieczorek M, Lange S, Sticht J, et al. Susceptibility to HLA-DM protein is determined by a dynamic conformation of major histocompatibility complex class II molecule bound with peptide. J Biol Chem (2014) 289:23449–64. doi:10.1074/jbc.M114.585539

Zacharias M, Springer S. Conformational flexibility of the MHC class I alpha1-alpha2 domain in peptide bound and free states: a molecular dynamics simulation study. Biophys J (2004) 87:2203–14. doi:10.1529/biophysj.104.044743

Zarling AL, Luckey CJ, Marto JA, White FM, Brame CJ, Evans AM, et al. Tapasin is a facilitator, not an editor, of class I MHC peptide binding. J Immunol (2003) 171:5287–95. doi:10.4049/jimmunol.171.10.5287

Zarutskie JA, Sato AK, Rushe MM, Chan IC, Lomakin A, Benedek GB, et al. A conformational change in the human major histocompatibility complex protein HLA-DR1 induced by peptide binding. Biochemistry (1999) 38:5878–87. doi:10.1021/bi983048m

Zhou Z, Callaway KA, Weber DA, Jensen PE. Cutting edge: HLA-DM functions through a mechanism that does not require specific conserved hydrogen bonds in class II MHC-peptide complexes. J Immunol (2009) 183:4187–91. doi:10.4049/jimmunol.0901663

Zhou Z, Jensen PE. Structural characteristics of HLA-DQ that may impact DM editing and susceptibility to type-1 diabetes. Front Immunol (2013) 4:262. doi:10.3389/fimmu.2013.00262

Zhou Z, Reyes-Vargas E, Escobar H, Rudd B, Rockwood AL, Delgado JC, et al. Type 1 diabetes associated HLA-DQ2 and DQ8 molecules are relatively resistant to HLA-DM mediated release of invariant chain-derived CLIP peptides. Eur J Immunol (2016) 46:834–45. doi:10.1002/eji.201545942

Zou Y, Stastny P, Süsal C, et al. Antibodies against MICA antigens and kidney-transplant rejection. N Engl J Med 2007; 357:1293.

INDEX

www.ingramcontent.com/pod-product-compliance
Lightning Source LLC
LaVergne TN
LVHW062221200926
848484LV00006B/1446
9781787151093